PATIENT SATISFACTION

BOOKS IN THE SERIES

PATIENT SATISFACTION

A Guide To Practice Enhancement

WENDY LEEBOV, Ed.D
MICHAEL VERGARE, M.D.
GAIL SCOTT, M.A.

The Einstein Consulting Group, a
subsidiary of the Albert Einstein
Healthcare Foundation

MEDICAL ECONOMICS BOOKS
ORADELL, NEW JERSEY 07649

Library of Congress Cataloging-in-Publication Data
Leebov, Wendy.
  Patient satisfaction: a guide to practice enhancement/Wendy
Leebov, Michael Vergare, Gail Scott
  Includes index.
  ISBN 0-87489-546-4
  1. Medicine—Practice—Quality control.   2. Consumer satisfaction.
I. Vergare, Michael.   II. Scott, Gail, 1946-   .   III. Title.
  [DNLM: 1. Consumer Satisfaction.   2. Practice Management, Medical.
3. Private Practice—organization & administration.   W 80 L482p].
R728.L39   1989
610.69′6—dc20
DNLM/DLC
for Library of Congress   89-8255
                                                                              CIP

ISBN 0-87489-546-4

Medical Economics Company Inc.
Oradell, New Jersey 07649

Printed in the United States of America

Contents

About the Authors

Wendy Leebov is President of The Einstein Consulting Group, a subsidiary of the Albert Einstein Healthcare Foundation in Philadelphia. She provides consulting services to hospitals, ambulatory care centers, and medical practices. She is the author of *Service Excellence: The Customer Relations Strategy for Health Care* (AHA Publishing, Inc., Chicago, IL, 1988). Wendy Leebov has a doctorate in human development from the Harvard Graduate School of Education.

Michael Vergare, M.D. is Associate Chairman, Department of Psychiatry at the Albert Einstein Medical Center in Philadelphia and Associate Professor of Psychiatry at Temple University Medical School. He is active in teaching residents in Einstein's residency programs to address the emotional and interpersonal challenges involved in providing quality medical care. Michael Vergare is Board-certified in Psychiatry and Psychiatric Administration. Having received his M.D. degree from Hahnemann Medical College and Hospital of Pennsylvania, he then completed a one-year residency in internal medicine and a three-year residency in general psychiatry at Hahnemann Hospital. He maintains a private practice in psychiatry.

Gail Scott, M.A. is Director of Consultation and Training for The Einstein Consulting Group. She consults with healthcare organizations nationwide on service management, team-building, and organizational revitalization. Gail Scott has an M.A. degree in communications from Beaver College.

The Einstein Consulting Group is a subsidiary of the Albert Einstein Healthcare Foundation in Philadelphia. Begun in 1985, this nationally recognized consulting firm helps healthcare organizations nationwide to develop the spirit, systems, and skills that constitute excellence in service and customer satisfaction. It also helps caregivers and other personnel to develop the harmonious relationships needed to achieve quality care, effective performance, and job satisfaction. For information, call or write: The Einstein Consulting Group, York and Tabor Roads, Philadelphia, PA, 19141, (215) 456-7065

Acknowledgments

We want to thank the many people who helped us create this book:

To the exemplary physicians who articulated their views, insights, and skills in in-depth interviews: Doctors Allen Arbeter, Randy Beame, Jose Castel, Lillian Cohn, Harris Gerber, Marvin Gershenfeld, Richard Greenberg, Howard Elefant, Gary Levine, Sandra Magos, George Manstein, Dahlia Sataloff, Mark Singer, Courtney Snyder, Marjorie Stanek, Margo Turner, Robert Weinstock, and Shahriar Yazdanfar.

To Liz Dunn, Ph.D., who designed the physician interview protocol, conducted interviews, analyzed the data, and wrote the chapter on "Interpersonal Skills of Successful Physicians." And to Allan Geller for his skillful interviewing.

To the practice enhancement innovators who generously shared their success stories: Benjamin Bierbaum, M.D., and Alice Eiseman, Ed.M, from Longwood Orthopedics in Massachusetts; Robert DiTomasso, Ph.D., and Dick Almond, M.D., of Tatem-Brown Family Practice Center, New Jersey; Robert Pearl, M.D., and Joyce Reynolds, Ph.D., of Kaiser Permanente Medical Center in Santa Clara, California; Paul Alpert, M.D., and Geraldine Alpert, M.D., from Kaiser Permanente Medical Center in San Rafael, California; Charles H. Ewing, M.D., Medical Director of Rydal Park complete care facility in Rydal, Pennsylvania; and Rachmel Cherner, M.D., of Jenkintown, Pennsylvania.

To Linda Schroeder who shared her family's real, often painful experiences with the healthcare system—experiences we used to illustrate sensitive aspects of the physician-patient relationship.

To Linda Schroeder, Sandy Tafler, Sheila Wallace, Silvia Bloise, Marlene Whalen, George Frascatore, and Nikki Gollub who provided the extensive clerical support we needed to produce a coherent, readable manuscript.

To Marion Silverman and Florence Rosenthal of the Albert Einstein Medical Center's Luria Library who beat the bushes and the computer lines for important reference material.

To The Einstein Consulting Group staff for their patience, expertise, and moral support: Susan Afriat, Katie Buckley, Jack Fein, Allan Geller, Gail Murphy, Diane Walker, Silvia Bloise, George Frascatore, Bill Johnson, Jeanne Joseph, Lori Goldstein, Jana Griffith, Wesley Hilton, Gary Reed, Joan Theetge, Loren Shuman, Kelly Yeager, and Virginia Yeager.

To Tina Phipps, Ph.D., for sharing resources and expertise related to the behaviors and issues key to effective patient–physician relationships.

To Holly Tubiash for her ideas, feedback, and encouragement.

To Barbara Mattleman, Liz Dunn, and Judy Stofman for their astute feedback and editorial suggestions.

To the dedicated physicians on the Physician Image Committee at the Albert Einstein Medical Center in Philadelphia.

To Martin Goldsmith, President of the Albert Einstein Healthcare Foundation, who continues to nourish and support the creativity and productivity of The Einstein Consulting Group.

To our own families whose experiences with an array of physicians have helped to sensitize us to the nuances of the physician–patient relationship and to the patient perspective on medical practices.

Preface

You say you entered the healthcare profession to *care* for people. But lately, with the technology explosion, increased competition, reimbursement cutbacks, and the liability crisis, is your commitment to patient care masked in paperwork, bureaucracy, and machinery? Well, you're not alone. Increasingly, physicians report a need to reemphasize the service dimension in order to revive their own enthusiasm and career satisfaction as well as to act on their commitment to their patients.

But that's not all. The current emphasis on excellence in *service* and deliberate striving to satisfy patients also generates additional benefits that make it a compelling priority—one that you can't afford to overlook.

In the good old days, physicians only had to worry about attracting patients when their practices were fledglings. Once established, a steady flow of patients was assured. Physicians rarely thought of patients in the same terms that businesses thought of their customers. The good old days!

But today, in our new atmosphere of competition and changing healthcare utilization and technology, physicians who don't place a high priority on patient satisfaction may find their practices gradually eroding. Physicians who ignore the power of patients to make or break their practice may find themselves losing patients to the practice down the street.

According to a survey of 500 physicians by the National Research Corporation and *Physician's Marketing Newsletter,* more than 50 percent of today's physicians are emphasizing "guest or customer relations" in their practices and spending time, attention, and resources on practice improvements that give their practice a "service advantage" (*Healthcare Marketing Report,* 1 (12), December 1987, p. 7).

Given the new competitors on the healthcare scene, physicians need to take *active* steps to secure their current share of the patient market. In fact, with shrinking reimbursement and the growing glut of physicians, many physicians need to take aggressive action to expand patient volume just to maintain their current income levels.

We intend this book to help.

We'll present what we believe is an unequivocal case for the leaders of medical practices to take conscientious, deliberate action to enhance their practices for the sake of patient satisfaction as well as for the sake of their own professional success. We'll go beyond the reasons and tell you nuts and bolts about how to enhance your practice—how to achieve patient satisfaction *by design*. We'll explain why excellence on service dimensions is never an accident, and why it requires painstaking attention to your patients' wants and expectations. And we'll help you discover how, given your resources and practice philosophy, you can best meet your patients' needs.

We'll share with you the practical nuts and bolts of moving your practice up the service-excellence continuum to gain a competitive edge and pride advantage. We'll present a framework for evaluating your practice on patient satisfaction dimensions, and tools for soliciting feedback from patients, improving staff behavior, improving ambience, making your office systems more user-friendly, and upgrading your environment.

And because every physician's relationship with the patient is the crux of your practice's success, a significant portion of this book focuses on the quality of this pivotal relationship. We describe physician behaviors that make a difference to the patient's satisfaction and likelihood not only to be loyal to your practice but also to spread the good word to others.

Our expertise on service excellence in health care is solidly grounded in hands-on experience. Since 1982, we have helped more than 130 hospitals, ambulatory care centers, and medical practices nationwide to institute comprehensive service excellence strategies, all designed to heighten patient satisfaction.

We emphasize *options*. Every practice is different from every other practice. So, we can't in good conscience offer you an exact formula for the perfect practice. Instead, we offer you tools for analyzing your practice and its effects, and for tailoring service improvements to your specific needs. For every key dimension involved in patient satisfaction, we spell out concrete options, which you can consider and choose from to make your practice a perpetual success in attracting and retaining a loyal patient following.

I
The Patient Satisfaction Imperative

Deliberate strategies to achieve patient satisfaction are increasing in popularity—and for good reason.

Part 1 provides a comprehensive backdrop for the nuts and bolts that come later. Specifically, you'll find in Chapter 1 the history of the rising trend toward practice enhancement and ten compelling reasons why strategic efforts to cater to patients is key to a thriving practice.

In Chapter 2, we address the question, "What do patients want?" We explore the criteria they use to judge medical practices and physicians and to shop among them.

In Chapter 3, we present a powerful model you can use to generate a conscious and conscientious strategy for your practice in order to achieve patient satisfaction and a loyal patient following.

In Chapter 4, we examine practice enhancement within the framework of "internal marketing"—your key strategy for keeping your spoken *and* unspoken promises to patients.

1

Focus on Patient Satisfaction: The Trickle That Became a Wave

What makes patient satisfaction imperative for your practice? The fact is, both solo and group practices need to realize the power of the patient, and develop a conscious and conscientious strategy for achieving satisfaction among their patients as well as other key customers.

DARE WE SAY "CUSTOMERS"?

Consensus is certainly lacking about what to call the variety of people whose satisfaction determines the success of your practice. We could continue the incumbent term *patient,* except that this term does not cover every constituency whose satisfaction and decisions matter to your practice's future. Specifically, it excludes thinking of referring physicians, of a patient's family and friends, and even of your employees as people deserving of excellent service by all associated with your practice.

Most of the time, we will be talking about patients and can call them just that. But sometimes we need a generic term. We considered *guest,* since many hospitals use that term in their efforts to strengthen their organizations on service dimensions. But we rejected that because, to us, this term fits hotel users but not healthcare users. The term *guest* implies too much of a voluntary relationship, as Table 1–1 shows.

In the newsletter *Guest Relations in Practice* (1 (1), February 1986, p. 2), readers responded to a survey about their preferred term for healthcare "users". Their responses did not resolve the nomenclature dilemma, but instead revealed the complexity of the problem:

> We have continued to call our users *patients*, even though the term *client* has been suggested. *Client* has the connotation of a legal or business relationship. *Customer* implies a business or purchasing relationship. Although the term *patient* may seem old fashioned, I believe it still stands for that special relationship between users and providers of healthcare. Perhaps its time we asked our users which term they prefer. (Helen DeSautel, R.N., M.S., Director of Patient Relations, Baptist Hospital of Miami, Miami, FL)

> My suggestion for a term to designate how we regard our *patients*, *guests*, or *customers* is *Guest-omer*—a customer who is also our guest. This is to recognize the needs of both. We treat guests in our home differently than we would treat customers at our business. *Guest-omer* recognizes the more intimate relationship we have with our customers in a hospital (healthcare) setting. (Deborah McMann,

Table 1–1. Hotel vs. Healthcare Users.

IN HOTELS	IN A MEDICAL PRACTICE
Most people want to be there.	Most people don't want to be there.
Most people are in good spirits.	Most patients feel nervous, worried, even frightened.
Guests expect hospitality.	Patients expect clinical competence, technological know-how, *and* compassionate treatment.
Personnel need to be courteous, solicitous, and helpful	Personnel need to be precise, skillful, safe, caring, responsive, gentle, quick, and much, much more.

Asst. Director, Patient Relations, University Hospital of Jacksonville, Jacksonville, FL)

The most accurate and realistic term . . . should be *victims*. Most consumers of health and medical services have no real choice as to "whether"—only "which." Obviously, preventive services are excluded, but then such services are more concept than reality. Unfortunately. (Richard Gamel, President, MD Search, Inc., Memphis, TN)

The discussion concerning the appropriate nomenclature for the 'new' patient/client/customer is so relevant to the issue that I too have spent creative think time trying to come up with an alternate title. It reminds me of the still unresolved "boy/girlfriend/live-in-/roommate/housemate/posslq" debate. Perhaps we need to consult an anthropologist/linguist. (Sylvia Wessel)

Given no optimal solution, we have decided that, when we can, we will use the term *patient*. But when we need a generic term for all the people whose satisfaction matters to your practice's future, we will use the term *customer*. We realize that to many people in healthcare, the term *customer* is offensive because it reflects only an economic relationship. Certainly in healthcare, the relationship between the patient and the physician is more than economic. To some, the term *customer* does not convey the human ingredient of healthcare that involves healing, caring, and compassion. It feels perhaps cold and mechanistic.

But the fact is, patients and referring physicians choose your practice from an array of alternatives and their choices have economic implications. At least that's clear. Other terms like *client, consumer, constituent* and *guest* are less clear and don't really solve the connotation problem.

Realizing that every term has strong advocates and strong opponents, this book sometimes uses the term *customer* as the generic term to mean any person whose satisfaction is key to your practice's success, including patients, their family and friends, your employees, referral sources and even third party payers.

WHO ARE YOUR CUSTOMERS?

Key customers for most medical practices are many: (1) patients, of course, (2) their friends and family, (3) professional referral sources, (4) the community at large, and (5) your own employees. The practice that succeeds is the practice that keeps all of these *customers* or constituencies satisfied by providing distinctive service. That's not easy, but definitely possible if you take strategic steps to enhance your practice.

Patients

Obviously, the first and foremost customer or user group key to the success of your practice is patients, the group with the most direct and intense experience with you, your staff, and services. For four main reasons, you need to concern yourself with patient satisfaction:

The humanistic reason: Patients deserve quality of care and service because they are more often than not vulnerable—sick, worried, pained, concerned, and anxious about their physical, emotional, and economic well-being. "Am I well? Can I get through this emotionally? Can I afford this?"

The economic reason: Patients are customers. They think like customers; they have options that they ponder more carefully than ever; and they expect value for their money.

The marketing reason: Patients are a public relations and sales force. They attract other people to your practice or away from it. They control the grapevine that influences future business.

The efficiency reason: Satisfied patients are easier to serve; dissatisfied patients, especially those who complain, consume valuable staff time—time that could be better spent serving more people more thoroughly.

Family and friends

The patient's family members and friends are your second key customer group. When they accompany the patient to your practice, staff frequently overlook them, since the staff's primary concern is with the patient. Yet, the patient's family and friends also have firsthand experience with your practice. They want their presence and importance to be acknowledged by you and your staff; and they appreciate comforts, amenities, and updates that help their waiting time pass more quickly. They may feel edgy, because they feel powerless to help their loved one. Concerned and anxious, they need information and reassurance. They also act on their protective instincts, scrutinizing your staff's behavior toward the patient, zealously advocating on the patient's behalf. If family and friends are favorably impressed with their own and their loved one's experience with your practice, they might consider patronizing your practice themselves when in need of similar services. But, whether impressed or not, they are credible and vociferous participants in the grapevine that spreads the word about your practice to the rest of the community. Family and friends provide powerful, free advertising. You control whether that advertising is good or bad.

Professional referral sources

Another customer group critical to the future of your practice are professional referral sources. Depending on the nature of your practice, these referral sources may include other physicians, insurance companies, HMO (health maintenance organization) or PPO (preferred provider organization) referrers, physician referral services run by hospitals, psychologists, day care workers, school nurses, and a whole plethora of other human service professionals or organizations. The individuals who make referrals for these organizations typically have reason to communicate with your staff—perhaps to follow up on a patient, to ask a question, to obtain information for accounting or further referral. Your practice's relationship to these people is powerful, since these people channel patients directly to your doorstep. The probability that they will continue to refer to your practice depends not only on their perception of your service to patients but also on the service you extend to the referrers themselves. Yet, staff in your practice might not be providing these referral sources with red-carpet treatment. Not only do staff rarely view these people as customers, they tend to find their questions and telephone calls a nuisance. This is a problem, since every contact may result in a future referral, to your practice or someone else's.

The community-at-large

An elusive but nonetheless powerful customer group for your practice is the community. Public opinion, or the reputation of your practice in the community-at-large, frequently determines whether patients will first use your practice or avoid it. There are many opportunities for physicians to work on their own behalf in the community. Many social, educational, and religious groups appreciate physician speakers on medical topics. Health fairs or other large gatherings present opportunities for you and your staff to provide free blood pressure or other simple screening procedures. The good will generated by such activities can considerably boost your practice's reputation.

Employees

Your own staff wear two hats: service providers and also customers. In their role as service providers, their mutual respect for one another is evident to your patients and other customers. As customers, employees may use your practice for healthcare, recommend it to family and friends, and field questions about it from community members. Because of their status as "insiders," any comments your employees make about your practice carry considerable weight with public opinion. What do your employees say about your practice on the bus-ride home, at family gatherings, at community meetings? Given their status as trusted information sources, employees must also be treated as potential customers and referral sources. They deserve to be on the receiving end of services, benefits, and information that will enlist their loyalty and support.

Customers—patients first, family and friends, referral sources, the community, and employees.

So many people to please.

WHY CONCENTRATE ON SATISFACTION?

Ten powerful factors

Ten factors empower your customers, particularly your patients, to an unprecedented extreme, making efforts to heighten patient satisfaction a strategic necessity.

1. Human Nature and Compliance.   The first reason for excelling in patient satisfaction is a matter of mission and tradition. The mission of medical professionals is to heal, to comfort. This is the core of medical practice that attracted most people to become physicians. When people are sick, they are vulnerable and often scared. They deserve, and increasingly expect, gentle handling. Clinical expertise isn't enough to soothe anxieties unless accompanied by concern, respect, courtesy, empathy and compassion. It's the behavior of the physician and staff that makes the point, "You're in capable and caring hands."

And effective physicians know that effective interpersonal skills are key to patient compliance with treatment regimens—how you explain medications and treatments, how you check for understanding, how you develop the quality of trust and confidence, so that your patients follow those recommendations you determine to be in their best interests.

2. Technological Similarity.   Physicians in almost any specialty can assume that other providers in their area have similar training and access to similar state-of-the-art technology and treatment protocols. America's superior medical education and stringent peer review systems have helped to assure patients that adequate technological services are available from many sources.

Medical anthropologist Irwin Press points out that the culture of the medical profession feeds into development of similarity among doctors:

> To a large degree, all physicians look alike to the patient, whether the MD be surgeon, internist, endocrinologist, or what have you . . .
> Their paradigm, identical training, and dependence on outside invented and standardized technical wizardry makes physicians largely

indistinguishable from one another. ("Witch Doctor's Legacy: Some Anthropological Implications for the Practice of Clinical Medicine," in N.J. Chrisman and T.W. Maretzki (eds.), *Clinically Applied Anthropology,* D. Reidel Publishing Co., 1982, pp. 193–194.)

The consumer sees many alternatives that look medically alike and, until proven wrong, assumes equivalent competence from every provider source. The competitive edge, then, the way to be different and better, is not clinical or technological. The competitive edge lies in the ability of your practice to offer its consumers *distinctive* service. You can stand out from the growing crowd of other physicians if you offer the magic of a caring, satisfying patient-doctor interaction and the kind of service that takes people aback because it exceeds their expectations.

3. New Providers. Competition is fierce and on the rise. Just as hospitals are facing new competitors such as surgicenters and imaging centers, so are physicians faced with new competition from urgicenters, free-standing nurse practitioners, and others. The competitors are at both ends of the spectrum, big corporations and solo practitioners in newly licensed categories. Many of these new providers perceived opportunity in the market place precisely *because* they saw service inadequacies and inconveniences in other available medical practices. They expect to seize market share because they offer the patient not better technique, but superior convenience, access, sensitivity, and compassion. The established practices that want to maintain their share of the market have to compete on customer service dimensions with these new entrants.

United Technologies ran an ad that makes the point:

> We no longer live in an era of caveat emptor; this is the era of caveat vendor. The lesson is clear: the vendor who fails to provide excellent service loses to a competitor who does—a competitor who has listened better, heard better, and had the courage to act even when such action necessitated change.

4. New Intermediaries. The healthcare insurance business has spawned its own set of new competitors. These new intermediaries such as HMOs and PPOs are competing vigorously with traditional indemnity plans. All types of intermediaries are seeking ways to reduce the costs of medical service while retaining quality technical care. However, the most savvy and successful plans are also advertising the superior service of their affiliated providers. Example: HMO-PA, one of the US HealthCare plans, advertises that its Service Excellence plan obtains care for children "as though they were the Medical Director's own."

Insurance plans attempting to distinguish themselves from the pack will seek out practitioners who not only provide competent care, but excel in customer relations. The volume of patients controlled by some of these contracting intermediaries or "macrobuyers" can make or break a practice by one decisive action—choosing other practices, not yours. All predictions are that the influence of managed care plans will continue to grow.

5. The New Breed of Consumer. While doctors face burgeoning competition, consumers are fast becoming a new breed. They are increasingly knowledgeable and discriminating. They *shop* for doctors or managed care plans, and, when they find them, they know they are paying dearly for healthcare and they expect value for their money. Once viewed with some degree of awe and distance, doctors are now more likely to suffer intense scrutiny by a discerning public. As a result, the rate of people who are changing physicians is on the rise. And, once you've lost a patient, you've lost not only that patient but all those whom that patient might have referred.

> When medical care is involved, *Credat emptor* (i.e., "Let the buyer trust") has now been replaced by *Caveat emptor* (i.e., "Let the buyer beware").

These watchful consumers have power to affect the physician's success and livelihood. The consumer has the power to initiate the doctor-patient relationship—and to terminate it if the practitioner loses the patient's confidence. The result: doctors have a stake in taking seriously the qualities that patients look for in a "good" doctor.

What does this discerning public want? What are the qualities that patients look for? Certainly more than medical expertise. After all, consumers, unschooled in the esoteric knowledge held by the doctor, are largely incapable of evaluating their physicians' technical competence. Market research (e.g., Harris research organization in a study commissioned by Pfizer, 1986) indicates that customer service factors, not technical competence, are cited as the major contributors to patient satisfaction.

In another national study reported by Tom Schleff and Maggie Shaffer ("How do consumers select physicians?", *Medical Group Management 34*, (3), May-/June 1987), 1,000 consumers were asked to cite the factors most important to them when choosing a physician. The top four responses (with percent responding "*Very important*") were:

Time and explanation given by physician	91%
Ability to obtain an appointment when needed	90%
Courtesy of office staff	76%

Physician keeps appointment on time   72%

The consumer who is dissatisfied with a doctor increasingly has the power to select an alternative. At the 1985 National Healthcare Marketing Symposium in Kansas City, John Cotillion, Vice President of Planning and Marketing for South Community Hospital in Oklahoma City, cited a study which showed that 68 percent of customers who don't go back to a care provider don't because they were upset by bad employee attitudes that resulted in mistreatment.

Consumers select and evaluate doctors based on service criteria which they know how to judge because of experience—not on the basis of clinical competence.

6. *The Powerful Grapevine*   Doctors face increasing scrutiny by consumers, and those consumers spread the word about what they see and experience. The word they spread, depending on its nature, quickens or slows the flow of patients to the practice under scrutiny. Delphi Forecasts (Healthcare Marketing Trends, Nashville, TN, January 12, 1987, p. 4) conducted a study of how consumers select physicians. Forty-five percent of both urban and rural consumers depend on word-of-mouth recommendations from friends and family. Healthcare is reportedly one of the top three topics of conversation among friends, family and co-workers. The result: the grapevine is a powerful referral source or deterrent. The word about a particular physician spreads like wildfire. Doctors who want to be survivors need that grapevine to work in their favor, attracting more patients, not turning away would-be customers to other care-givers.

7. *The Negativity Obsession.*

> The most important thing to know about intangible products is that the customer usually doesn't know what he's getting until he doesn't get it. Only when he doesn't get what he bargained for (and paid for) does he become aware of what he bargained for. Only on dissatisfaction does he dwell.
>
> Satisfaction is, as it should be, mute. Its prior presence is affirmed only by its subsequent absence. (Theodore Levitt in *The Marketing Imagination,* (New York City: Free Press, 1983, p. 105)

The powerful grapevine gives disproportionate air time to people's negative experiences. Perhaps it's human nature to dwell on the negative. The Technical Assistance Research Project (TARP) in Washington, D.C. (1985) conducted a massive study of consumer behavior in service industries. TARP found that the average consumer tells five other people about positive experiences they've had with a service organization. On the other hand, they tell 20 people about their experience if it was negative. So consumers speak to four times as many friends, relatives, and co-workers about negative experiences or dissatisfactions with a service provider than they speak to about positive experiences. The result: a practice has to satisfy four people for every one it disappoints just to stay even in terms of public image and reputation.

You've undoubtedly witnessed this negative mindset among patients who have complained about a hospital visit. When a hospital staffer is grumpy for two minutes out of an hour, many patients will view the person as irritable and rude. They focus on the irritating two minutes, not on the congenial 58.

According to Tom Moody, Vice President and General Manager of The Marketing Prescription, more than 21% of the people who switch doctors do so for negative reasons, that is because of disaffection or dissatisfaction rather than for a neutral cause such as relocation. *(Healthcare Marketing Report,* Volume 5, (#2), Feb., 1987).

track!

8. The Stereotype of the Greedy, Disinterested Physician. Aren't you tired of the negative stereotypes perpetuated about the typical physician (Figure 1–2)?

Consider the immortal words of two literary greats, Ambrose Bierce and William Shakespeare.

> Physician: *one upon whom we set our hopes when ill, and our dogs when well.* (Ambrose Bierce, *Devil's Dictionary*)

> Reputation, reputation, reputation! O! I have lost my reputation. I have lost the immortal part of myself, and what remains is bestial. (Shakespeare, *Othello,* II, iii).

The age of doctors on pedestals that can't be brought down is no more. According to David Mechanic ("Physicians and Patients in Transition," the

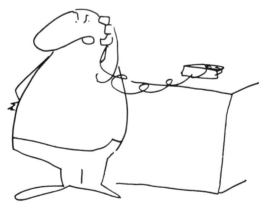

"Your chest cleared? Good—I'll prescribe the same medicine for your check."

Figure 1–2. Cartoon from *Funny Bones*

Hastings Center Report, Volume 15, December, 1985), a recent AMA analysis suggests that the public believes that "doctors don't care as much as they used to," that they don't spend as much time with their patients, and that they are more motivated by money and prestige than by a desire to help people. According to the AMA, these attitudes underlie the erosion of patient confidence.

Anthropologist Irwin Press says it eloquently:

> The physician today who believes that patients view him (*sic*) as selfless servant of the community's health needs, is severely misled. A deep well of resentment and distrust underlies many patients' attitudes toward the medical profession—even while many of these same patients are totally committed to the biomedical paradigm and its technological wizardry. Indeed, this very commitment underlies the resentment. Modern biomedicine is the ultimate monopolistic 'phone company'." (Irwin Press, "Witch Doctor's Legacy: Some Anthropological Implications for the Practice of Clinical Medicine," in N.J. Chrisman and T.W. Maretzki (eds.), *Clinically Applied Anthropology*, D. Reidel Publishing Co., 1982, p. 193).

The popular media have undoubtedly contributed to doctor bashing. The stereotype of doctors as arrogant, greedy, disinterested, heartless brutes is an image reinforced by the fact that malpractice, medical treatment atrocities, fraud, and other physician offenses are newsworthy in a way that the quiet, well-functioning, caring physician can never be. Victimized by stereotypes, physicians who want and deserve a positive image and reputation have to bend over backward to overcome the suspicion and distrust widely held by consumers.

These physicians and everyone in their practices have to pay painstaking attention to the humanistic ingredients of care, and provide care so sensitive and respectful that it contradicts people's negative stereotypes of physicians dramatically enough to be noticeable. Serving the patient well enough to avoid being perceived as offensive is not enough. The winning practice works to impress the consumer. And this doesn't have to be done by the physician alone. All staff must be recognized as diplomats and ambassadors of goodwill who extend the efforts of the physician to heighten patient satisfaction.

On a continuum of service quality from "poor" to "excellent," it's not enough to be "adequate" or "good." "Excellence" is what makes the wary consumer take notice.

> The four A's required of a physician to develop a practice are ability, affability, availability, and affordability. . . .Another "A", arrogance, is certainly not one of them." (Mitchell Karlan, M.D., "Arrogance: A Malaise That Needs a Cure," *American Medical News*, June 20, 1986, p. 28).

9. The Liability Crisis.   From a patient:

> I was hospitalized, sick, terrified, and more than anything I wanted a
> kind word, the touch of a hand on my shoulder, some reassurance,
> some reason to believe that everything might be all right . . . What I
> got instead was a cold fish in a white coat who told me that I had
> cancer, that things didn't look too good, that he didn't have time to
> explain it in detail to me, but that he would 'try' to stop by later in
> the day. . . .I told him not to bother. Is it any wonder that doctors are
> being sued in record numbers? It's the only way that ordinary people
> have to strike back. (Darrell Sifford, "Medical Malpractice Suits
> Stir Up Doctors and Patients," *Philadelphia Inquirer*, January 15,
> 1987, p. 5-D).

The fact is, if people can't find doctors who will listen to them, they certainly
can find lawyers who will. The wary public is quick to sue—to seek legal
remedies for dissatisfaction with their doctors, for whatever reason. The AMA
estimates that the number of malpractice claims tripled between 1975 and 1983,
and that the rate of claims increased from 3.3 per 100 physicians before 1978 to
8.6 in 1984 (Mechanic, "Physicians and Patients in Transition," *Hastings Center
Report*, Volume 15, December 1985). Malpractice premiums continue to climb.
Most doctors have faced increases of 25 percent to 50 percent or more of their
insurance premiums every year (Roy Petty, "A Disease in the House of Medicine," Health and Medicine, Winter 1986, p. 27). Doctors cannot afford malpractice suits in terms of expense or reputation.

Irwin Press, Professor of Anthropology at Notre Dame University, claims (in
a 1986 speech) that a prime factor in determining whether people launch malpractice suits against their physicians is their perception of that physician's attitude and manner toward them. Paul Sommers, Ph.D. ("Malpractice Risk and
Patient Relations," *J. Family Practice*, 20, (3), 299–301) cites the evidence that
demonstrates that the more positive the relationship with the physician, the
lower the malpractice risk. "Reduction of such liability can be easily facilitated
by providing patient-oriented services" (p. 300). According to Sommers, when
patients believe that their doctor is interested in them and intent on meeting their
needs, the patient remains undaunted in support and trust for the physician.
People don't like to sue a nice, well-intentioned person, even a doctor. And
there is evidence that, given equal severity of medical outcomes, people sue
physicians they perceive as well-intentioned much less frequently than they sue a
physician perceived as cold, impersonal, insensitive, or uncaring. Physicians can

make malpractice suits less likely by strengthening their own and their staff's interpersonal and communication skills. (Robert Bianco, "What Turns a Patient into a Plaintiff," *Int. Ophthalmol. Clin.*, 20(4), Winter 1980, pp. 43–52)

10. The High-Tech, High-Touch Tightrope.

> Medical knowledge has rapidly expanded in recent years, but medical care has in certain crucial ways deteriorated. (Edward Dhorter, *Bedside Manners: The Troubled History of Doctors and Patients*, New York: Simon and Schuster, 1986, p. 19)

Fancy devices, newfangled diagnostic procedures, esoteric jargon, machinery, buzzers, and beepers play an increasingly important role in medical practice. These technological tools, innovations, and even miracles, while producing new hope for diagnosis and cure, tend to distance the care-giver from the patient.

Thomas Ferguson, in his Presidential Address at the Sixty-Second Annual Meeting of the American Association of Thoracic Surgery (Phoenix, AZ, May 3-5, 1982), describes "an inverse relationship between medical miracles and medical esteem, a gap which seems to widen with each new medical advance."

While high-tech devices and services indeed impress patients and give the impression that treatment is state-of-the-art, these same devices and procedures also intimidate. Caregivers walk a tightrope between use of the best of contemporary technology and humanistic, personalized care. To alleviate or prevent the patient's apprehension in the face of mystifying and sometimes frightening technology, physicians and their staffs need to consciously complement high tech with the high-touch elements of caring, warmth, explanations, comforts and personal attention, in short, service factors.

Patients: an appreciating asset

Physician practices face unenviable marketplace pressures—pressures that can be tackled with effective results if you confront the fact that your practice is a service business. For humanistic, marketing, and financial reasons, you can augment clinically excellent healthcare with keen sensitivity to consumer needs and wants regarding service. The result: the ability to attract and retain a loyal patient following.

In interviews with successful physicians, we asked, "How do you think physicians are perceived today compared with 20 years ago?" Here are the highlights:

> Twenty years ago, the physician was revered. Patients were more accepting and grateful. Patients today don't blindly accept what doc-

tors tell them. Physicians must provide more information and more in the way of interpersonal support, because patients demand it. (Dahlia Sataloff, M.D.)

I think physicians are seen more as human beings and not being deified as they used to be. What the doctor said was law. But today, people are questioning more. The pedestal is no longer there. (Jose Castel, M.D.)

Patients are more aware that they have the option to shop for a different opinion and a different style. For the first time in history, significant numbers of patients are interviewing their doctors as much as being interviewed by their doctors. (Lillian Cohn, M.D.)

Physicians used to be looked up to as people who healed; that was all they did. Now, it's much more in the open that medical practices are businesses in some ways, and they have to operate for profit. (Margo Turner, M.D.)

Themes loom large:

- Because physicians are not idealized, their patients challenge and question them to an unprecedented extent.
- Patients now explicitly "shop" for physicians, using stiff criteria.
- Patients are increasingly aware that the physician's practice is a business.

In short, physicians seem to agree that this is a new age of the empowered patient and the demystified doctor. The age of M.D. as the short form for "medical deity" is largely gone. Physicians who recognize the increasing scrutiny they're under are taking active steps to achieve impeccable quality care and service in their practices.

Well-served patients are key. They are appreciating assets who give your practice stability, continuity, and strength.

2

What Do Patients Want? Key Factors in Practice Enhancement

The crux of the matter is *patient* satisfaction, since satisfied patients return to your practice, they compliment a referring physician for sending them to you, and they spread the good word to family, friends, and community.

To satisfy patients today, you need to go the extra mile to meet their ever-rising expectations (see Figure 2–1).

Patients today want an unprecedented level of *service* from the medical practice they patronize. But what constitutes service when a consumer is talking about medical care? What criteria do patients care about and use to judge your practice along service lines?

You probably know from experience. Think of a place in your own life where you were an extremely satisfied customer, a place that you thought offered you and its other customers great service: A great restaurant? A particular hotel that rolled out its red carpet? Disney World?

Now think about what happened there that made you conclude that the service was terrific. Chances are you thought about people who were warm, friendly, and took initiative to make you feel special and cared for. You probably also

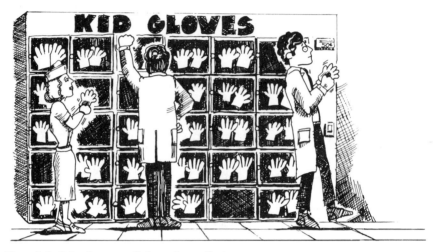

Figure 2–1. Going the extra mile for patient satifaction.

thought about conveniences and other gestures you would have liked to see extended to you to reflect that, to the service provider, you and your needs are important and primary.

It's not very different in your practice. On the average, patients look for the same reflections of service distinction in their doctor's office that they look for at Disney World, on the plane, at the Ritz, or at their favorite restaurant or supermarket. They just care about service more in the doctor's office because they are typically nervous, sometimes fearful. And the stakes are higher.

Ironically, the growing body of research on what patients look for in evaluating healthcare providers indicates that medical expertise, although important, is *not* the central determinant of patient satisfaction. In fact, patients evaluate a physician's practice along six dimensions:

- Medical expertise
- The environment
- People skills
- Systems
- Amenities or "extras"
- Affordability

While the relative importance of one dimension compared to another varies with different populations, all six determinants have been shown repeatedly to be critical success factors. As factors amenable to change, they therefore suggest areas for improvement if you want to enhance your practice's ability to attract and retain patients. Now, more about what is meant by each factor.

THE COMPETENCE FACTOR: MEDICAL EXPERTISE

Traditionally, in the healthcare industry, technical competence, including that of the doctor as well as that of the lab tech, the receptionist, the nurse, and every other staff member, has received the most attention from healthcare providers—whether a diagnosis is right, whether lab tests are accurate, or whether the maintenance worker can fix the air conditioner. Because of the necessity for quality standards applied to the consequential business of medical care, this emphasis is unquestionably important. However, as far as customers are concerned, it is not their only consideration. Perhaps because of the excellent medical education and peer review systems in this country, customers have come to expect clinical/technical competence from their healthcare providers, unless they have specific reason to doubt it. In reality, the consumer is least able to judge technical competence, and instead uses surrogate measures to judge a medical practice. Marketing-oriented healthcare providers realize that other factors must be in place in order to meet the public's heightening expectations for medical service.

While patient satisfaction does not rest heavily on the provider's clinical/technical expertise, research conducted by the Cleveland Clinic Foundation (Frank Weaver, Division of Public Affairs, 1986) suggests that, when the consumer draws conclusions about their provider's medical expertise, they base their judgments on the following factors:

- The examination skills of their doctors
- The likelihood of being cured
- Medical treatments used
- Medical technology available
- Types of medical problems the doctor handles
- The doctor's involvement in medical research
- The medical skills of nurses and other staff

These are important to the patient, but not as important as other service factors, since patients know they don't have the background to judge physicians on their medical expertise. Trust is required, and trust is a function of the strength of other service factors.

THE AMBIENCE FACTOR: THE ENVIRONMENT

The *physical* environment of your practice also merits attention. A conducive, comfortable, relaxing, professional environment is important, although most patients don't think environmental factors are as important as other service features. Obviously, other things being equal, patients are attracted to upbeat, soothing, clean, safe environments. Frustration about parking, lack of accessible transportation, and other physical access problems turn patients to other providers. Practices located in dilapidated, unkempt, or unsafe buildings dissuade patients from returning. Also, the immediate environment of your offices where people spend the most time affects their comfort and their perception of whether they are in good hands.

The Cleveland Clinic research pointed to five environmental factors that particularly affect patient satisfaction:

- Cleanliness of the facility
- The condition of the building
- Ease of finding your way
- The size of the facility
- The surrounding neighborhood

Cleanliness is critical. People in the airline industry know that when the customer sees a dirty tray table, they wonder how the company takes care of its engines. In a doctor's office, if the building is dilapidated, the furniture moth-eaten and the restrooms anything short of spotless, patients question the cleanliness of the office, and it makes them wonder about your attention to instrument sterilization and infection control. Patients want to feel safe and confident in the good, clean hands of their doctor. Disarray, dirt, and maintenance problems all affect patient confidence in their medical treatment.

Doctors who want to draw patients from a wide geographic area also have to compensate for the distance barrier by creating a haven of comfort and cleanliness that makes the patient feel the trip was worth it. And, if the immediate neighborhood is a barrier to use of your office, your office needs to exude "quality of life," so people focus on how nice it is to be on the inside, instead of how uncomfortable it was to get there in the first place.

How comfortable can a patient and their companions feel, and how energetic do physicians and other staff feel in an unappetizing environment? The physical environment, its accessibility and aesthetics deserve consideration in practice enhancement. A comfortable, attractive environment instills confidence in patients and their companions as well as energy and the ability to concentrate by physicians and other staff.

THE KID GLOVES FACTOR: PEOPLE SKILLS

Think back to a time when you were the customer left angry by your interaction with a particular business. Most likely, you were angry because you were ignored, or treated with disrespect or a lack of responsiveness by a human being. That's the service factor that most affects the satisfaction of most patients, more than any other factor. If you're typical, when you think of the place where people were rude, short-tempered, or inattentive, you would, if you have other choices, probably hesitate to go back. And you probably would tell your friends not to go there either.

For these reasons, the burgeoning interest in patient/guest/customer relations for healthcare has focused primarily on "people skills," and specifically on the courtesy, care, and concern that personnel in the practice extend to patients and their companions. No doubt, people skills have a dramatic impact on consumer satisfaction, the reputation of your practice that spreads through the grapevine, and consumers' future choices about where to go for care. The receptionist who blurts out, "I *said* I'd be with you in a minute! Can't you see I'm busy!" can turn away a patient faster than a vague diagnosis, access problems, or even a long wait explained apologetically. Interpersonal skills and behavioral reflections of a positive attitude are critically important to patients. Patients can evaluate these factors expertly, since they feel the consequences firsthand and immediately. That curt line or irritated tone of voice can undo positive expectations and generate instant distrust of office staff and physicians. Also, the more subtle indignities during a patient visit create long-lasting resentment that affects the probability that your office will ever see that patient again.

The Cleveland Clinic research again pinpoints seven interpersonal skill components that matter to patients:

- The doctor's demonstration of concern for the patient
- The doctor's willingness to communicate with patients and family
- Time spent by the doctor with patients
- Meeting of the family and patient's emotional needs
- The nurse's concern for patients and family
- Helpfulness of receptionists and other staff
- The friendliness of receptionists and other staff

These factors are all important to the patient and therefore to your practice's resilience in the healthcare marketplace.

SYSTEMS: THE MAZE FACTOR

Problematic systems drive people crazy—patients and employees alike. Long waits for appointments, long waits in the waiting room, long waits in the exam room after hearing "I'll be right back," sitting unclothed while being talked to, misplaced charts, billing errors, faulty equipment, frustrated efforts to reach the office and the doctor by phone, long delays when trying to reach the doctor in an emergency—all of these signal systems problems in your practice. Is it any wonder that the consumer public concludes that the doctor values his or her own time more than he or she respects the time of the patient? Hopefully, it hasn't happened to you, but more and more doctors are receiving bills from patients charging the doctor for the time they were kept waiting after they showed up on time for an appointment. The consumer has had it with long waits, and the only doctors who continue to get away with these long waits on a regular basis are ones who have a corner on a specialty and can, because of supply and demand, get away with it—but still at the expense of the patient.

Systems problems also impede staff performance with the result that patients suffer. Consider the example of Harper Medical Associates (a fictitious name). Harper patients had complained of staff rudeness and a reticence about catering to the patient. The practice manager of Harper arranged for its 22 employees to experience an extensive 16-hour patient relations training course. Employee behavior toward patients improved, but only temporarily. With their heightened customer relations skills, employees had no tolerance for the congenital systems problems in the Harper practice. Specifically, Harper had a very poor scheduling system. Patients inevitably waited and waited, getting very frustrated in the process. They complained to staff. Over time, staff came to "shut off" toward patients, so they wouldn't have to explain and re-explain and take the flack for the long waits required of increasingly irritable patients. When Harper provided training in "people skills," the staff perceived this as a cosmetic effort to put a band-aid on systems problems that the physicians were unwilling to tackle. And the staff were angry. It seemed to them as if the management blamed patient dissatisfaction on employee skill deficits, when employees saw the main barrier to patient satisfaction as being an obsolete and unexamined scheduling system that victimized staff and patients alike. In this case, the practice enhancement strategy adopted was incomplete, negligent of the causes of staff distance from patients. The result: it failed to change, and in fact exacerbated, the situation.

Wonderful "people skills" are short-lived unless underlying systems support them. The friendly employee gets very frustrated apologizing for the same inconveniences day after day, year after year. Staff resent underlying systems problems, inconveniences, senseless or problematic practices that interfere with their ability to extend themselves to your patients and their families. Employees want your practice's systems to *enable* them to serve your patients well. When these systems interfere with what employees know to be humane patient care, they are understandably resentful. Patients, too, express intolerance of cumbersome procedures, obscure forms, confusion over scheduling and the like. They look for user-friendly systems and procedures.

The fact is, patients want convenience. They want your office systems to go like clockwork—so smoothly that they don't even think of your systems. Smooth, streamlined, efficient systems, patients believe, respect their time, and also reflect an organized, efficient, "managed" practice. And this translates to a perception of quality service.

The Cleveland Clinic research points to four systems factors that stand out in importance from the patient's point of view:

- Efficient provision of service
- Ability to get appointments quickly
- Time spent waiting for the doctor
- Time spent waiting for tests

AMENITIES AND EXTRAS: GESTURES THAT SAY "PATIENTS FIRST"

Remember the old days when the family doctor gave all the kids a lollipop after an office visit, or made home visits? Do you dispense free sample medication, hand out samples of health promotion materials, free thermometers, booklets on smoking, nutrition and exercise, do you offer free refreshments in the waiting area, or provide a child's play area with play equipment for half-pints?

No doubt, there are "extras" or amenities that a practice can provide to its patients and their companions to make them feel comfortable, special, and appreciated: coffee in the waiting room, trinkets and a play area for the kids, "Walkmans" in the dental chair, prescription starter packages, discount parking, jigsaw puzzles, VCRs, video games and personal computers in the waiting room, valet parking, and more. Patients report appreciation for these amenities, because they suggest that the people steering this practice value their time and have taken extra steps to make their experience more pleasurable, or at least less tedious or nerve-wracking.

But attention to amenities can be dangerous if your practice has deeper service weaknesses that you neglect. Freebies don't make people forget rude words by a nurse. Extras don't make people forgive disrespectfully long waits. If systems and people skills are in place, then amenities are noticed and appreciated, bringing comfort and amusement, making the time go faster. Otherwise, they are resented as smoke screens for problematic people and systems. Patients perceive them as efforts to appease or distract, so the patients won't notice the more significant service weaknesses. Amenities, from the point of view of the patient, don't tend to compensate for other service deficiencies. Patients know that a pile of magazines and fresh coffee in the waiting room may make the time pass quickly, but they do not make up for tediously long waits caused by systems problems, and they do not make up for rude employees noticeably lacking interpersonal skills or care.

AFFORDABILITY: THE MONEY FACTOR

The importance of cost is controversial. Many people question the competence of a practice that doesn't charge much, believing "You get what you pay for." Recent studies have shown that bargain rates at the doctor's office aren't the number one factor that attracts or repels patients. But, in the face of frustration with other aspects of your services (long waits, a rude receptionist, an office visit during which the patient sat naked on the exam table for 15 minutes while you audibly talked to another patient on the phone)—when these kinds of things happen, many patients do focus on cost—as an insult. The high price you charge suddenly becomes an affront, the symbol of the patient's oppression. Patients point to high price as adding insult to injury. They feel cheated.

ADVANCING FROM "GOOD" TO "EXCELLENT"

Six factors matter most to patients. Perhaps you think these factors are already working for you. Perhaps they are. But, in observing many medical practices, we found that the outstanding practices are ones where the leaders value, not mediocrity or getting by, but excellence—straight out "there's always room for improvement" excellence.

The fact is, the competitive edge is excellence when it comes to practice enhancement. Consider the continuum in Figure 2–2. When a service dimension is "lousy," or poor, everyone can pinpoint the problem, and it tends to be clear what can be done to improve on it. But most practices aren't lousy on any dimensions. Most have relative weaknesses that are sometimes easy to tolerate unless they have reached horrendous proportions.

THE SERVICE CONTINUUM

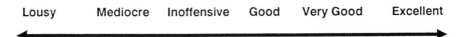

| Lousy | Mediocre | Inoffensive | Good | Very Good | Excellent |

Figure 2–2. The service continuum.

Take "people skills" as an example. When a receptionist is blatantly rude, it's clear that something has to be done about it. If an office manager or physician confronts the receptionist, describes the problem and states the need for improvement, improvement may indeed occur. But improvement might merely move that receptionist's behavior up the continuum from "lousy" to "inoffensive." When the behavior reaches inoffensiveness, the office manager and physician might feel relieved that the behavior problem is solved. But inoffensiveness is a far cry from excellent behavior. Excellent behavior is going way up the continuum past inoffensiveness and seizing the previously missed opportunities that make the employee's behavior truly excellent, even impressive, from the patient's perspective. Let's say the receptionist initially ignored patients who entered the office and acknowledged their presence only after the patient cleared her throat for the fifth time, and then looked somewhat put out by the "interruption." That's offensive behavior in a frontline person. After being confronted by the office manager who fielded several complaints about coldness at the front desk, the front desk person acknowledged patients sooner and said, "Yes? May I help you" in a lukewarm tone. Her behavior moved from lousy to inoffensive, probably eliminated complaints from patients, and even gave you a warm glow of success at having conquered one service problem. But, although improved, that employee's behavior certainly didn't impress anyone. It was better but not great!

The fact is, to enhance your practice, the goal cannot be solely to achieve a consistent level of inoffensiveness such that patients do not complain outright. The challenge is to identify and seize opportunities that move you to "excellence." Only when patients experience excellence do they feel perhaps mildly shocked, but certainly impressed, and likely to go and tell the world about how *wonderfully* they were treated within your practice.

The competitive advantage in practice enhancement comes from making a perpetual series of incremental improvements on key service factors that move your practice from "good" to "excellent" on every aspect of service and patient care.

3

Patient Satisfaction by Design: A Model

Knowing the elements that constitute excellent service from the patient's perspective, you can enhance your practice by systematically building on your service strengths and tackling your service weaknesses. Not just a service orientation, but a *deliberate practice enhancement strategy,* can help your practice thrive.

AN ARCHITECTURAL APPROACH

Patient satisfaction is never an accident.

When a person looks for an architect, he or she usually defines the job in terms of the effects he or she wants the architect to create by design. For instance, let's say you want to design a new waiting area that is welcoming, nonintimidating, and generates an upbeat, not depressed, feeling among patients. You know the effects you want to create on each patient who enters, and you ask the architect to create a design that produces these effects.

Architects then have several variables to maneuver in order to create the effects you want. They can experiment with color, light, texture, space, and more. They make a combination of decisions about these variables that they believe will create the desired effects. If their decisions don't work, they can change them, choosing different colors, lighting, and textures.

The same goes for you in devising your practice enhancement strategy. You want satisfied, even impressed patients. You, too, have variables to maneuver in order to create satisfaction among your patients. To enhance your practice, you need to examine and reexamine these variables with an eye to making improvements in patient satisfaction. You are the architect who can combine elements by design that result in heightened patient satisfaction.

The Einstein Consulting Group has developed an analytical tool called "The Practice Enhancement Matrix" to help physicians devise a strategy for strengthening the service side of their practices. The Practice Enhancement Matrix defines six variables that you can maneuver to strengthen patient satisfaction. In the matrix below shown in Table 3–1, the six variables are listed on the left. The matrix is structured to invite an analysis of your practice's current strengths and weaknesses related to each variable.

To use this matrix in planning a practice enhancement strategy, you need to assess your practice on all six dimensions, identifying the strengths to build on

Table 3–1. The Practice Enhancement Matrix.

SERVICE FACTOR	STRENGTHS	WEAKNESSES
Medical Expertise		
Environment/Surroundings		
Staff Courtesy/Responsiveness		
Office Systems/Procedures		
Amenities/Extras		
Affordability		

Source: The Einstein Consulting Group. ©1988 and reprinted with permission.

and the weaknesses to attack in order to improve patient perceptions and heighten their satisfaction.

PLANNING IN THREE STEPS

Consider this three-step analytical process that translates into more satisfied patients and a competitive edge:

Step 1.   Know your patients—their preferences, perceptions, and expectations.

Step 2.   Evaluate your practice along the six service dimensions as they apply to your patients. Use the Practice Enhancement Matrix.

Step 3.   Generate a phased strategy for heightening patient satisfaction by building on your practice's service strengths and overcoming your practice's service weaknesses.

Step 1: Know your patients

The first step is to collect information about your own patients' preferences, perceptions, and expectations. In your quest to satisfy your patients, remember that they are your best consultants. Focus groups, brief surveys, telephone interviews, and a host of other techniques from simple to complex, from costly to cost-free, can yield this information.* Your internal staff or professional marketing and evaluation consultants can collect this important information. The key is, when you want to know more about your patients, ask them. Without input from your patients about their needs, concerns, preferences, and expectations, you are hard-put to set service objectives for your practice. Also, your own assessment of your practice, in the absence of patient feedback, runs the risk of being biased by perhaps unchallenged assumptions among your staff about what patients want.

Chapter 5 (See Your Practice as Others See It) provides an array of feedback devices that you can use to learn more about your patients, so you can tailor your practice to better meet their needs and expectations.

Step 2. Evaluate your practice along the six dimensions key to patient satisfaction

Knowing what patients want and value, you now need to scrutinize your practice using the Practice Enhancement Matrix. You, your staff, your patients and their families and friends all have perceptions of your practice's strengths and weak-

---

*The Einstein Consulting Group also performs one-day "Service Audits" for medical practices that accomplish this purpose.

nesses on service dimensions. After inviting people with multiple perspectives on your practice to express their perceptions, you can develop an accurate picture of what's working and what isn't in your quest for patient satisfaction. Chapter 5 also includes tools for soliciting perceptions of your practice on service dimensions.

Step 3. Generate a phased strategy for enhancing your practice on service dimensions

Based on a thorough assessment using the Practice Enhancement Matrix, you can then prioritize areas needing improvement and generate plans for making these improvements reality. If your assessment results in identification of multiple needs, that's normal. Achievement of service excellence needs to be a frequent, incremental process, not a one-time burst of activity. Attending to service improvement should be a way of approaching your business; it should not be a discrete event. It requires repeated efforts to understand the degree of satisfaction felt among patients, to consider possible improvements (their costs and benefits), and to make incremental improvements and refinements as needs and perceptions change.

Some practices, especially larger ones, devote quarterly meetings or sometimes annual retreats to take stock of their practice on service dimensions and set goals for improvements. When we serve as facilitators in retreats with this purpose, we engage physicians, office managers, and all other staff in synthesizing feedback results, adding their own perceptions and setting service improvement goals, priorities, and implementation plans.

DELIBERATE PRACTICE ENHANCEMENT PLANNING: ONE EXAMPLE

In getting concrete, consider an example of one practice that went through this process together and generated a conscious strategy to enhance their practice.

Holman and Starker is a two-doctor group practice in internal medicine, located in a medium-sized Midwestern city. Drs. Holman and Starker were not satisfied with the rate of growth of their patient population. They guessed that the grapevine controlled by their current patients was not enthusiastic enough to attract new patients.

Holman and Starker developed a patient survey that their receptionist asked patients to complete and return by mail after their visit. The survey simply asked these questions:

- What do you like about receiving your medical care from our practice?
- What don't you like about receiving your medical care from our practice?

- What can we do to meet your needs better when you use our services?

In a 2-week period, approximately 50 patients returned the survey in the confidential return envelope. The results were clear.

- Patients found the physicians competent.
- Several patients didn't like having to sit in the waiting room for several minutes before anyone noticed their presence.
- People didn't like the way they were asked for money *before* their office visit.

When asked to suggest ways Holman and Starker's practice could be improved, the 50 patients offered more than 70 suggestions.

Holman, Starker, and their entire staff held a three-hour meeting on a Saturday to examine the results and decide what to do about them. The meeting began with a review of the patient feedback information. The group then added their own perceptions of the practice's strengths and weaknesses using the Practice Enhancement Matrix as an organizing structure.

After filling out a large matrix on the wall, Dr. Starker asked the group to divide into trios and have each trio pretend to be the consultants who would recommend a specific step-by-step plan for enhancing the practice. After the groups presented their proposed plans, the entire group discussed elements they particularly liked and built a grand plan (See Table 3–2).

After developing this plan, the group designated deadlines and assigned responsibility for pursuing the various tasks. They also agreed to meet every two months to take stock of progress and new problems.

It doesn't take fancy expertise to develop a Practice Enhancement Plan like this, it just takes a decision on the part of your practice's key players to pay deliberate attention to the service side of your practice and take steps to strengthen elements that will result in more satisfied patients.

Table 3–2. Practice Enhancement Plan.

	JULY–OCT.	NOV.–FEB.	MAR.–JUNE
Medical Expertise	No Problem	Add a doctor to staff; assess better equipment options	Upgrade equipment
Environment	Fix holes in chairs; clean rug	Paint; buy nicer art.	Rebuild front desk area for confidentiality
People Skills	Set clear expectations of staff	Hold skill training for staff; monitor skill transfer to job	Patient survey on staff behavior
Systems	Investigate computerizing scheduling; design system for follow-up calls to patients	Install computer scheduling; start follow-up calls system	Evaluate scheduling; survey patients on callbacks; fix
Amenities	Survey patients on preferred magazines; subscribe to top five; get bottled water; keep cups available	Develop patient education library on most frequent ailments	Work out transportation options for older patients
Affordability	Call other doctors; study comparability of charges	Fix charges, if needed; educate staff to explain charges	Survey patient perceptions

4

Practice Enhancement Is Internal Marketing

THE WAITING ROOM SHUFFLE

Mr. Jones is 58 years old and has come to SuperPractice for an appointment. He *knows* something is wrong with him, and after much denial, he's finally come for a checkup. He waits. And he waits. He is not told how long he must wait, he is not asked if he is warm enough, comfortable, bored, thirsty, or whether he needs a bathroom. Alone, he has only his own apprehension for company.

Busy staff hurry by; no one stops to tell Mr. Jones what he can expect, explain what's happening, or see if they can do anything to make him comfortable. He still has not been told why he is being kept waiting, how much longer the wait will be, who will see him, or what will be done first.

After another interminable wait, he goes to the front desk where he asks timidly if perchance he might have been forgotten. The receptionist sighs, claiming that he will be taken when they're ready—shortly. She reminds him that he is not the only person waiting.

A few minutes later, Mr. Jones is directed to an exam room. After waiting there for more than ten minutes, a nurse finally comes in, updates his chart, and tells him that the doctor will be right in. Still no explanation and no apology. The doctor arrives and examines Mr. Jones. Throughout, Mr. Jones feels irritable, and the doctor finds him difficult. Sure enough, the doctor suspects that Mr. Jones has a stomach ailment, perhaps serious, that merits further tests. The doctor tells him that any information would, at this point, be guesswork, and that tests are the right next step. Mr. Jones says he'll call back to make test arrangements. He leaves. He doesn't call back. He doesn't trust these people. He asks a friend for the name of her doctor.

LOST BUSINESS

Family practitioner Harold Samson didn't depend on the rudeness of others to repel his patients; he did it himself. His annual income plummeted by 15 percent in the two-year period between 1986 and 1988. Dr. Samson's discouraged staff pointed to the physician's manner as the cause. According to them, Dr. Samson was curt with patients and rarely took time to talk with them about their concerns. Since he was always running late, he felt he had a good excuse.

Many of Dr. Samson's patients change physicians, since they expect from their physician and staff more personal attention and more respect for the value of their time.

QUICK, LET'S DO SOME MARKETING!

Drs. Hand, Wall, and Cort find their practice declining in patient volume. They're concerned. They decide to jump on the marketing bandwagon. They run a series of ads in the local paper focusing on new services they're providing. The ads all include the line, "Our staff is caring and responsive to your needs. Call us."

New to the community, Hannah Harper is looking for a doctor. She sees the ad and decides to call for an appointment. She calls and listens while the phone at Hand, Hall, and Cort rings at least 15 times. She hangs up, deciding she'd better ask a neighbor to refer a doctor.

Leslie Starr sees the same ad and, after failing to get an early appointment with another doctor he used once before, he decides to try this "caring and responsive" practice of Hand, Hall, and Cort. He calls. The receptionist responds with, "Hello. Please hold" Mr. Starr waits and waits, gradually feeling forgotten. He hangs up, stewing about the irony of the discrepancy between the ad's claim about "care and responsiveness" and the undeniable reality.

MISGUIDED MARKETING

Sound familiar? The stories are endless. The problem from a marketing stand-point: these medical practices neglected to stand behind their claims. They didn't keep their promises to patients. They neglected "internal marketing."

These anecdotes are not fiction. Ask consumers. Increasing numbers of physicians are employing marketing strategies in an effort to attract patients and referring physicians to their practices. Yet, some retain rude receptionists, keep patients waiting interminably, give inadequate explanations, make phone access frustrating, and expect patients to tolerate it all. Small wonder, then, that their medical practices have problems attracting and retaining patients.

PRACTICE ENHANCEMENT AS "INTERNAL MARKETING"

Marketing has begun to gain popularity among physicians. While there's no question that advertising, promotion and public relations are often necessary to attract patients and referring physicians, it's not enough. In fact, these methods of external marketing backfire unless every patient's experience *inside* your practice produces a high level of satisfaction. Deliberate attention to the quality of people's experience—particularly along service dimensions—is the mission of internal marketing. Practice enhancement, which is what internal marketing is all about, keeps people coming and coming back. Poor internal marketing, which means complacency about your patients' experience, is usually a result of neglect, not strategic error, and can drive an otherwise high-potential practice into the ground.

Getting concrete

Because of the intensity and quantity of interaction that patients, their family, friends, and other external customers have with your practice, you need employees and physicians who are *customer-oriented* and *sales-minded*. And you need a deliberate practice enhancement or internal marketing *strategy* as part of your practice's overall marketing plan to insure that an impressive service-orientation and sales-minded people are part and parcel of your practice's marketing strengths.

Better more than less

External marketing is, for most doctors, no longer a four-letter word. While it used to be that the thought of advertising summoned the image of huckster in many people's minds, that's not as true today. As Katie Tyndall explains in "Doctors Drum Up Business Success" (*Insight*, September 29, 1986), in today's competitive arena, "advertising is fast becoming a way of life for health care providers who wish to keep a practice afloat in a market that is overstocked."

But internal marketing through practice enhancement needs to come first, before external marketing. It's logical. Before you can make an important impact on your bottom line through external marketing, you need to insure that your house is in order, that your employees are selling your services and that a service orientation pervades your practice.

Specifically, you have to make sure that you meet or exceed patient expectations.

> It's far better to underpromise and overdeliver than the other way around.

Imagine needing a bank loan quickly. You call Bank A. The loan officer there says he'll have your loan ready for you by 2:00 PM that afternoon. You arrive at 2:00 PM for the check, only to discover that it won't be ready until 4:00 PM. You probably get really irritated, since Bank A failed on its promise, causing you to waste your valuable time. What conclusions would you draw about this bank's service?

Now consider Bank B. When you called Bank B for a quick loan, they said they would have your loan ready by 5:00 PM that day without fail. You arrive at 5:00, and your check is there to greet you.

In absolute terms, Bank A was more responsive to your need for a quick loan than was Bank B. They readied your check one hour faster. But even so, you probably developed a better opinion about the service at Bank B because they had your check ready *when they promised it.*

The same dynamic affects your patients—in clinical interactions as well as on service issues like waiting for an appointment. If a patient is going to have surgery that will be painful, clinical wisdom says it's better to tell them so that they know what to expect. When they have the pain, they won't be surprised. If it turns out to be less painful than you predicted, the patient will be relieved and grateful. On the other hand, if you understate the pain and the surgery proves agonizing, the patient might become panicky and even distrusting of you, because the pain is greater than you led them to expect.

Violated expectations also cause havoc to people's perceptions of the service quality extended to them by your practice. Consider the person who arrives in your office for an appointment. If you've made promises about short waiting time and then keep the person waiting, your patient gets annoyed. If you are honest about the wait time or even overestimate it, your patients will be much more satisfied, or at least much less dissatisfied. It's human nature. It does little good to purchase expensive brochures and ads if the quality of services, and your employees' helpfulness and spirit expressed toward your patients, are not also selling your practice—from the inside out. Patients faced with unfriendly, indifferent or uninformed staff will not develop loyalty to your practice, no matter how fancy and state-of-the-art your technology, and no matter how glitzy your ads.

Practice enhancement is not a supplement to external marketing. It is not concurrent with external marketing. It is a prerequisite.

The fact is, external marketing makes promises, while internal marketing through practice enhancement keeps promises. You need to make sure you can keep your promises before you make them. Otherwise, your external marketing efforts are no more than puffery, and your credibility is at risk. Figure 4–1 illustrates how this happens.

If you install an effective practice enhancement strategy, the dynamics of patient flow reverse (see Figure 4–2).

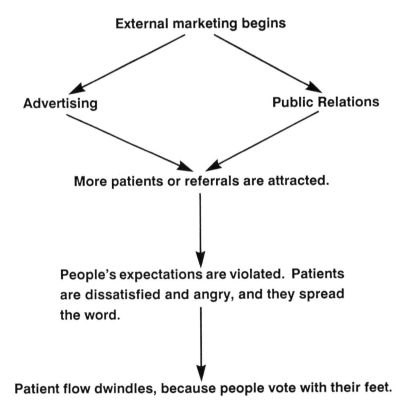

Figure 4–1. How patient flow dwindles.

Practice enhancements -- your internal marketing strategies are implemented. They heighten patient satisfaction.

External marketing spreads the word.

More patients and referrals are attracted.

People are satisfied and spread the good word.

Patient flow increases, because people vote with their feet.

Figure 4-2. How patient flow expands.

Bud Thieman, head of the Service Bureau for Doctors in Louisville, Kentucky ("The Doctors Most Likely to Get Hurt by Competition," *Medical Economics,* February 1, 1988, p. 102) summarizes the situation:

> It doesn't take a prophet to see what's in store for doctors over the next few years. Competition will continue to get more intense. Patients and referring physicians will continue to grow more demanding. Some practices won't survive. But those that do survive, and prosper, will thrive because the doctors who run them have honed their internal marketing skills to give patients and referring physicians what they want

In summary, you need a practice enhancement strategy and maintenance plan in order to control the quality of your patients' actual experience with your practice.

II
Your Environment, Systems, and Procedures

Just as architects vary lighting, color, texture, materials, space, height, and more in order to achieve their objectives, so can you also arrange or rearrange many variables purposefully in order to achieve your practice's patient satisfaction goals.

One influential trigger of patient satisfaction or dissatisfaction involves your practice's environment, systems, and procedures.

If you admit to weaknesses or missed opportunities in your practice related to the above areas, this section will help. We identify aspects of your environment, systems, and procedures that have an impact on patient satisfaction and present options for improvement.

In Chapter 5, we describe feedback devices that enable you to see your practice as others see it, and gain guidance in improving it.

In Chapter 6, we tour your office environment and examine the features and options that create ambience.

In Chapter 7, we address the sticky issue of money and how to deal with collections in a sensitive, caring manner.

In Chapter 8, we present an array of patient communication devices that reflect your commitment to patient satisfaction.

In Chapter 9, we examine the power of the telephone and offer alternative ways to use it to advantage as well as to avoid turning people away out of frustration.

In Chapter 10, we consider the omnipresent power of time, access, and convenience, and how to harness these factors to work for, not against, patient satisfaction.

5

See Your Practice as Others See It: How to Invite Feedback from Patients

Ask yourself, in your practice:

1. Do you really want to make your practice better based on feedback? (See Figure 5–1.)
2. Do you monitor patient satisfaction?
3. Do you monitor satisfaction of your referral sources?
4. Do you assess the satisfaction of the family and friends who accompany your patients to appointments?
5. Do you monitor staff satisfaction?
6. If you monitor satisfaction, do you do so regularly?
7. Do you feed back the results to everyone involved in your practice?
8. Do you make decisions about practice enhancements after examining the results?
9. Are your methods helpful?

Are you open to expert free consulting on how to enhance your practice? Such consulting is available to you in abundance if you're willing to invite

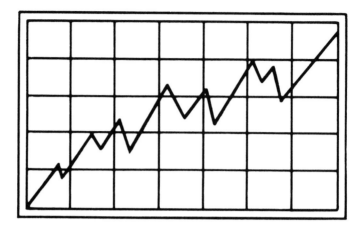

Figure 5–1. Graph indicating increasing patient satisfaction.

feedback from patients and their companions, and from your staff, that is, from the people on the receiving end of your practice's services.

These days, patients are thought to be increasingly demanding and knowledgeable. They scrutinize doctors and their practices for signs of malfunction, malpractice, and malice aforethought. You might view this scrutiny, on the one hand, as a debilitating pressure. But it doesn't have to be. The fact is, you can *use* the patient's observant nature to improve your practice, if you invite, or even encourage them to share their perceptions with you.

WHY DON'T MORE PHYSICIANS INVITE FEEDBACK?

In a recent phone survey of 35 medical practices in the Philadelphia area, we discovered that only two out of 35 practices did any sort of evaluation of their practices from the patient's perspective. People in 33 out of 35 practices were quick to explain why they don't solicit feedback from their "customers." In the course of these interviews, we identified eleven reasons (see Table 5–1). With which do you agree?

If you agree with many of these statements, feel normal! But examine your assumptions, some of which might be questionable. If you disagree with most of the statements, perhaps you just don't know easy ways to invite feedback. This chapter will provide an array of alternatives.

Let's examine for a moment the validity of the eleven reasons why doctors don't solicit feedback.

Table 5–1. Reasons Physicians Gave as to Why They Do Not Solicit Feedback from Patients.

	TRUE	FALSE
1. I already know what's best for my patients. I have nothing to learn that I don't already know.	T	F
2. We try as hard as we can to satisfy our patients, and can't do any better.	T	F
3. You can't trust what patients say.	T	F
4. Some patients are complainers and will never be pleased by anything.	T	F
5. If people complain, my staff will feel depressed or criticized, and less motivated to work.	T	F
6. If we ask for feedback, we'll cause people to bring their dissatisfactions to a conscious level, and therefore feel more dissatisfied than they would have if we hadn't asked.	T	F
7. I'm a doctor, not a researcher. I don't have the expertise to assess patient satisfaction.	T	F
8. We're busy and don't have time to get feedback.	T	F
9. If they're upset, they speak up. We don't have to ask for it.	T	F
10. Ignorance is bliss. If I don't hear about problems, I won't have to change the way we do things here.	T	F
11. I am who I am. The people who like my style find me. Those who don't like my style will find another doctor anyway.	T	F
TOTAL:		

1. "I know what's best for my patients."

You might be right. Or you might not be. In "Physician Perceptions of Patient Satisfaction: Do Doctors Know Which Patients Are Satisfied?" (*Medical Care*, 22 (5), May 1984), William Merkel, Ph.D., describes a study that revealed no relationship between actual patient satisfaction and physician perception of patient satisfaction. In Dr. Merkel's interpretation in this careful study, he suggests, "High technology medicine and the traditional, passive patient role may both interfere with physicians' ability to make accurate assessments of patient response" (p. 453). Also, there are or could be choices and alternatives available to the patient in terms of your services. By spelling these out to the patient, he or she can feel a greater sense of control over the outcome by expressing preferences. And you can show your openness to patient opinion.

On "service" issues, this point is particularly important. The only judge of patient satisfaction is the patient. To be frank, it's presumptuous to assume that you know what's most satisfying to your patients without asking them.

People associated with a practice get accustomed to the way things are. But as consumers get tougher in their expectations of a medical practice, you had better stay in touch with their changing expectations. Your "hallowed traditions" might become obsolete, but you might be too used to them to notice. By inviting feedback, you can put an important check-and-balance system on your assumptions about patient likes and dislikes. If you learn nothing new, you can feel affirmed in your sensitivity and astuteness. If you learn something new, you can enhance your practice.

2. "We try as hard as we can to satisfy our patients, and can't do any better, so why ask for advice?"

Just because you're used to doing things in certain ways doesn't mean there aren't better ways. By asking outsiders, you will inevitably get great ideas—in fact, inexpensive, simple ideas—for enhancing your practice. And why not try for free consulting. After all, you don't have to take any advice you don't want to take.

3. "You can't trust what patients say."

This attitude is dangerous. You have immunized yourself against taking seriously what your patients (your customers) think and feel about your practice. Patients are hypersensitive or even allergic to this attitude. When they choose another physician because you didn't value their thoughts, then will you believe what they think?

4. "Some people are complainers and will never be pleased by anything."

That's certainly true. But most people aren't *perpetual* complainers. If you solicit feedback and find that the vast majority of patients are happy with certain aspects of your practice, you can feel free to ignore the opinion of the never satisfied minority. But, on some service dimensions, you might find that many people (more than the typically complaining minority) are bothered by something. By asking for feedback and discovering a problematic pattern, you now have the chance to fix the problem.

5. "If people complain, my staff will feel depressed or criticized, and less motivated to work."

If people complain *and you don't do anything about their complaints*, you're right that your staff would become depressed, because nobody wants to be part of a practice that is blatantly unresponsive to its customers. But if people complain and you emphasize that their complaints give you the chance to fix the problem, your staff will, we promise, feel elevated and relieved. After all, they have complaints, too.

6. "If we ask for feedback, we'll cause people to bring their dissatisfactions to a conscious level, and therefore feel more dissatisfied than they would have if we hadn't asked."

Market research has shown this way of thinking to be grounded in false assumptions. First of all, if people are dissatisfied with your practice, they are dissatisfied whether or not you invite them to voice their dissatisfactions. If they are dissatisfied and you ask them to express themselves, they are impressed, because they realize that your intention is to satisfy them. If they are satisfied and you ask them to express themselves, they are also impressed that you cared enough to ask.

7. "I'm a doctor, not a researcher. I don't have the expertise to assess patient satisfaction."

Fortunately, you don't have to be a market researcher to solicit useful feedback from patients. Later in this chapter, we'll present a smorgasbord of simple, homespun methods that the typical intelligent physician can use to generate patient feedback.

8. "We're busy and don't have time to get feedback."

The issue here is commitment. If you want to enhance your practice, then you have to devote some energy to getting your patients to guide you in this process. It does take some time, although it doesn't have to take much time, since you can build simple feedback methods into ongoing activities and procedures.

9. "If they're upset, they speak up. We don't have to ask for it."

False. Here's the shocking statistic that refutes this belief. *Nine out of ten* people who are dissatisfied don't complain. Some feel at their doctor's mercy and are afraid to complain. Some don't have the self-confidence to speak assertively. Some are afraid they will hurt your feelings. And others feel that their physician is probably not interested in what they think. For this whole host of reasons, *most* people don't voice their complaints. But here's the crux of it. Just because they don't complain, it doesn't mean they're satisfied. It just means they didn't voice their complaint. Yet, if you can *get* the dissatisfied patient to complain (to you, not to their neighbor), they are *90 percent* more likely to be loyal to your practice. This suggests the need to invite, even beg and plead, for complaints.

10. "Ignorance is bliss. If I don't hear about problems, I won't have to change the way we do things here."

This is true. You won't have to change anything, in fact, you don't have to change anything even if you do invite feedback. But if you have problems and you decide not to change anything, you can expect to experience consequences, such as a dwindling patient following and a grapevine about you that would make you wish you were hard of hearing.

11. "I am who I am. The people who like my style find me. Those who don't like my style will find another doctor anyway."

The people who would tend to like your style may indeed find you. If that group is large enough to sustain your practice, so be it. However, these days, most physicians target a mix of patient types. They develop a diversity of styles so that they have the potential to serve a variety of people effectively. And many find that it is absolutely possible to expand their repertoire of styles to cater to various kinds of people—especially if they solicit and learn from feedback.

Lots of reasons exist for not welcoming or soliciting feedback. You need to ask yourself whether these reasons, many of which fly in the face of reality, outweigh the potential benefits of the opposite action, that is, taking deliberate steps to generate feedback.

THE BENEFITS OF FEEDBACK

Feedback can help you do the following:

- *Know*, not guess, the level of satisfaction among your patients, their companions, and your staff.
- *Monitor* satisfaction over time, so you have the chance to respond to downward trends.
- *Identify* the aspects of your practice that foster high satisfaction, so you can feel good about them, continue them, compliment staff who contributed to them, and even build on them.
- *Pinpoint* the aspects of your practice that interfere with high satisfaction, so you can acknowledge these weaknesses, fix them, or if you can't, then compensate for them in some way that minimizes their detrimental effects.

- *Reinforce* a service orientation among staff by having individual staff members ask questions of patients about their satisfaction and then see the results.
- *Heighten accountability* for patient satisfaction. Have the means to confront yourself, your colleagues, and staff about the effects of their actions on patients.
- *Measure* the results of innovations and changes you're making to see if they're having the desired benefits.

The point is, if you don't measure it, you can't manage it or control it. And given the fact that *staff* respects what management inspects, if you don't solicit feedback, you will have a tough time holding staff accountable for results.

It boils down to this:

You can't tell if you're winning without a scorecard!

ELEVEN ALTERNATIVE METHODS

If you want to understand your patients' perceptions, methods abound. Ideally, you should mix methods, since you'll capture new information with each new method.

This section describes 11 different methods that can be used mix-and-match to get a solid, ongoing, helpful grip on patient perceptions, concerns and preferences. The methods are:

- The simple paper-and-pencil survey
- The post-appointment telephone interview
- The patient focus group
- Interviews with companions: While-U-Wait feedback
- Perceptions among your referral sources
- "Patient drain" tracking
- Formal surveys by a pro
- Ask your employees
- The good, old-fashioned suggestion box
- The service audit
- Complaint tracking

Method 1: The simple paper-pencil survey

You can develop a printed patient survey that you distribute to patients after their appointment. You can invite them to fill it out and leave it in a box near the exit, or you can provide a stamped, return envelope that they can use to mail back the survey to you within the next few days (see Table 5–2).

Or consider a survey form used by Valley Health Center, an ambulatory care center in Santa Clara, California (see Figure 5–2):

Figure 5–3 shows another great example from Barbara Lewis, "How To Develop and Use a Patient Questionnaire" (from *Physicians Management,* 26(2), February 1986, pp. 164–65.)

Here's a brief, simple tool that asks open-ended questions:

1. What did you like about your visit with us today?

2. What didn't you like about your visit with us today?

3. How can we improve any future experiences you might have with our practice?

Method 2: The post-appointment telephone interview

A wonderful source of rich, qualitative information is a telephone interview one to three days after a person's appointment. This can double as a way to follow up on the patient's condition and, at the same time, invite comments about their satisfaction and complaints related to the service they received.

Some physicians have the office manager or nurse conduct these interviews. Others have all staff (including the physicians) conduct a few interviews, thus getting everyone involved and developing a stake in patient satisfaction. How might such a method work?

Dr. Strand has a group practice with six other physicians. Dr. Strand, her office manager, and their receptionist met to develop the interview protocol. Dr. Strand then held a "training session" for all staff and physicians associated with the practice. She shared her belief that the future of their practice rests on happy patients. She expressed the view that every person involved in their practice should listen to patient feedback and participate in enhancing the practice to produce a level of patient satisfaction that would make them all proud. She conveyed her plan to engage everyone in a patient satisfaction study the last week of every month. Specifically, each person would be assigned four patients to call on the phone and ask about their experiences with the practice. Dr. Strand handed out a list of the questions that her committee had developed. She divided people into pairs and asked them to try the questions on one another. Afterward, the group refined the questions and discussed ways to handle resistant people, people who didn't seem to have much to say, and so on.

The interview protocol looked like this:

> Hello, this is _____ from Dr.'s _____ office. How are you feeling? *(Listen and be responsive. Then, move on.)* I wanted

to know how you're doing, and I also have another reason for calling. Several of us from our office are calling patients who visited our office during the last month to ask a few questions about how they viewed their experience with our practice. We're trying to make whatever changes we need to make in our practice in order to give our patients the service they deserve . . . I'd like to know if you would be willing to answer a few questions about your experience with us? . . . I'd like to arrange for a five-minute, *confidential* interview with you at a time convenient for you . . . now or at a more convenient time. Would you agree to that? (Now or another time?) . . . Great! I really appreciate your taking the time . . . Let me begin . . . .

1. What did you like about your last visit to our office?
2. What bothered you about your last visit to our office? Please feel free to mention anything big or small, since that will help us make things better.
3. What can we do to make our service better for you?
   (Push here for many suggestions, a wish list.)

Closing: Mrs. _____, I really appreciate your willingness to answer these questions so frankly. It helps us know what we're doing right and what we need to work on in order to give you the quality of service you deserve. Thanks so much and I hope you *(feel better? continue to feel better? continue to feel well?* etc.)

Dr. Proctor has a different way of implementing the idea of telephone interviews with patients. He pays his receptionist for four extra hours per week to make evening phone calls to patients.

The Washington Medical Group *alternates* the responsibility for post-appointment phone calls among its 12 staff people. One person makes 12 calls per month, summarizes the results, and reports back to the staff at a monthly "stock-taking" meeting.

Haskins Associates has a pizza dinner once a month after which people sit at phones (telethon style) and call patients. The next day, they have a protected, scheduled meeting at which they compare results and identify problems they want to solve in order to strengthen the service features of their practice.

All of these practices value patient feedback. All devote time and resources to staying "close to their patients" and using feedback to make their practices better.

Table 5–2. One-Minute Check-Up.

You came in for a checkup. now, I'm asking you to give me one. I'm concerned about the quality of medical care and service I provide for you. I would appreciate it if you would take a minute to complete this checkup and return it to me in the enclosed, stamped envelope.

I care what you think and will consider your feedback carefully so I can serve you better.

Kindest personal regards,
M. Doctorly

****

ARE WE MEETING YOUR HEALTH CARE NEEDS?

Please take a few minutes to complete our questionnaire. This is strictly confidential, so please let us know your honest evaluation. It is our hope to serve your healthcare needs better. Thank you.

1. How satisfied are you with the courtesy you receive when you phone our office?
   _____ very dissatisfied   _____ somewhat dissatisfied
   _____ somewhat satisfied   _____ very satisfied
   If not satisfied, why not?_____

2. How easy or hard is it for you to obtain convenient appointment times with us?
   _____ very easy   _____ somewhat easy
   _____ somewhat hard   _____ very hard

3. How promptly does the doctor see you?
   _____ a long delay   _____ a short delay   _____ right on time

4. How pleasant and comfortable do you find our reception area?
   _____ very uncomfortable and unpleasant
   _____ somewhat uncomfortable and unpleasant
   _____ somewhat comfortable and pleasant
   _____ very comfortable and pleasant
   How would you improve it? _____

5. How well does our staff explain policies and procedures to you?
_____ very well   _____ somewhat well   _____ not well at all
Comments_____

_____

6. How reasonable are our fees?
_____ very   _____ somewhat   _____ not at all

7. How well do we explain our fees?
_____very well   _____ somewhat well
_____ somewhat poorly   _____ very poorly
Comments_____

_____

8. When you leave the office, how well do you feel we have explained your medical problems and reasons for prescribed therapies?
_____ very well   _____ somewhat well
_____ somewhat poorly   _____ very poorly

9. Would you recommend our practice to your family and friends?
_____ YES   _____ NO

10. Please share your advice about how we can satisfy you better.

_____

_____

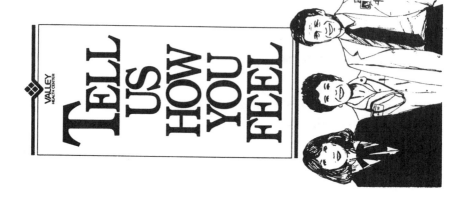

Dear Patient:

As a patient, you have seen Valley Health Center from the most important perspective. We hope you'll take a few minutes to tell us about your visit to our health center. Your comments and suggestions will help us meet our number one goal: providing our patients with the best care and service available in Santa Clara County.

Thank you for your assistance.

Sincerely,

Robert Sillen
Executive Director

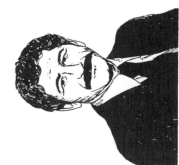

Figure 5–2. Survey form used by Valley Health Center, Santa Clara, California.

VALLEY
HEALTH CENTER

About your visit...

1. Were you scheduled for an appointment within:
   - ☐ One (1) week
   - ☐ Two (2) weeks
   - ☐ Three (3) weeks
   - ☐ Four (4) or more weeks
   - ☐ Urgent visit, same day

2. When you arrived for your appointment, was your paperwork handled promptly?
   - ☐ Yes
   - ☐ No

3. How long did you wait in the waiting room before you saw the physician?
   - ☐ Less then 15 minutes
   - ☐ 15 to 30 minutes
   - ☐ More than 30 minutes

4. Was the staff friendly?
   - ☐ Yes
   - ☐ No

5. Please list any Valley Health Center staff you came in contact with during the visit who deserve special recognition for exceptional service.
   _____
   _____
   _____

6. Please also list any Valley Health Center staff you came in contact with during your visit who were unfriendly or insensitive to your needs.
   _____
   _____
   _____

7. Did the doctor...
   seem courteous and interested in you
   - ☐ Yes
   - ☐ No
   spend sufficient time with you
   - ☐ Yes
   - ☐ No

provide you with adequate information about your treatment
   - ☐ Yes
   - ☐ No

8. If you were unhappy with your visit, please explain
   _____
   _____

9. Did the facility look clean and well-maintained?
   - ☐ Yes
   - ☐ No

About our other services...

10. Did you receive service in X-ray?
    - ☐ Yes
    - ☐ No

11. If yes, prior to your X-ray did you receive
    - ☐ adequate instructions
    - ☐ no instructions
    - ☐ didn't need any instructions

12. Did you use the Pharmacy?
    - ☐ Yes
    - ☐ No

13. If yes, did the Pharmacist give you
    - ☐ adequate instructions about your prescription
    - ☐ no instructions

14. Did you receive service in the Laboratory?
    - ☐ Yes
    - ☐ No

15. Were you seen promptly in these areas?
    - ☐ Yes
    - ☐ No
    If no, please explain
    _____
    _____

Overall...

16. Would you rate our services at the Valley Health Center as
    - ☐ Excellent
    - ☐ Good
    - ☐ Average
    - ☐ Needs improvement
    - ☐ Poor

17. Would you recommend Valley Health Center to a friend?
    - ☐ Yes
    - ☐ No

18. How was payment for your bill handled?
    - ☐ Self or family
    - ☐ Valley Health Plan
    - ☐ Blue Cross
    - ☐ Other Insurance
    - ☐ Worker's Compensation
    - ☐ Medicare
    - ☐ MediCal
    - ☐ Ability To Pay Determination Program (APD)
    - ☐ Other _____

19. Did we miss an area you would like to comment on? Any suggestions?
    _____
    _____
    _____
    _____
    _____
    _____
    _____
    _____

SAMPLE PATIENT QUESTIONNAIRE

Dear patient:

Based on your experience and feelings, please rate each of the following questions. Mark the box that best expresses your judgment. A 5 is the equivalent of "excellent" — a 1 is "poor." If a question is not applicable, simply draw a line through the five boxes.

	Excellent 5	Above average 4	Average 3	Below average 2	Poor 1
When you telephoned, how promptly were your calls answered?					
How courteously and efficiently were your questions or requests handled?					
How quickly were you able to reach me in an emergency after office hours?					
When you visited my office, how welcome were you made to feel?					
In terms of comfort and attractiveness, how do you rate the reception room?					
How comfortable and attractive was the examination room?					
How would you rate the amount of time I spend with you during our initial meetings?					
How do you rate the thoroughness of the examination you received?					
To what degree of satisfaction and understanding did I explain the results of your examination and recommendations?					
Before surgery, how was your understanding of what would be done, details of the postsurgery period, and what the final results were likely to be?					
How helpful were the printed materials you received from me?					
How well were the fees and costs for care explained to you?					
How easily understood were the billing statements or insurance forms?					
How much to your convenience was the day and time of your surgery?					
Was the amount of time and care after surgery sufficient for you to recover?					
How comfortable and attractive were the postsurgery facilities?					

Source: Steve Ollan, CPBC, Practice Management Concepts, Burlingame, California.

Figure 5–3. Sample patient questionnaire.

	5	4	3	2	1
Please rate the degree of privacy in the office during each of the following: Examination and consultation					
Financial discussions and arrangements					
Before and during surgery					
Immediately after surgery					
How satisfied were you with the results of your surgery?					
How do you rate the patience, warmth, and understanding you received from me?					

	Yes	No
Did you ever call my office, and the telephone was <u>not</u> answered? If "yes," at what time of day? _____		
Did you ever have a long wait to see me? If you did wait a long time, were you given the reason?		
Do you feel the need for additional information to aid your understanding of surgical procedures, their effects and their results?		
When you visited my office, was parking convenient?		
Do you feel the need for information and services concerning skin care, make-up, and diet as part of your care?		

Would you take a moment to reflect on the various staff functions and rate certain qualities, using the scale of 5 as "excellent" to 1 as "poor":

	Courteous and pleasant?					Helpful and patient?					Professional and efficient?				
	5	4	3	2	1	5	4	3	2	1	5	4	3	2	1
Receptionist															
Office nurse															
Surgery nurse															
Bookkeeper															

Any other suggestions or comments you might have will be greatly appreciated. Please feel free to jot them down on the lines below, and use the back of this page as well. Thank you for your help.

_____

_____

Method 3: Patient focus groups

Dear Ms. Stone,

   I am interested in making my patients' experiences with our medical practice as positive as possible.

   On June 13th, Susan Afriat from The Einstein Consulting Group will be holding a "focus group" dinner with several patients who use our practice. We invite you to be our guest at dinner. Also, we will provide you with a $25 honorarium for you to help defray your transportation, childcare, or other expenses involved in attending this gathering. The purpose: to invite people to share their views on our practice, its strengths, weaknesses, and how we can improve it to achieve greater patient satisfaction. I won't be there, because I want people to feel very free to speak up. In fact, all of your comments will be held in strictest confidence. I don't want my presence to inhibit any comments that might prove very useful in making our medical practice better.

   Will you join Ms. Afriat and several other patients for this dinner discussion?

   Time: 7–9 PM

   Place: Ming Dynasty (Chinese Restaurant), 2nd and Bainbridge
        Streets, Philadelphia

   Please call my office at 444-4444 to R.S.V.P. I hope you can make it. If not, I want to encourage you to share your views and suggestions about our practice with me or any of our staff, so we can give you the quality of health care and service you deserve.

   Thank you very much.

                        Sincerely,
                        Mike Fine, M.D.

Ms. Stone would probably be surprised to receive an invitation like this, pleasantly surprised. Increasing numbers of doctors are instituting periodic group discussions or "focus groups" to invite qualitative feedback about how to enhance their practices. Focus groups are "focused" discussions structured and led to evoke perceptions and suggestions from the people your practice is designed to serve. Focus groups are also used to solicit reactions to plans and ideas you have, so you can debug and refine them *before* you institute them. The reason some people prefer focus groups over individual interviews is that the participants trigger memories and suggestions in one another. The result is often a very high quality of in-depth feedback and even creative suggestions about how to enhance your practice, because people piggyback on one another's views and ideas.

Some practices hire a professional focus group facilitator to conduct focus groups. Other practices use a person on staff (e.g., office manager, congenial receptionist, one of the doctors) who has the congeniality, the ability to listen without getting defensive, and skill in sparking open discussion. If you use a professional (available from market research and patient satisfaction assessment companies), this person works with you to:

- Identify what you want to learn
- Make all the arrangements
- Take a patient list you provide and call people to secure a large enough participant group
- Conduct the group discussion
- Send thank you's to the participants
- Develop for you a rich report that details what people said and the facilitator's conclusions and recommendations

Some practices hire a professional focus group facilitator to conduct one focus group. An appropriate member of your staff can watch and then learn how to conduct future groups.

With the results of focus groups in hand, you or you with your staff can generate a service improvement plan based on patient feedback. If one of your own people conducts these groups, you save money, but you have to make sure that they have the skills to invite openness and concrete, helpful responses. Some practices try an in-house person first to see if they can make that approach successful. If not, then they seek the help of professionals.

Here's an example of two Focus Group Question Protocols. The first was designed to tap overall perceptions of one medical practice. The second was designed to *pre*-test on consumers key aspects of one group's proposed practice enhancement strategy.

Focus Group Protocol #1: Tap Patient Perceptions.

1. Introductions; your experience with our practice: number of years, who in your family, how you heard about it initially.

2. Think back to the last time you had some kind of interaction with our practice. Could we go around and have people say a bit about the situation and how you felt about it?

3. In your experiences with our practice, what have you liked?

4. In your experience with our practice, what haven't you liked?

5. Can you think of specific situations you wish the staff had handled differently?

6. Can you think of specific situations you wish the doctor had handled differently?

7. How do you feel about the office environment? What could improve it?

8. How do you feel about office systems, like scheduling appointments, phone, billing, etc.? What could improve these?

9. (Give out sheet of rating scales. Ask people to fill it out and then talk from it. Collect these, so you can tally results.) e.g., How would you rate this practice on:

- Amenities or extras provided to make you feel comfortable?
- Personalized attention and responsiveness to you as a person?
- Staff courtesy?
- Physician attention?
- Convenience?
- Access to the doctor when you want it?
- The way people handle billing/money situations?
- And more.

10. If this were your practice, how would you improve it?

Focus Group Protocol #2: Pretest an Enhancement Plan.

The leader starts: "You've been using this medical practice for more than 2 years. The physicians are planning to make some changes in this practice that they believe will serve you better. But they want to get patient reactions to these proposed changes before they institute them, to make sure the changes will, from the patient's point of view, make things better. That's why you're here. I've been asked to describe these changes to you and get your reactions and suggestions"

Leader then presents key features of practice enhancement plan, e.g.,

- new waiting room layout and color scheme
- new office hours and scheduling system
- two options for patient education resources
- optional amenities—which would patients prefer?

Leader ends by asking, "You're the most valuable consultants we could ever get. What other suggestions do you have for how people in this medical practice could be made to be better for its patients?"

Method 4: Interviews with companions: while-u-wait feedback

Many people go to the doctor with a friend or family member. That companion sometimes goes into the exam room or consulting room along with the patient. Other times, that person sits and waits in the waiting area. In both cases, this observer is collecting valuable information about your practice. Typically feeling protective of their loved ones, they scrutinize what's happening and see it all. They tend to be keenly astute because of their inclination to be advocates for the right treatment for their loved one.

Why not take advantage of the time they are spending sitting around watching how your practice functions? If you invite their perceptions and suggestions, not only do you have the chance to learn a lot but you simultaneously make their waiting time go faster by occupying them. You're also communicating the message that you don't think they're invisible, but instead, important.

You can tap their views by providing a short written survey or having a member of your staff sit down with them for a few minutes and ask a few questions. A survey might look like this:

> Dear Friend,
>
> Here you sit—waiting. While you're waiting, you have a chance to see how we function here. And you know how our office and people make you feel. Would you be willing to share with us your opinions of this medical practice, based on your own observations and anything you might have heard about us before? Your views will be confidential. You don't have to put your name on this form, and you can drop it in the box by the door along with everyone else's. We really want you to be frank with us and not be concerned about anyone here knowing who said what!
>
> 1. What's good about this medical practice—anything at all? (environment, staff, doctors, getting here, waiting area, other facilities, etc.)
>
> 2. What don't you like about this practice? (same probes as above)
>
> 3. What would you change here in order to make this the ideal medical practice?
>   Please drop this card in the box near the front door. And, thank you very much for helping us better satisfy our patients.

Similar questions can be asked of people by office staff. Or, you can identify specific questions about aspects of your practice you particularly want to learn more about. An example follows.

Here you sit, waiting for your friend or family member. Would you be willing to share your views about the experience you're having waiting in our waiting room? It will help us make future waiters' waits more tolerable.

1. Regarding the physical environment in this waiting area, how do you feel about:
   - the colors you see
   - furniture arrangement
   - chair comfort
   - sounds you hear
   - air temperature
   - things available to do to make the time go faster
   - staff behavior toward you

2. Please share any suggestions or ideas you have about how we can make the experience of waiting here more pleasant.
   - any amenities or conveniences we could provide
   - environmental improvements
   - etc.

   Please drop your comments in the box by the door. And thank you *very* much!

Method 5: Referral source perceptions

If your practice receives referrals from other physicians, community agencies, or other professional groups, consider asking them for feedback about what they see and what they hear secondhand about your practice. Referral sources are, after all, customers whose referrals help build your practice. Try a semiannual letter to referrers or quarterly phone calls to a selection of referrers. Ask questions like these:

1. What have you heard about our practice?
2. What have you heard about our positive features?
3. What have you heard about our weaknesses or negative aspects?
4. How do you feel about our relationship with you as a valued referrer? Do we communicate well enough? How could we communicate better? Do we refer patients back to you at the appropriate point in their treatment? Do you have any suggestions?
5. What suggestions do you have for making our practice more responsive to you and the people you tend to refer to practices like ours?

Method 6: "Patient drain" tracking

Some patients move away. Some pass away. Some join an HMO without your practice as a participant. Others select a competing doctor because of something that happened or didn't happen that made the patient angry. You need to know why patients leave your practice, since, if you choose to, you can do something about many of their reasons.

One of the most valuable sources of feedback comes from patients who patronized your practice, but, for one reason or another, decided to take their healthcare business elsewhere. You really shouldn't let these people just go away. You should send them a letter at the very least, or better yet, have someone call them to solicit their reasons for abandoning your practice. Some physicians say, "You win some; you lose some. If they didn't like me, then who needs them?" But people might have been turned away by aspects of your practice that you can *fix*—if you know what they are. So, when someone calls to cancel an appointment and doesn't schedule a new one, train your staff to press for reasons. If someone calls or writes to have his or her medical records transferred, train your staff to find out *why*. At the end of each month, summarize the results. Show how many patients left for each major reason; then ask, "Knowing these results, how can we reduce patient drain?"

To a lost patient:

> I understand you called to have your medical records transferred to another physician. We're interested here in making changes to better achieve patient satisfaction. I would appreciate it very much if you would share with me why you've decided to change doctors.

If the reason has nothing to do with your practice (e.g., the person moved too far away), ask for their views about your practice anyway. If their reasons seem to have something to do with the care, treatment or service received from your practice, then pump for feedback and suggestions, and thank the person profusely, being careful not to get defensive or try to talk them into giving your practice another chance.

Here's a possible telephone scenario (reprinted with permission from "The Doctor's Office" Newsletter, November 1986, p. 4):

Mrs. Wells, Patient: Hello.

Linda, Office Manager: Mrs. Wells? This is Linda, the office manager at Dr. Fargo's office. We have your message to cancel your appointment, but there isn't a reason. Is everything all right?

Mrs. Wells: Well . . . I am feeling better, but that's not why I cancelled.

Linda: I'm glad to hear you're feeling better. But I would like to know why you cancelled. You see, Mrs. Wells, you've been a patient of Dr. Fargo for a long time and when you cancelled your appointment without a reason, we were concerned . . . .

Mrs. Wells: Well . . . I'd really rather not say.

Linda: Sure, I understand. If it's something personal . . . you know, we do think of you as a friend. If there's something you'd like to say, I can promise you the same confidentiality you always get from Dr. Fargo.

Mrs. Wells: Well . . . the last time I was in . . . someone said something about my weight. It was that blonde-haired nurse . . . the pretty one. Why couldn't she just write it down, instead of announcing it to the whole world!

Linda: I'm very sorry, Mrs. Wells. I don't know why that happened. . . . we certainly don't want that to ever happen here. But seriously I'd hate to think this incident could destroy the good relationship you've had with this practice for so many years. I surely wouldn't want the continuity of your care to suffer because of something like this.

Mrs. Wells: Well, I was just so embarrassed . . .

Linda: Mrs. Wells, I'd like to apologize to you for the practice. I'll see that it doesn't happen again. Do you think we can start over?

Mrs. Wells: Well, if you're sure it will never happen again . . .

Linda: Dr. Fargo and I will speak to the nurse you mentioned. We really are very sorry that this happened. Would you like to make a new appointment with Dr. Fargo?

Mrs. Wells: Well, I am feeling better . . .

Linda: Well, that's just great then . . .

Mrs. Wells: But there was another problem I'd been meaning to ask Dr. Fargo about. Maybe I should come in . . .

You might also ask if the patient would like to, or be willing to, talk with the doctor personally about why they are leaving the practice. This is especially important if there's a chance that behavior on the part of other staff might have been a contributing factor.

Or consider this example of a written communication that you send to a patient who has requested a record transfer ("The Doctor's Office," November 1986, p. 5).

Dear Mrs. Wells,

You've been a good patient and a welcome friend of this practice for _____ years, and we want you to know we value the relationship we've had with you. That's why we were especially concerned when we received your request to have your records transferred. We didn't know that you were unhappy with your treatment here, and we were puzzled.

If you've moved or if you've found a practice you feel can serve you better, then we wish you all the best. But if there's another reason you made this request, we'd like to know what it is, so we can avoid making the same mistake in the future. If you're upset by something we've done or failed to do, please take a moment to call and tell us about it. Just call us at 000-0000 and ask to speak to one of the doctors or to me.

Or, in case you're not comfortable discussing it on the phone, we've enclosed a readdressed envelope you can use to express your feelings in writing. Thank you again for being a long-standing friend and patient of this practice, and we look forward to having you as a friend for many years to come.

Sincerely,
Linda Esh
Office Manager

Also, institute a method for tracking all exiting patients, so you know the trends regarding your growth compared with your losses of patients. Leave a simple tracking form at the front desk, accessible to everyone on the staff likely to learn of exiting patients. If certain reasons keep showing up, like inconvenient appointment times, difficulty reaching the doctor by phone, long waits, and so on, you have your work cut out for you.

This kind of practice of pumping lost patients for feedback is a no-lose strategy. You might get some valuable information. But most certainly, if you don't ask for feedback and the person is angry at you or your practice, they will tend to spread this negative word to many, many people. If you invite feedback and thank them, without being pushy or angry, they might tell friends they switched doctors, but they tend to add, "But they know they have problems and are working to fix them. In fact, they even asked me to tell them what I thought of them."

Method 7: Formal surveys by a pro

Of course, you can hire a market research or patient satisfaction assessment company to conduct patient satisfaction studies for you. Some practices do this every two years. Others hire a pro once and have a staff member apprentice to this person in order to learn the method for the future. They believe it's worth the money to have a thorough, controlled study done that gives them relatively more objective feedback from patients than they could get themselves. Studies like these can also involve other practice's patients and, more significantly, patients who used your practice but left it.

If you want to engage outside help, ask around for people who know the healthcare field. Interview prospective research vendors and make sure they have the experience and the methods needed. Ask for a specific proposal with prices. Or ask your local hospital's marketing department for help.

Method 8: Ask your employees

You can be sure that people in your service area make comments and cracks to your employees about your practice—on the street, at the supermarket, at family gatherings—anywhere, in fact. As a result, your employees pick up scuttlebutt about people's experience with your practice.

Provide a protected way your employees can express what they hear about your practice. If what they hear is bad, it demoralizes them and dampens their commitment to work. You benefit from inviting them to share the grapes from the grapevine, so you can know what they heard, *and* can know if employees are likely to be demoralized about the word on the street about your practice. They are part of your practice, and your reputation reflects on them.

If you have positive relationships with your employees, just come right out and ask what they hear on the street about your practice. If you suspect that employees might not feel free to share all that they've heard, use a more protected method. One such method is a group meeting (without you present) where people make a long group list of everything anyone heard about the practice in the last two months. Who said what is not relevant or apparent. Another approach is to develop a form like the following:

Scuttlebutt Report

"If we hear the scuttlebutt, we'll
know what we need to fix!!"

Staff,

Please write or type below anything you heard about our practice from anyone outside of it, including:

1. questions anyone asked you about us and our ways,
2. comments anyone made about our practice or any of us.

Thanks.

Method 9: The good old-fashioned suggestion box

Place a box inviting "Complaints and Suggestions" in one or two prominent places around your offices (e.g., waiting area, bathroom, hallway near exam room), and encourage people to use them. Attach to each box a pad of paper and pencils, so people don't have to fish through their belongings to be able to submit a suggestion or complaint. Read through the results every week and you'll get great ideas for practice enhancements. If people signed their names to their entries, send out a thank you note.

Method 10: The service audit

Finally, by calling in outsiders with a fresh perspective, you can gain additional feedback about your practice. Hotel managers or members of the marketing department of the hospital with which you're affiliated, or consultants, can visit your practice, walk through your systems, observe, talk to people, and give you comprehensive feedback about your service strengths and weaknesses and recommendations for improvement.

The daughter of one physician formed a "user-friendly committee" consisting of her father's patients. She met with this group and asked them to meet with one another, revisit the offices, examine the details, and develop recommendations about how the patient experience with her dad's practice could be enhanced. They read the pamphlets in the waiting area; they looked at the quality and wording of signs hanging here or there around the office; they examined the forms patients have to fill out and recommended plain-English ways to get the same information; and more. Not only did these patients enjoy this process; it yielded more than 20 suggestions for improving the practice. The same process would work with volunteers, college students, students in hotel management school, and so on.

Method 11: Complaint tracking

Without being asked, some people voice their complaints to you or other members of your staff. Instead of listening to these complaints and then forgetting about them, institute a tracking system that everyone uses to record complaints and identify patterns that warrant attention. You might consider keeping a form at the front desk that tracks the date of complaint physician or staff involved, nature of complaint, follow-up and results.

SEQUENCED APPROACH TO MEASUREMENT

If you want feedback so that you can enhance your practice, try the following sequence:

- Measure perceptions on many service dimensions

- Identify the *key* service attributes

- Invite whatever complaints people might be harboring

- Develop a long-range satisfaction tracking plan based on knowing the service attributes valued by your patients.

Remember the Patient Satisfaction Matrix presented earlier? It identifies six major dimensions of excellent service:

- Medical expertise
- Environment
- Interpersonal skills
- Easy-to-use, convenient systems
- Amenities/"Extras"
- Affordability

You can invite *ongoing* feedback about these dimensions to keep you on track.

The bottom line

Consider five points:

1. Feedback is the seeing-eye dog for a practice. When you're used to doing things a certain way, and you do it that way day after day, you run the risk of becoming blind to its effects and the alternatives. Feedback from your patients and their companions, and your staff and referrers, gives you a different perspective that enables you to target your strengths and weaknesses and take deliberate action to make your practice more effective and more successful.

2. Ongoing is better than one-shot. It's easy to forget to get feedback. That's why many enlightened physicians are building feedback-gathering into their practices on a systematic basis—monthly, weekly, quarterly—on a systematic, regular, nonhaphazard basis. Then, you don't forget.

3. Don't worry about using methods that are research, pure or unobtrusive. The methods described here have proven to be effective in evoking valuable, usable information. Also, when you are blatant about what you're trying to learn, you not only gather usable information, you also communicate to your respondents that you care what they think and are dedicated to making your practice meet their needs—even to the point of inviting negative comments. Regarding obtrusiveness, the more you and your staff ask for patient satisfaction feedback, the more your minds will be focused on taking all possible steps to achieve patient satisfaction. The questions implant in your mind a service orientation that tends to attune you to patients and their needs. It's all to the better if the existence of these questions makes you more responsive to patients before you get a chance to measure their perceptions. The goal is to optimize satisfaction every which way.

4. Involve your staff in the criteria, in order to raise their awareness.   Everyone in your practice needs to act on the results of patient feedback. People are more likely to act on feedback if they asked for it. That's why it helps to get your staff together to generate the questions your feedback devices will ask. Your staff will be more invested in seeing and acting on the results. If you don't involve your staff in generating or refining or asking the questions, you run the risk of having them feel that you're checking up on or judging *them* when you seek patient feedback. And make sure you feed back the results to staff in meetings, memos, and newsletters.

Good News

Patient ratings are up! Of those who responded to last month's survey, _____% said they are happy using our practice and plan to continue using us. This compares to only _____% the month before. Here's a sampling of their suggestions:

(add a few comments here)

Thank you for all you're doing to make our group a star among medical practices!

5. Don't ask if you're not going to listen, believe what you're hearing, and act.   Some people invite feedback in order to convey an *image* of responsiveness. The fact is, if you don't act on feedback, people know that you invited their views only for image reasons, not because you really cared to improve your practice. That's why you have to make sure you review the results of whatever feedback devices you use and generate plans of action based on them, even if you only strengthen one thing at a time.

6. Be patient if there's much to fix; start somewhere.   Some practices ask for feedback and hear about a whole array of problems they feel compelled to fix. You can create a sequenced agenda for enhancing your practice. You don't have to do everything at once. A slower enhancement plan, in fact, often works best because after you implement one change, you can monitor its effects and ripple effects, making sure your next steps still make sense. View your practice as a sculpture that you carefully, methodically chip away at in order to make it a work of art.

6

Ambience:
The Environment and
Patient Satisfaction

Most people become nervous just thinking about a doctor's office, let alone an impending visit, even if the doctor is gentle and personable. Through simple conditioning, people imagine and expect negative experiences replete with problems, painful injections, illness, bad news, discomfort, fright, and expense. While the reality is often more benign than the expectation, the typical healthcare consumer is at least a bit overwrought on the way to the doctor, suffering such symptoms as a quickening pulse, rapid breathing, cold hands and sweating.

Symptoms such as these are so common that some have even been given special names, like "white coat hypertension," which is the term for the elevation of blood pressure found to occur *only* when the doctor is measuring it.

While anxiety is somewhat inevitable due to the nature of the medical transaction, the doctor who takes deliberate action to counteract or minimize this anxiety or stress impresses the patient and his or her family. People notice and appreciate it.

That's why more physicians than ever are taking a new look at their office's physical environment and taking conscious and sometimes costly measures to rebuild, renovate, rearrange and adorn the environment so that it alleviates patient stress, confusion, and discomfort.

IT'S A JUGGLING ACT

The fact is that if you want an optimal environment, you have to juggle a number of sometimes competing specifications. You have to create an environment that accommodates the technology you need, technology that frequently changes and therefore makes space flexibility a must. Some practices must also have space flexible and/or large enough to make diverse activities available simultaneously, from routine exams to tests, to time-consuming procedures, to emergencies. You have to take into account the needs and preferences of the physicians who probably vary in terms of what they want to the left and right of them, in one room versus another room, and so on. You need a location that is accessible, convenient, and close to related services. You need space that allows for efficiency on the part of your medical and nonmedical staff, all of whom have preferences regarding lighting, color, room size and arrangements, relative locations of treatment, exam rooms, offices, and more. Also, you have to consider privacy, confidentiality, sanitation, cost factors, and security, and undoubtedly that's not all.

A juggling act it is, to create and sustain an environment that is healthy and nurturing for patients as well as healthy and nurturing for staff. With so many factors to keep in balance, it's not unusual to give too little thought to the patient's experience of your environment. What do *they* see, hear, smell, and feel when they're on your premises? Taking the patient's point of view is the key to manipulating the environment to heighten patient satisfaction. If you ask patients, they cite repeatedly certain critical aspects of your environment: for instance, your directions to your office, the comfort of the waiting area, availability of a rest room, and issues of cleanliness.

The challenge is to make sure that your environment meets your needs for technological flexibility and efficiency, while sending to the patient an unequivocal "We care about you" message. Grounded in years of research, environmental factors that affect patient satisfaction are known. And fortunately, the features that satisfy patients (like color, seating arrangements, windows, etc.) are the very same features that have been shown to be therapeutic (D. Canter, and S. Canter, "Creating Therapeutic Environments," in D. Canter, and S. Canter, (ed.), *Designing for Therapeutic Environments*, New York: Wiley, 1979; R. Mathews, "The Psychological and Social Effects of Design," *World Hospitals*, 12(1), March 1976, pp. 63–68; and R.E. Petrie, "Patient Well-Being Is Designer's First Concern," *Michigan Hospitals*, 16(9), 1980 September, pp. 12–13).

This chapter identifies critical points along the patient's path through a medical practice and identifies environmental issues that affect the patient's satisfaction. Specifically, we will address:

- Finding the way to your office
- Stairs, elevators and hallways
- The waiting and reception area
- The exam, treatment, or diagnosis room
- Environmental amenities
- Needs of special patient groups

WHAT MATTERS TO PATIENTS?

The answers are not surprising. According to J. Reizenstein Carpman, M. Grant, and D. Simmons (*Design That Cares,* Chicago: AHA Publishing, Inc., 1986, p. 19), for patients, the following environment-related needs dominate:

- Way-finding
- Physical comfort
- Privacy and personal territory
- Symbolic meaning

Wayfinding. Patients experience stress when they have any sort of problem finding their way to the office. They feel insecure, frustrated, and sometimes helpless. Graphics and signs help, but they could also interact with other environmental elements that contribute to or impede finding one's way without impediment or confusion.

Physical Comfort. Chairs, lighting, room arrangements, color, smells, noise, textures—all affect the patient's comfort level. If these variables are arranged with an eye to comforting the patient, you can ease patient anxiety.

Privacy and Personal Territory. People tend to want to control the extent to which they interact with others. When you go the doctor, do you like to talk to other patients in the waiting room or sit by yourself? Do you mind if other patients see you when you have nothing but a gown on, or don't you care? Do you mind being overheard when you're explaining your symptoms to a caregiver or discussing financial problems? Since people vary in their responses to these questions, the optimal environment allows for people with different preferences to find a way to honor their preferences without having to assert themselves or buck the system. For instance, some people going to the doctor want to sit quietly and not have to talk to anyone while they're waiting. Others would just as soon *schnooze* with a waiting room full of people to make the time go faster. The question is: does your office design allow both people to find a conducive position for themselves, so they can follow their inclinations and not fall victim to interactions you've caused to happen by office design?

Symbolic Meaning. Beyond issues of comfort and privacy, all features of your office environment combine to convey an overall image that patients perceive as either caring and responsive to their needs or the opposite. The patient looks around, walks around, and concludes that he or she is either important to you or not.

The needs that patients have offer valuable clues about how to enhance your practice. If you accept these patient needs as needs that must be served in positive ways, then you have a sense of direction for generating ideas and strategies that will enhance your practice from the patient's perspective.

OPTIONS, OPTIONS, AND MORE OPTIONS

To address each need on the part of patients, you have many options. If you want to revamp your environment in major ways, we strongly recommend that you read *Design that Cares: Planning Health Facilities for Patients and Visitors* by Carpman, Grant, and Simmons (Chicago: AHA Publishing, Inc., 1986). This book, devoted to the subject of creating therapeutic, comfortable environments for patients, offers an in-depth treatment of environmental considerations that heighten patient satisfaction. However, here we will describe several of the more salient considerations at each point along the patient's pathway through your practice: (1) wayfinding, parking, arrival, and departure; (2) waiting and reception area; and (3) exam and treatment rooms. We will also discuss the environmental needs of special groups that merit attention.

Wayfinding, parking, arrival and departure

Getting there is easy for you and your staff because you're used to it. But, especially when patients are anxious, many obsess about whether they can find your office on time, without getting lost, delayed, or frustrated. They worry about whether they can find a parking space. Are you aware of the fact that many patients actually rehearse the trip to their doctor's office by actually going there a day or two before their appointment, just to reassure themselves that they can find the way? This attests to the anxiety created by the trip itself.

When people have trouble finding their way, some feel incompetent because they blame themselves for what they believe is their own stupidity or confusion. But many more become angry and anxious and some miss or arrive late to their appointments (see Figure 6–1).

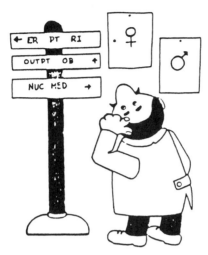

"Do you suppose any of this means Bathroom?"

Figure 6–1. Easing the patient's way.

You can ease the patient's path from their world to your registration desk in several ways:

Maps. Your Patient Information Booklet and your New Patient Information Letter/Kit should include a map to your office. Since some people are visual and some people are spatially oriented, the map should include verbal and pictorial directions from key points north, south, east and west of your offices. The point is to describe the trip to your office from various points of origin. Some physicians include a photograph of the building to make it easier for new patients to recognize. And make sure you describe public transportation options, favorite taxi companies and other ways to access your office.

You should also have a map that shows patients who are *exiting* your office how to get to the major ancillary service points your practice tends to use, such as labs, hospitals, outpatient treatment facilities, and the like.

Helpful Signage. Once the traveler approaches your office location, he or she (and, in fact, all passersby) should be able to easily read clear words and/or symbols that identify your building. *Medical Offices* is clearer to patients than *Medical Pavilion*. *Walkway* is clearer than *transitway* or *overhead link*.

If you own your own building or occupy an entire building, you have a great deal of control over this aspect and can post tasteful, attention-getting signs that reflect the image you want for your practice. If you wonder whether you need to improve your signage, ask a few patients, especially new patients. Or ask friends who don't use your practice to visit and be a "user-friendly consultant" who tells you ways you can make way-finding clearer and easier. Ask them about best colors, print size, and the direction the signs should face, so you reap advice of the prospective user, and get unstuck from the point of view of you and your staff who are "on automatic" on their way to the office.

If you rent or lease, you might ask your patients how big a problem building identification is, and if it is a big problem, join with other tenants to lobby for a bold sign to be hung outside the building so people know they've found the right place.

What makes a sign effective? That's debatable, but, if you design your signs to meet the patient's need for information and the doctor's need to market the practice, here are guidelines that seem to work: (1) make your signs big enough, bright enough, and positioned so that it can be easily read from the road; (2) include as much information as possible that tells about your practice, e.g., the name, doctors' names, logo, specialties, special services, and office hours (if they are more convenient than other practices' hours); (3) light it up so it can be seen 24 hours a day, and (4) make sure your signs fit with your building's exterior and style. (A high-tech sign outside of a log cabin office makes the consumer wonder.)

Transport Service. Increasing numbers of medical practices have begun to provide transportation services to and from their offices. Some provide taxi vouchers, and some contract with a local van service that remains at their beck and call. Especially if you have a high percentage of elderly patients, you might want to consider this powerful benefit that pays for itself in terms of marketing. So many people today, especially ailing and/or older people experience or expect to experience transportation hardships on the way to the doctor. Also, if your building is in a moderately trafficky location, you can probably arrange for a taxi stand nearby, or a direct-line phone to a taxi service, to make taxi calls quick and easy.

Parking. Parking is so often *the* deciding factor when prospective patients are doctor-shopping. If you can provide sufficient, safe, comfortable, convenient, and accessible parking, you ease patient and their companions' fears about getting to your office hassle-free. In this age, we daresay, if you lack access to decent parking for your patients, it might be time to consider moving, unless there are powerful compensating factors.

To make parking easier to find, be utterly clear about it. Clarify in writing (in your information brochure and your New Patient Kit) where parking exists, the best way to get there, the number of minutes it takes to walk from the parking to your office, and the price. If you offer a parking discount, subsidy voucher, or provide free parking, communicate this loudly and clearly, since these extras are known to attract patients and help them over the parking hump.

Patients also express concern about the security of parking facilities. Figure out all the reasons why your parking facilities are secure and tell the patient. Is the lot open-air? Does it have a video monitoring system? Can patients call a certain number and get escorted in and out if they choose to?

Easy Drop-Off.   Many patients, especially those with constraints on their mobility, will be dropped off for their appointment by a friend, family member, or transport service. Ideally, your building should facilitate a safe, simple drop-off by providing a protected area where people can get out of the drop-off vehicle slowly and without fighting traffic. A circular drive is ideal, or a No Parking area close to the entrance from the parking area, or at least a protected curbside location. And patients appreciate it if you post a sign that identifies the Drop-Off area.

Pay the Fine When It's Your Fault.   When people use metered or other short-term parking and you keep them waiting, they become irate at *you* if they find that their car has been ticketed. Your staff can prevent this outrage (that's what patients call it) by: (1) asking registering patients where they parked and identifying short-termers, and offering to monitor time and send a runner to put more money in the meter if the patient outstays their parking allotment; and (2) telling patients that, should they receive a ticket, your office wants to foot the bill, since the length of their visit was not their fault. Expensive? Yes, if you sustain long waits and develop no back-up system whereby your staff help patients manage their parking problems. But it's more expensive to lose a patient.

Information Desk.   Particularly in large buildings, a staffed Information Desk is seen by patients as a great aid to wayfinding and security. If you're office-shopping, you might want to give this factor consideration.

"You-Are-Here" Map.   Once people enter your building, especially if the building is large, you should post (or have the landlord post) a "You-Are-Here" map. These maps orient the patient and their companions to where they are standing and helps them find your offices quickly and without frustration.

Waiting and reception area

Ambience begins here. If patients experience frustration in reaching your office, they carry that frustration through the door even if they don't blame you for it. But there is no doubt that, once a patient enters your office, they attribute their comfort or discomfort to your practice, because they know that you created the environment that now impinges on them.

And, in many practices, patients begin their visit by waiting, and sometimes waiting and more waiting. Fortunately, through careful attention to creating a conducive environment, you can counteract some of the negative effects of unavoidably long waits. Specifically, you can arrange the environment so that patients and their companions:

- Don't start wondering if they've been forgotten
- Feel comfortable
- Can talk to other people if they choose to, but not if they don't
- Have access to amenities that matter, like phones, restrooms, water, and things to do.

Fortunately, you can take steps to insure that the environment in your waiting and reception area is aesthetically pleasing, comfortable, respectful, and that it provides for conveniences that meet the variety of patient needs that arise when people are anxious and essentially powerless to make their appointment happen at will.

Starting at the Door.   The patient arrives. Do you have several doors to your offices? Is it clear to the patient which door is the right door for entry? Many medical offices have installed glass walls, windows, doors, or windowpanes so that incoming patients can see the waiting area and the Registration Desk from the hallway, and know they're headed in the right direction. This might seem trivial until you think of the feeling of uncertainty that most people experience when they are about to open a door without knocking. Also, when people knock and, upon entry, discover a waiting area full of patients, they feel embarrassed. The transparent entry solves the problem. People inside see them coming, and the entering patient sees the inside activity.

Also, on the subject of doors, do your patients have to struggle to open the door to your offices? The force needed to open a door should not exceed eight pounds and yet many medical office doors require much more. A too-heavy door that requires upper body strength calls the patient's attention to their weaknesses and also creates an access barrier to your practice. These are details—details that matter.

A Place To Put Things.   For the patient's sake, your office should clearly indicate where the patient and their friends might hang their coats and store their bags. Coat-racks, or better yet, closets within view of the receptionist, are ideal because patients feel they are relatively secure.

Explanatory Signs and Orientation Aids.   Signs and other orientation aids help people orient themselves to their environment. If your practice is small, you might be thinking that you don't need these. But, small or large, practices benefit their patients by making clear where the facilities are and how things work. People would rather not rely on staff to answer what they think are mundane questions, like "Where is the restroom?" They would rather find out what they need to know without having to bother anyone. And that keeps your staff freer as well.

Make sure you have signs on exterior doors inside your building, like *Men, Women, Exit, Reception Area, Private.* Many practices post a welcome sign that explains the registration procedure. Some hang a sign with the name of the person at the desk a la the Manager-on-Duty sign in McDonald's, and another sign that explains your payment procedures and key facts about insurance filing. Some also provide a brochure or fact sheet about the practice and a letter or flier that poses and answers questions frequently asked by patients.

Positioning of the Front Desk. If you ask patients, they will tell you that they like to see the receptionist as soon as they enter the office. That suggests that, where possible, the front desk should be positioned so that it faces people as they enter. And, in case several patients and companions accumulate at the front desk at once, there should be space between the front desk and the seating area so that neither is cramped by a cluster of people simultaneously ready for front desk attention.

Since the front desk area is so important, pay attention also to the image it conveys about your practice. Does the desk and the visible area behind it appear cluttered or disorganized? Does it look barren and boring, showing nothing to indicate that the people there are interesting (like family pictures, indications of interests, a favorite—but tasteful—cartoon)?

User-Friendly Features. Does the reception area look people-oriented or metallic, sharp-edged or high-tech? Do you make it easy for patients to read and write when they need to (e.g., nonglare lighting, wide counter space, clipboard with working pen, etc.)?

Privacy and Confidentiality. Confidentiality is an urgently felt patient need. Soon after they arrive, you need to gather information from them, about their history, symptoms, condition, financial status, outstanding bills, or whatever. Patients want to be able to communicate this information privately. They think it's no one else's business. Consequently, you need to arrange the environment and/or offer systems that make it possible for patients to perceive these conversations as confidential. You can achieve this in a number of ways. Ideally, you can offer a separate room for registration and information-gathering, or a carrel or cubicle that feels private. If not, consider the room arrangement that places other people's chairs as far away as possible and preferably with people's backs to the patient conversing with your staff. Also, if sounds carry in your office, invest in acoustical tile or sound-absorbing dividers. These do wonders in cutting down on noise, dampening sound overall, and making privacy possible in even small rooms shared by other people. Dividers (if not separate rooms) also buffer areas meant to serve different functions (e.g., work, waiting, collections and interviews).

Clocks. In a recent survey of 15 medical offices (an admittedly uncontrolled study), we found that only five had clocks visible to people in the waiting area. When questioned, staff pointed out that if people see a clock, it calls their attention to how long they're waiting and makes matters worse.

Real patients, when questioned, say this reason is a myth. First of all, when people are waiting, and especially if they're nervous, every minute feels like an hour. So, a realistic view of time passing tends to be less detrimental to patients' impatience than an uninformed perception would be. Also, if other people are in the waiting room, the curious person will ask aloud for the time, and everyone will have his or her attention called to it, even the people who have, in some way, become absorbed in making the time pass quickly.

People need to see a clock—to have a realistic view of how long they're waiting, to know if they need to call the children, or to put more money in the parking meter.

If wait-time in your office is so lengthy that you want to eliminate clocks, you have a very deep service problem that you can't compensate for by environmental amenities. You need to tackle those problems *and* hang a big clock visibly in your waiting area.

Decent Chairs. Since people spend most of their wait-time sitting, the quality and quantity of chairs deserves attention. After reviewing studies of seating comfort in waiting areas, Reizenstein, Carpman, Grant, and Simmons give this advice about chairs:

Guidelines for Comfortable Seating

- Provide seating that will accommodate a wide range of users, including children, pregnant women, heavy or tall people, elderly people, and the physically weak.

- Whenever possible, provide seating that has backs and arms, and supports thighs, lower back, upper back and neck.

- Avoid seating that has sharp edges.

- Select seating material that will be comfortable, neither scratching users nor causing them to perspire.

- As an aid in rising and in sitting down, provide seating with firm support at the front edge, room for the sitter's feet to tuck under the front of the chair, and arms that extend out to or slightly past the front edge of the seat.

- When seats are placed next to each other, use armrests on some to give people a sense of separation from their neighbors. (*Design that Cares*, AHA Publishing, Inc., 1986, p. 11)

Amenities that Comfort and Entertain. Demographer and lifestyle trend expert Faith Popcorn, in her speech at the Eighth Annual Symposium for Healthcare Marketing (1988), describes a burgeoning trend among consumers to appreciate "small indulgences." Popcorn describes how consumer choice and purchasing behavior now favor restaurants that provide creme de menthe after-dinner mints and warm hand-towels, hotels that welcome you to your room with a personalized fruit basket, and so on.

Healthcare providers aware of this trend are increasingly offering patients and those waiting for them clever and special patient-pleasers, such as things that help the time pass: puzzles and games, VCRs, special treats, a fish tank, and the like—all catering to this new consumer infatuation with small indulgences.

People want and deserve access to restrooms without having to embarrass themselves by asking aloud for all to hear. You should also provide at the very least a drinking fountain, although many practices now also offer tea, coffee, juices or other popular and hopefully healthful beverages.

Whether you keep patients waiting or not, their companions will have to wait for them. While waiting, some people like to stare into space, but most prefer doing something to make the time go faster. Help them by providing diversions, such as these:

- Arrange some, but not all, of the chairs so that the people who like to chat with others can sit in a position that fosters conversation.

- Some people like to do nothing much. For these people especially, provide plants, nice pictures on the walls, and perhaps an aquarium, sculptures and other aesthetically pleasing visual stimuli.

- Provide books, magazines, and other things that make quiet activity possible. Lately, increasing numbers of medical practices make available small jigsaw puzzles already set up on little tables, crossword puzzle books, art-and-craft supplies, toys and a play area for the kids, radios, tape recorders (with tape library) and even VCRs, all with earphones so some people can tune in to whatever they choose without disturbing others.

- Display patient education materials on health promotion and illness, some written by the doctors in your practice (*that*, you can be sure, builds credibility), along with pamphlets available at little or no cost from organizations, such as the American Heart Association, the American Cancer Society, and the like.

• Almost everybody prefers a room with windows so they can watch traffic and people, and feel a part of, not cut off from, the world outside.

Exam and treatment rooms

Typically, especially in small medical practices, the same spaces are used for multiple purposes, including examination, diagnosis, treatment, and consultation. Usually, patients move from the waiting area to the exam room where they wait for the doctor. Sometimes the patient undresses before seeing the doctor and sometimes not. Patients might be examined, undergo a treatment or procedure, get dressed, and then discuss the results, and follow-up, and questions with the physician—often in the same room. Larger practices might have separate rooms for dressing, exams, special function treatments, tests, and offices.

No matter what your room configuration, patients have certain basic needs that they carry with them through your spaces. They need to travel from the waiting area to their first room. They need to change their clothes with privacy and convenience; they need to feel protected and dignified while they're clothed only in a gown; they need to endure their treatment or diagnostic process; they need to talk confidentially with the physician to understand their condition, what they can expect, and what they should be doing as follow-up. They then retrace their steps through this sequence of events until they are ready to leave.

This section identifies patient needs that are salient during this trek through your system, needs that must be met by you within the constraints of the space you have. Some practices must accommodate more equipment and apparatus than others. Here, we address the space considerations that apply to exam and treatment rooms in most practices, since thorough treatment of specialty-related needs would require a book in itself.

The Key Is Flexibility.   You have many different kinds of patients to satisfy— patients who visit your practice in different states of illness and stress, with or without companions, with different degrees of fear and understanding about what they are likely to experience, and with needs for various kinds of treatments, examinations, and procedures. To accommodate this inevitable diversity, you need to ensure that exam and treatment rooms are somewhat flexible, so you can cater to individual needs.

Disrobe, Please!   Although most patients realize they'll need to get undressed for many types of medical visits, the mere thought of it is anxiety-provoking. If you ask your patients, most will tell you that, when they undress, they feel vulnerable, having crossed the bridge from being the business tycoon or tennis player that they are in the outside world to being a body to be examined and treated. People also can cite times when other patients or inappropriate staff saw them undressed; they believe this embarrassing situation could have and should have been avoided. When an inappropriate person sees a patient undressed and says, "I'm sorry," it tends to make matters worse. It calls attention to the fact that they saw what they saw. If the patient feels embarrassment or shame, the apology accentuates it. The key, then, is prevention.

If your practice is small, your patients probably disrobe in the same room where you examine them. In larger practices, special rooms or cubicles might be available. Fortunately, in either setting, you can, through environmental creativity communicate your determination to treat every patient as a valued adult and an individual who deserves dignity, convenience, and respect.

When patients are asked to identify what helps them through the undressing and dressing experience, they cite these environmental features:

- "Make it possible for adults to lock the door, and provide a 'readiness latch,' to indicate to their physician that they're ready to be seen." The technology for this could barely be simpler. Picture the lavatory door and latch on airplanes. The occupant can push the latch so that it reads to an outsider *Occupied* or *Unoccupied*. Patients would breathe easier if there were a clear system for handling what is, for most, a few minutes of uneasiness. Many people, in fact, report that they undress at top speed, to decrease the chance that someone will enter before they're ready. Some even report accelerating blood pressure during these few minutes. And all that uneasiness could be prevented by instituting a simple readiness signal.

- If you provide a separate changing room, then make it possible for the patient to lock the door or hook it shut from the inside. If you have a group changing area, consider replacing curtains with doors (even saloon-like), since patients feel much less exposed with solid doors.

- Make sure that patients can travel from the changing area to their next destination without being seen by hordes of people, especially people in street clothes waiting in the reception area.

And, within the changing room, make it easy for people:

- Make sure cubicles are big enough to navigate in, without getting shoulder cramps.
- If possible, provide a chair, so people can sit if they prefer.
- Have some areas with room and a chair for the patient and their companion-helper, since some patients may want physical help undressing or just moral support.

- Make sure the room is warm enough, so that people don't get chilled when they disrobe.
- Hang a floor-to-ceiling mirror, so people of every size can use it.
- If you have separate dressing areas, consider carpeting these, since cold feet appreciate carpet, and most people who go to the doctor have cold feet!
- Make it convenient to store and hang things by installing hooks, shelves, racks, lockers or baskets.
- Clarify for and with the patient what exactly they're supposed to do when they're finished undressing. Tell people what to do, and, if you have a standard procedure for people to follow after undressing, reiterate it on a sign. Are they supposed to sit there and wait, open the door, move to another area, or what? And tell them approximately how long they should expect to wait for the next action in your typical sequence of events.
- Figure out some way to assure the security of patient belongings if you're moving patients away from their possessions for the exam. Reassure patients that their things are safe. Consider lockers, locked cubicles with a key, or an area guarded by a staff member.
- If you have a group waiting area for your patients, see whether you can partition the area so that males and females can sit apart from one another.
- Regarding gowns: more colorful, less revealing gowns are preferred by patients. Assertive patients have increasingly come to question the need for flimsy gowns that barely cover them. If you provide such gowns, ask yourself whether a more protective coating would severely interfere with your practice, and consider the alternatives that many vendors now provide. Some physicians now provide terry cloth robes!

The issue here is dignity. Medical staff get so accustomed to seeing one patient after another in scant clothing or none at all, that we get used to it. Patients don't. Because they expect to feel vulnerable around the experience of undressing, if you take steps to minimize their discomfort, you impress the patient with your sensitivity.

The Exam Room. Basics do the trick. They include: an exam table, the equipment and supplies you need, a mirror, something nice to look at on the walls, soothing colors, a chair or two for the patient (and a companion if appropriate), and diversions like music, a scrapbook, or magazines to help the time pass if people are likely to wait more than three minutes.

When patients are asked to discuss what makes them comfortable in exam rooms, they tend to respond with what they recall making them *uncomfortable*. Patients are uncomfortable when they hear conversations through the walls, because they imagine that their doctor's conversation with them can be heard reciprocally. They complain about a configuration that allows other patients and staff to see them when the door is opened. They also point out the discomfort they feel with cold instruments and apparatus, which you can avoid by using warmers, and intense or glaring light which you can control by using dimmers or soft lighting supplemented by focused lighting for use during procedures.

Consultation Rooms and Offices.   If you have the space for it, know that most patients prefer a separate room for consultation and discussion. They comment that the move from the exam or treatment room to a consultation or office-like room gives them a chance to collect themselves, adopt their most adult mindset, gather their questions, and face the physician as adult to adult.

If you have a separate consultation room (in many cases, your office), don't hesitate to have the physicians hang their degrees and certificates there as well as any other photographs, memberships, or awards that enhance credibility. Patients want to have immense confidence in the medical professionals that serve them, and the consultation room environment can be arranged to build the physician's credibility. Patients tend to prefer a professional environment in the consultation room, with soothing colors and a warm atmosphere that makes discussion easier.

On Noise.

> Noise, *n*. A stench in the ear. Undomesticated music. The chief product and authenticating sign of civilization. (Ambrose Bierce, *The Devil's Dictionary*)

Distracting, unwanted sounds fill our everyday experience. At home . . . dishwashers, blenders, beaters, fans, TVs, and radios. On the streets—the blare of cars and trucks, horns, sirens, lawnmowers, children yelling, the neighbor's power drill.

In the medical office, people expect it to be different—*quiet*. The degree and nature of noise in your office contribute to ambience.

Research has shown that noise in medical settings causes adverse effects on patients and reduces staff productivity. And *voices*, not equipment, are largely responsible; it's *people* noise—loud talking, yelling down the hall, outbursts, and heavy footsteps.

When patients are asked to distinguish between tolerable and intolerable noise, they describe as tolerable the noise that they think is "necessary" (equipment, deliveries, patients talking loudly, staff talking softly). But they resent unnecessary noise like doors banging, loud talking, and boisterous laughing.

• Noise *increases* a patient's perception of pain.

- Noise interferes with relaxation and rest which, in turn, interferes with recovery.
- Noise leads to irritability and anxiety.
- Noise triggers high blood pressure.
- Noise insults patients; they find it intrusive and inconsiderate.

What can you do about noise? A lot. Most noise comes from people. But fortunately, you can reduce noise *without* sacrificing the normal healthy sounds of people. Recommend these tips to your staff:

- Be aware of how loud, how long, where and when you talk. Make a *conscious* decision about it.
- Hold conversations where *appropriate*. Ask yourself if your conversation is appropriate in the elevator, or so near a waiting room filled with anxious, impatient people.
- Avoid calling out, yelling down the hall, or shouting. Get *reasonably* close to the person you're talking to so you don't have to raise your voice.
- See if you can move, place, open, close, pull, push, set down, roll, wheel and slide things gently, and *quietly*.
- Take extra pains to avoid banging, bumping, slamming, dropping, and rattling. Such sounds are particularly irritating to patients.
- Adopt a "library voice" that shows respect for others who might be concentrating on other things.
- Have the guts to be an advocate for quiet. Say to people, "I think we're getting too loud" Or, "Let's hold this conversation later" Or, "Let's talk over here; I'm concerned we're too close to the waiting room."
- Answer phones quickly. Turn down the volume of the phones, if possible.

If you think your offices might suffer from noise problems, consider doing a noise audit. To do a noise audit, have a person sit down in an unobtrusive place and listen intensely to any and every sound that surrounds them, including the humming air conditioner, the phone tone, breathing, voices, and so on. If three or four people do this at various times of day and your office has a problem with unnecessary noise, the auditors will not only become more aware of noise problems, they will also be able to identify noise reduction strategies that will enhance your patients', and probably your staff's, satisfaction.

SUMMARY AUDIT

Have your staff or, better yet, your patients complete this environment audit to identify ways your practice's environment can be improved to the benefit of patients. This works best if you have multiple individuals complete this audit and then compare the results.

Environment Audit

☐ Is the name of your building obvious and easy to read from several angles?

☐ Is parking clearly marked, close-by and well-lighted?

☐ Are there special spots available close-by for people with handicaps, casts, bad backs, or other conditions that warrant special convenience?

☐ Is it easy and safe for someone to drop off a patient?

☐ Is the drop-off location accessible to the front door?

☐ Are the drop-off area, the main entrance, and route to your office barrier-free?

☐ Are there taxis available nearby or a method for calling taxis as needed?

☐ Once people enter your building, is the way to your office clearly indicated?

☐ Is your office clearly marked in the hallway, so people know when they've arrived?

☐ Is you reception desk positioned so that your staff are quick to see people entering?

☐ Are work surfaces and equipment unrelated to registration invisible to people in your waiting area?

☐ Do you have nonglare lighting and nonglare coverings on counters and surfaces?

☐ Does your reception area have shelves, hooks, or closets for the personal items of patients and their companions?

☐ If possible, do you provide specially designed areas conducive to reading, child's play, and conversation?

☐ If you have a play area, do you have play materials that are durable, safe and usable by more than one child at a time?

☐ Does the waiting area have windows to the outside and to the hallway?

☐ If you have a TV in the waiting area, is it positioned so that not everyone has to watch or hear it?

☐ Are chairs arranged so that people can sit alone or in comfortably close groups, as they choose?

☐ Are your chairs comfortable for children, heavy people, tall people, pregnant women, older people, and weak people?

☐ Do your chairs provide support to people's backs and arms?

☐ Is the material used on your furniture comfortable, insofar as it does not stick to people or scratch them?

☐ Do you have chairs that are easy to get out of?

☐ Is there a phone available for use by patients and their companions?

☐ Do people find your waiting area to be comfortable during a long wait?

☐ Do you have soothing artwork in your waiting area?

☐ Do you have patient education materials easily accessible to people who are waiting?

☐ Do you have trash receptacles available in your waiting area?

☐ Do you have easy-to-read clocks in waiting and exam rooms?

☐ When people check in, can they do this out of earshot of others in the waiting area?

☐ Are locations where staff interview patients conducive to communication and self-disclosure?

☐ Do furniture arrangements facilitate eye contact between people talking with one another without barriers?

☐ Do you have private offices, cubicles or partitions that control noise and provide privacy?

☐ Do rooms where people undress have doors the patient can lock or ways the patient can indicate *Occupied—do not disturb?*

☐ Do you have a convenient bathroom and water fountain for use by people in the waiting area *and* patients who are gowned?

☐ Are exam and treatment rooms where people might be unclothed kept slightly warm?

☐ Do you have a mirror in rooms where people dress?

☐ Do you have a place for people to put their clothes and personal items when they undress, such as hooks, hangers, shelves, or hampers?

☐ Are exam and treatment room doors, exam tables, and curtains arranged to protect the patient from view from the hallway when someone opens the door?

☐ Do you have privacy curtains where appropriate, and do you insist that staff use them?

☐ Are examination and treatment rooms soundproof, so people can't hear what's happening from one room to another?

☐ Do you have an extra chair in exam rooms in case the patient brings a family member or companion?

☐ Are your exam and treatment rooms decorated in a way that is comfortable, colorful, and noninstitutional?

☐ Do you have ways of protecting patients from contact with cold instruments and equipment?

AMBIENCE MATTERS

Patients and their companions care about the environment since it affects how they feel while they're in your hands. The environment also affects staff productivity, morale, and pride in being part of your practice. This chapter describes the multitude of ways to enhance your office ambience, whether your practice is large or small.

The overarching point is: When it comes to your environment, excellence is in the details.

7

Money Matters

Would that healthcare were free and that staff in medical practices were on a generous subsidy for providing quality care to people in need. Alas, such is not the case. That raises the thorny issue of money and how to handle it, or more specifically, how to collect it, without embarrassing, angering, or alienating patients.

There is no perfect solution. The best you can do is to take a look at your practice's ways of charging patients and collecting money, check out the effects of your ways on patient satisfaction, and explore options or alternatives that might better satisfy the patient's needs and yours simultaneously.

THE PHYSICIAN'S ROLE

Most physicians go to great lengths to avoid having to talk money with patients. This is too bad, because patients expect to pay and they tend to accept charges better if the physician is the first to mention them. Many physicians mention the total cost of a service and leave it to their business agent or billing person to break down the charges into their component parts. And, if a patient questions payment or the payment schedule, the physician suggests that the patient sit down with the appropriate staff member to work out terms. The physician reassures the patient that "I'm confident that you and Mary can work out terms convenient for you. And whatever terms you work out will be fine with me"

Hopefully, your office practices can be well defined and debugged so that the physician rarely needs to discuss money matters at any length. But how about the situation where the treatment the physician is suggesting costs more than the patient believes he or she can handle, and the patient doesn't understand the extent to which their own insurance covers the forthcoming charges. In this case, the physician or staff member should begin with a discussion of the cost and the degree of insurance coverage in advance of the person's decision to proceed with the treatment. This shows respect for the patient's intelligence and tends to keep them loyal to you. In the discussion, you should then

- Confirm the patient's feeling that the treatment is costly, instead of arguing the point.
- Clarify the issue—that the cost of not treating the health problem is probably greater than the money needed to pay for it.
- Close the deal, e.g., "So, let's get started today," Or, "Are you prepared to go ahead with it or would you like to think it over?"

EXPEDITING COLLECTION

There are certain steps you can take to speed up the influx of income without jeopardizing patient satisfaction.

Will that be Cash, Check or Credit Card? First of all, make it easy and convenient for people to pay you. If you haven't done so already, add credit cards to the payment options you offer to patients. People are used to paying with credit cards, knowing that they have time to cover their charges. If your patients can't pay with plastic, know that they can at the practice down the street, and patients consider it a convenience. But also, know that if you arrange to enable patients to pay by charge card, you are offering your practice and the patient a valued service. You tend to collect more effectively and more often on the spot, because people can pay you even when they have no cash or check. You will probably reduce your bad debts because, if patients don't pay their bills to the credit card company, it's that company's problem, not yours. The fee you pay to credit card companies for their service is far less than the fee you pay to collection companies! Also, patients *like* to pay by credit card. For psychological reasons, the bite of a bill just isn't so acute when people pay with plastic.

Insurance Fact Sheets. Also, join with the patient in a partnership to fight red tape that makes money matters worse. You can ease the burden on patients and diminish their fears of paperwork and getting lost in the insurance-government bureaucracy by making sure that you have a staff person who's a whiz at investigating and explaining insurance coverage. This is especially important for elderly patients and patients with coinsurance. Also, you can develop convenient, plainly written Insurance Fact Sheets. Well-designed, these can greatly demystify patients' insurance and the procedures they need to follow in order to take full advantage of their benefits. Patients and others who might be financially responsible for their healthcare deeply appreciate the caregiver's help in this area. And, in fact, if you don't help, they tend to blame you (the closest party) for the hassles they have to endure. By initiating Insurance Fact Sheets, you can achieve a reputation as a practice that is working *with* (not against) the patient to tackle their insurance problems.

Insurance fact sheets explain how a person's coverage works; they also explain your practice's policy toward that insurer's coverage, and how the patient can obtain maximum benefits. In so doing, the patient is clear about what to do, and you're likely to collect the patient's share of their bill *and* the insurer's share quicker, since the patient will be more able to complete the necessary paperwork.

Fact sheets aren't as hard to develop as you might think. Probably, most of the information is already known to your people. They probably know what Blue Shield, Medicare, and many private carriers cover and how they work—their deductibles, co-payments, coverages, and so on. And your people know which plans your practice participates in and accepts assignment from, what your expectations are regarding the patient's share of the payment, what your fees are, and how to complete forms. In other words, the knowledge and know how already reside in your practice, perhaps in your Office Policy Manual, regarding the filing of claims. The point is to rewrite these in a way that is user-friendly to patients. Share the information with them and help them use it to navigate better through the turbulent world of insurance.

Ideally, you'll have a separate sheet for each type of insurance which you can in many cases send to the patient before their appointment. You can have a stack of each on hand or, if your office is computerized, you can teach your computer to spit out the right sheet for each patient.

"The Doctor's Office" newsletter (April 1987, p. 7) presents this outline for an effective Insurance Fact Sheet:

Outline for a Typical Insurance Fact Sheet

A. Heading—Title each sheet as a *fact sheet* for a specific insurance program or carrier. When possible, include the mailing address and direct-dial phone number of the insurer's claim office.

B. *Participation*—This sheet lets patients know whether you "participate" by accepting the insurer's payment as payment-in-full for your fees and what this means to the patient, or whether you prefer to have the insurer pay its portion of your fee as benefits assigned directly to your office.

C. *Specifics*—Define terms such as *deductible* (the portion of your medical bills—$00.00 per year—that must be paid before your insurance coverage begins); *allowable* (the amount the insurance company considers "covered" for a test, exam, or procedure), and *co-payment* (the portion of your bill paid by your secondary insurance coverage). Explain what those terms mean in dollars and cents under that patient's program or contract, and give patients a formula to help them see how much their "share" of a typical procedure's fee would be.

D. *What to expect*—Honestly and openly, tell the patient when you expect fees to be paid at time of service, when the patient must pay just the co-payment at time of service, how long, and under what conditions, you will wait for the insurer to pay its share of your fee. Tell the patient what your billing procedure will be, from the time of service until the bill is paid in full.

E. *How to fill out a claim form*—This is really nothing more than a reminder to fill in all numbered spaces and to put emphasis on those spaces which are most important in getting the form through the claims office speedily. You might also tell patients that claim forms are a lot easier to fill out than most people think and that patients help keep office costs (and fees!) down when they are considerate enough to fill out their own forms.

BUILD STAFF UNDERSTANDING AND COMMITMENT

The fact is that, when the patient resists, any system of collection relies on *people* as collectors, and initially people on your staff. To be effective in the collections process, your staff need to accept and even feel committed to your office's charges and payment policies. Otherwise, they might not do all they can to expedite payment while also maintaining patient goodwill. Specifically, if some staff admit to the patient that they agree with the patient that your charges are too high, you have a problem. And if a member of your staff seethes about the unfairness of pressing an unemployed person to pay anyway, you're going to have another problem.

Enlightened physicians engage the commitment of staff to optimizing revenue *and* patient satisfaction by informing staff in detail about the policies regarding payment and, here's the rub, *the thinking behind these policies*. Sometimes this means squaring with staff about the expenses involved in running a practice, the prices for equivalent services charged by your competitors, the value you want patients to receive for their money, and so on. Many think this is a radical view, and perhaps it is. But if your staff are not invested in effective collections *and* in maintaining a loyal patient following, they, perhaps unconsciously, act in ways that interfere with these objectives.

PATOS: NEARLY EVERYONE'S DOING IT

First of all, make charges clear, and make clear your timing and systems for collections. Most practices today have a Pay-at-the-Time-of-Service (PATOS) policy which they make clear to patients ahead of time.

Imagine being a patient ready to leave the office. A receptionist stops you to set a new appointment time and then, within earshot of several others in the waiting area, suggests in a professional tone, "The charge now for today's visit is $40."

Taken aback and a bit embarrassed, you grope for your wallet, hoping you have enough cash or a check. Finding that you can't spare the cash you have, you say, "I'll mail it to you like I always do."

The receptionist says that's okay, but tells you that next time you're expected to pay at the time of your visit and to bring money with you.

Most people in this situation find themselves feeling angry and a bit humiliated, since the office assistant has put them on the spot, in front of others. Many people cancel appointments after an interaction like this. Some just don't show for their scheduled appointment. And many people change doctors.

It's estimated that billing a patient by mail and tracking the payment costs a minimum of $30 per patient by the time you consider typing, filing, tracking, staff time, supplies, and postage. That's why PATOS is, according to recent surveys, practiced in about three-fourths of all medical practices. PATOS saves the physician considerable money and cuts down greatly on record-keeping, tracking, and staff time.

But, being concerned about patient satisfaction, you know that many patients don't like the idea. It turns out that patients don't like the idea so much for the idea itself as for the way it's executed. Too many practices surprise people with their new PATOS policy instead of giving them adequate, respectful, advance warning.

If you're thinking about converting to a PATOS policy, think it over carefully before you do it. And if you do it, do it right. If you already have one, check to see that you've covered the necessary bases, to minimize patient discomfort and maximize the effectiveness of your PATOS approach.

How to do right by patients with PATOS

At least a month before you institute PATOS, notify your patients by mail. Explain your new policy, and tell the truth about why you're doing it (probably to cut down on billing costs, and alleviate the need for an immediate increase in your charges). Also, be sure to explain that the policy is for all of your patients, that the recipient of the letter has not been singled out because of a problematic payment history. Imply that there will be exceptions to the policy so that people feel, if they have a health problem and a payment problem, they'll know they should approach you about an exception to your rule, so they can get the treatment they need.

Karen Zupko, president of the management consulting firm Karen Zupko Associates, shares an example of such a letter in "Just Saying 'Please' Won't Collect Your Fee," Medical Economics (June 8, 1987, p. 129):

> Dear Patient:
>
> We find ourselves confronted with ever-increasing costs for almost every supply and service we use in rendering professional care to you.
>
> Rather than raise our fees at this time, we are asking your help in a new cost-cutting plan. Beginning on (date one to two months in advance), we will ask you to pay for your office call at the time of your visit. By asking you to do this, we can significantly reduce the costs of billing and bookkeeping.
>
> We understand that occasions may arise when it will be necessary for you to request a statement rather than to pay at the time of service. We will also continue to recognize the need to set up payment plans for patients who require extensive treatment.
>
> We want to explain this new system to you well in advance because your understanding and cooperation are so important. Please remember, if you have questions about this or any other office policy or procedure, we will be pleased to discuss them with you. We value you, our patient, and will continue to provide you with our best professional care.
>
> Sincerely,
> James L. Wethington, M.D.

Such a letter can be mailed to current patients and, for new patients, included in your Patient Information Booklet. The letter is a first step, but not at all the only way you need to alert patients to your PATOS policy.

If you prefer to notify current patients only when they are about to have an office visit, you might send an appointment reminder that alerts the patient to your PATOS policy. For example:

I look forward to seeing you for your next appointment on April 23 at 10 AM. As we mentioned in a previous letter to you, in order to keep our billing expenses down, we're now asking that patients pay for our services at the time of their visit. You're scheduled for a routine visit, so you can expect a fee of $40, unless lab tests are needed.

Also, consider posting a sign in the office that says something like:

To cut down on the cost of billing and keep our fees as low as possible, we ask that you pay at the time of your visit. Thank you.

But most important, work with your office manager, office assistant or who-ever is most likely to interact with patients about money. You need to decide up-front how important it is for you to have people pay at the time of their visit. If it's critical, you need to help the right staff people know exactly how and how hard to press for payment, and whether you want her or him to mention your payment expectations over the phone. If you do, and most physicians serious about PATOS do, then develop a clear message for use over the phone—a message consistent with the message you communicated in your letter and in your Patient Information Booklet.

Then, at the time of service, clarify the fee. While many practices state the fee aloud to the patient, practices that have the capability to computer-generated bills and receipts on-the-spot usually have a practice whereby staff hand the patient a slip of paper showing charges while stating the fee to the patient. Staff and patients tend to find this more comfortable than face-to-face communication during this often tense moment.

Sample of Charge Slip
  Patient's Name _____

  Fee for today's services $ _____
  Prior payment balance   + _____
  Total fee due today   = _____
  Payment received   − _____
  New balance   = _____

Staff intitials _____ *Date* _____

Also, you need to work out how you want your staff to handle people who refuse to pay on the spot. What exactly do you want them to say in a variety of circumstances? For instance, if someone says, "I never pay after my visit. I always send you a check." Do you want your staff to respond, "I can make an exception this time, but in the future, we're asking you to pay at the time of your visit." Or, "I realize we haven't asked you to do this before, but now we are asking people to pay at the time of their visit. Of course, if you feel you can't, Dr. _____ will still see you. And we can see what arrangements are possible for you regarding your bill." You need a predetermined policy that dictates how your staff should handle patients who really don't have enough money to pay their bill. A sliding fee scale? Payment spread over a period of months? The clearer you are, the more constructive your staff can be in handling the delicate matter of payment.

Another approach that will ease the pain of a PATOS policy occurs in the context of phone calls designed to confirm a patient's appointment. If you do such calls routinely, great! If not, you might consider instituting such calls at least in the short-run if you're instituting a new PATOS policy. When your staff member calls the patient, he or she can say, "Mr. Hart? This is Hilary Metcalf from Dr. Strong's office. I'm calling to confirm that you'll be coming in for an appointment with Dr. Parsons tomorrow at 3 PM. . . . *(After the patient confirms)* Mr. Hart, I also wanted to make sure you got Dr. Parsons' letter about our new payment system." If the patient did, he or she will be reminded to bring money and expect to pay tomorrow, or will have the chance to express irritation in private or ask questions. If they don't recall the letter, it gives your staff a chance to reiterate the new policy *before* Mr. Hart arrives and is taken aback by an outright request for payment.

Some physicians report that when staff remind the patient of the new policy, some patients say, "Forget it! I want to cancel my appointment, because this is offensive. I have paid reliably for years and I don't have to tolerate this!" You have to think through what you want your staff to say in this kind of situation so that they feel prepared for any contingency. Do you want your staff to apologetically hold firm or relent with a line like, "We certainly didn't mean to offend you with our new policy, and we have certainly developed trust for you over these years. This new policy is just Dr. Parsons' way of cutting the high cost of billing so our fees won't have to go up. But, in your case, I know Dr. Parsons will agree to have us continue to bill you for services as we always have."

A phone call like this, handled by *prepared* staff, tends to decrease no-shows, alert you to irate patients, and handle their feelings by phone, thus fending off a perhaps more difficult scene in the office.

COLLECTING BY PHONE

Who in your office makes phone calls aimed at increasing collections, or do you communicate only in writing and then give nonpayers to a collection agency? If members of your staff make calls to late payers, you need to make sure that they are phone-savvy—that their tact reflects a respectful attitude and that they have a repertoire of appropriate responses to various scenarios.

How do your staff rate when it comes to collecting money by phone? Have the person who does this dirty-work for you fill out the survey in Table 7–1. Also, have your office manager or another nearby co-worker complete it as well—answering the questions based on their perceptions of your money caller's behavior. Have the two people then get together and discuss any problems or situations that they think they might handle more effectively.

Test results and discussion

1. *True.* The patient deserves privacy and confidentiality when their finances are at issue. Also, the staff can concentrate better.

2. *True.* Both are necessary. Collecting money, but alienating the patient, is nearsighted. And so is failing to collect the money because of fearing patient feelings. The collector must feel that the practice has earned payment, while also treating the patient as gently and respectfully as possible, so that this patient remains loyal to the practice.

3. *False.* When you apologize, it's like saying, "We don't really deserve this money." The collector needs to feel comfortable that the practice deserves payment.

Table 7–1. Survey on Collecting Money by Telephone.

This is a True-False Test. Circle *True* or *False* to indicate your view of each statement.

1. I'm careful to make collection calls in a private, quiet place where I can avoid interruptions.	True	False
2. I have two goals: collecting money owed and keeping the patient.	True	False
3. I usually apologize when I request payment.	True	False
4. I'd rather get the patient to pay partially than not at all.	True	False
5. If a person claims more than once that they didn't get a bill, I send another return receipt requested and by certified mail.	True	False
6. I try to make friendly conversation with a patient before requesting payment.	True	False

4. *True.* You have to bend sometimes in order to succeed. This means that you should start by asking for and expecting payment for the full amount; but if you're getting nowhere, work on developing partial payment now and a predictable payment schedule for the remainder.

5. *True.* Why argue an unprovable point with a patient? It's best just to begin the transaction again, this time documenting your efforts.

6. *False.* This is a very controversial point, but we think it works best to be direct and go straight to the point. Unless the collector knows the patient personally and is genuinely concerned about knowing how they are, it's better to spill the beans on the nature of the call. Otherwise, patients believe they've been manipulated.

NONPAYERS

You need to have a clear approach to people who don't pay their bills, but it's not easy, because people's reasons vary depending on their circumstances.

Most practices already have different ways of handling typical nonpay situations. Some, of course, provide some services and charge nothing. Some bill the patient nothing beyond what their insurer covers. Most work hard with patients who can't afford payment outright to work out a gradual payment schedule.

And when all else fails, some give up, while others use collection agencies.

Do you use a billing company?

If you use a billing company, you might have had the experience of patient complaints about the treatment given them not by you, but by the billing company. Frequently, a billing company will automatically send the patient a monthly bill even after the patient has paid his or her bill. The patient gets annoyed at your staff, because they aren't necessarily aware that a separate company is billing them. And, if they are aware, they blame you anyway, since *you* selected that billing company.

Despite the fact that your office staff didn't cause the problem, they need to bend over backward to apologize to the patient as if your office *had* created the problem. They also need to intervene lickety-split with the billing company to get the problem solved, instead of leaving that onerous and infuriating task to the patient.

ON COLLECTION AGENCIES

If you use collection agencies, you should be sure to let your patients know at what point their payment is considered delinquent and will be referred to such an agency. Also, you need to do all you can to retain patients, monitoring the style and practices of your collection agency to make sure they are effective in collecting on receivables while not unduly jeopardizing patient relations. In *Winning at Receivables* (Franklin, WI: Eagle Press, 1988), David Zimmerman suggests regular monitoring of your collection agency's approaches, at least yearly review of their notices and letters; frequent visits to their office to listen to their collection staff collect on your accounts, and voicing intolerance of practices that impede your relationship with your patients.

That should help you secure the best possible effects on patients subjected to professional collectors' routines. However, you might want to consider escalating your efforts to avoid referring overdue accounts to collectors—for the sake of patient satisfaction and even your own financial interests.

If you've tried everything and the patient still pays nothing, you might think that the patient has in a sense earned the embarrassment of being confronted by a collection agency. But many still resent your resorting to this tactic.

Consider going to your patients before you send out their account for collection and offering them a last-chance cash discount—for the sake of goodwill. For instance, tell them that their account is being considered for outside collection, but that you want to extend them a chance to settle their account in full and take advantage of a 10 percent discount if they pay immediately. If the patient seems to want to settle but just does not have the money, you might increase the discount to 25 percent or even more. You still win because most collection services take between 40 percent and 50 percent of what they collect on your behalf. You collect more actual dollars and you're much more likely to retain the patient's satisfaction and loyalty.

WHAT IF THE PATIENT IS UNEMPLOYED OR UNINSURED?

Sometimes you find that a patient who has paid on time in the past and even referred new patients to you suddenly is not paying their medical bills. This often happens when someone becomes unemployed or uninsured. When people become unemployed, they tend to become anxious about that fact, but also anxious that their medical care might be interrupted or negatively influenced by their financial status.

This is a delicate situation in which you need to balance several needs: the need to remind the patient of their financial obligation, the need to contain your costs in carrying their account, the need to collect money, and the need to maintain their goodwill since they've been a valuable patient.

Here's one practice's policy regarding payment by unemployed patients:

> We are committed to continuing to see patients who find themselves unemployed or uninsured. We will not abandon them during this already stressful period. We will make special arrangements to

meet their healthcare needs and bend our payment expectations as follows:

- We will consider a sliding fee scale that makes immediate payment possible.
- Except in emergencies, we see the patient for cash-only until their outstanding bill is paid.
- We will contain our billing costs by temporarily eliminating this patient from our billing system and sending them a bill not monthly, but in three months.
- When billed after three months, the patient must: pay partially or agree on a payment schedule he or she and we can live with; or update us on his or her financial situation then and monthly thereafter until that situation changes.

If we don't hear from the patient after 45 days, we will call him or her to remind them of our agreement and then renegotiate terms. Because we want to stick by our patients during hard times, we will also, on a case-by-case basis, consider reduced fees for current visits during this period.

WHAT IF PEOPLE FALSIFY?

Some people might plead "hardship" more than reality warrants. If you find this to be the case (e.g., they are no longer unemployed, but they're still not paying your bills), re-enter them in your collection system and send them the appropriate collection letter that states in a tactful way your understanding that their situation has changed, and that you now expect payment.

However, most practices approach this patient with sensitivity and a frank discussion. They convey expectations that the patient will pay an affordable amount over time until their obligation is met. Often, they work out a written agreement or plan that summarizes the results of their discussion about reasonable, manageable terms.

THAT AWKWARD MOMENT OF COLLECTION

Most doctors use charge tickets to simplify the collection moment. They give the patient or their assistant a charge ticket to take to the person who does collections. They provide a private place for this awkward moment. You also need to train or coach your staff to handle this moment well. The language your collectors use is critical to making the collection moment smooth, not bumpy. Some staff say hesitantly, "Will you please pay your fee today?" This suggests to the patient that there are other alternatives that your office is used to. If you want payment on the spot, then your staff are better off saying, "Mr. Hart, the fee for today's visit is $45." Period. Or, better yet, give the patient options, "Mr. Hart, the fee for today's visit is $45. Would you prefer to pay cash or give me a check" Both options trigger payment.

Your staff also need to know how to communicate a large fee and a combination of fees that may be charged by different providers, e.g., the doctor, the lab, and so on. The key is to explain the situation to the patient so they'll know what to expect. For instance, "The fee for services you received today, Mr. Hart, is $100. That's $45 for the visit, $35 for the blood work, and $20 for the shot. You can expect to receive a separate $35 bill from the lab for the blood work. The total doctor's fee which includes the visit and the shot is $65, and that's due now." And perhaps on large fees, you will allow patients to pay partially at the moment and schedule payment of the remainder.

Of course, increasing numbers of practices are instituting payment by credit card. Another amenity you might consider is to offer the patient a "counter check." You can keep a supply of counter checks from each of the main local banks, so that, if a patient has no check, you can offer him or her a counter check from his or her own bank. Patients only need to fill in their name and account number, and if they don't know their account number, your staff can offer to call the bank for them then and there. Or, just write the patient's name and address on the check face and the bank will accept the check without the account number. It's less costly (and even quite thoughtful) to offer this amenity than to channel the payment through a typical billing process.

And there will be times when a patient just isn't prepared to pay and says, "I'm unable to pay today. This time, will you please bill me?" Even in this situation, you can prepare your staff to respond in a way that saves you on billing. For instance, "No problem, Mr. Hart, but instead of billing you, here is your bill with an envelope already addressed and stamped to make it quick and easy for you. Can you predict when you might mail payment?"

MONEY MATTERS ARE DELICATE

The fact is, money is sticky and uncomfortable to handle. Regarding patient satisfaction, the best you can do is think through and *test* language needed to handle your billing and collections process. The goal is to optimize a difficult interaction, so that you collect your fees in a way that makes the patient feel respected and trusted. After all, patients resist paying for healthcare, because rarely do they want to consume it in the first place.

8

Communication Devices that Reflect Your Commitment to Patients

- Do you communicate regularly with your patients whether or not they have a presenting medical need or appointment?
- Do you make your commitment to patients explicit in printed materials circulated by your office?
- Do you anticipate patient questions and attempt to preempt them by communicating information proactively?
- Do you supplement information you communicate verbally with written information, making it possible for patients to educate themselves and review important information?
- Do you distribute to all patients key information about your practice, your philosophy, your services and your availability?
- Do you communicate with patients in ways that will impress them that will make them stop and take notice of your consideration?
- When you communicate with patients through the mail, do you or someone in your office review the communication from the pa-

tient's point of view, making sure that the message is conveyed in a respectful, positive way?

If you answered "yes" to most of these questions, consider your practice as being among those progressive practices that take initiative to use written communication as a strategy to heighten patient satisfaction. Increasingly, physicians are realizing considerable power in creating and shaping the patient's image of their practice through carefully designed written communication—and lots of it.

We've talked with healthcare consumers and identified the kinds of written materials and devices that they associate with physicians they consider helpful and caring. In this chapter, we examine a variety of these that you might consider in your efforts to enhance patient satisfaction.

THREE UNDERLYING PREMISES

To make our case for escalating the written communication generated by medical practices for the sakes of patients, consider first the extent to which you agree with these three premises:

- To the patient, information is power.
- Proactive is better than reactive.
- Continuity of communication helps build loyalty.

First of all, consider the fact that, when one's health is involved, *information is power*. Increasingly, patients want information. In fact they believe they deserve it. If you communicate information richly and energetically, without having to be asked, patients are generally impressed, even if they don't read or absorb the information.

Second, patients today are aware of alternative healthcare providers. To shop among practices and to judge their satisfaction with their physician of the moment, they use as criteria for judgment the factors they know best—namely service factors. The practice that *proactively* takes steps to provide information that makes their practice more user-friendly is appreciated. Your efforts to orient patients to your practice, to make hours of access and phone numbers easy to find and read, to know without feelings of insecurity what to do before an appointment and what to bring to that appointment—all of these bits of information make a practice stand out as service-oriented and user-friendly. And patients notice.

When it comes to written communication, more is not necessarily better, because the quality of that communication matters. But generally, regular, planned communication goes a long way to stay in touch with your patients whether or not they have a presenting medical problem or need. When you communicate, you can choose the words, the images, the associations you want to stick in people's minds. And if you do this regularly, you're saying to the patient, "We consider you family and we don't forget you." Depending on the kind of practice you have, you might want a long-term relationship with your patients, a continuing relationship that you maintain through written communication between visits.

WHAT TO COMMUNICATE AND HOW?

A mix of standardized and personalized communication devices is ideal. Standard communication devices include such useful items as a new patient orientation guide, a hospital visit kit, patient satisfaction surveys, and newsletters. Personalized devices include anything from birthday or get well cards to thank you notes to mailing of personally relevant clippings with a note "Thinking about you . . . ." More details about some of the more popular options follow.

Guide for new patients

If you buy a new car, you receive a thorough guidebook that explains how the car works, how to take care of it, how to get optimal mileage, what to do in the face of one problem or another—in short, how to get the greatest satisfaction from your purchase. Why not provide similar information to your new or prospective patients. Provide a guidebook that details how the patient can obtain the best care and the best service from your practice.

Some practices hire public relations professionals to prepare a glitzy guidebook of this type, especially if their patients are in a particularly affluent market with high expectations and lots of competition. Others work with a local printer who has an in-house graphics person. Still others create their own guidebook at lower cost.

"Doctor's Office" newsletter (January 1987, pp. 10–11) describes a simple self-made guidebook with a four-panel cover, the likes of which you can purchase in a stationery store (although you might prefer a custom-printed or embossed cover with your practice's name and other important bits of information). Here's what they suggest for the sample cover letter:

Dear *(Patient Name)*,

We are looking forward to seeing you at *(appointment time, date)*. This appointment has been set aside especially for you, and it includes time for us to answer any questions you may have.

Please take a moment now to read our enclosed brochure. It answers many of the questions most of our new patients have on their minds.

It's also very important that we have certain facts before your first visit. Please be sure to (a) fill out the enclosed insurance and medical history forms and bring them with you when you come in, (b) sign the enclosed records release authorization and mail it to your previous physician as soon as possible.

We estimate that the combined fees for your initial visit will be $00.00. We generally request that the office visit fees be paid at the time you receive our services.

Thank you very much for the trust and confidence you've expressed in choosing this practice for your medical care.
Sincerely,

M.D., D.O., O.M., Receptionist

You can lay out the folder in the following way.

The Cover. You'll be faced with a smothering choice of paper (cover stock), colors, and design options. To narrow this choice swiftly, we suggest: (1) choose a cover stock just "heavy" enough to keep from appearing flimsy; (2) choose a color that ties in with your practice—white for surgeons and dentists, pastels for OB/GYN and other practices that serve mostly female patients, and bright colors for pediatricians and family practices, (3) use easy-to-read black ink.

The front panel will appear distinctive if you print merely your practice name, logo, address, and telephone number—large enough to be easily read, but not so large as to "scream" for attention.

The inside front may have a photograph of your doctor(s) and a brief statement of your practice's values and guiding philosophy. No matter what this statement says, it should begin by welcoming the patient to your practice and end with a sentence thanking the patient for coming to you.

The inside flap should call attention to the importance of the material inside the flap. A brief paragraph along these lines should do:

> Please read the enclosed material and call us at 000-0000 if you have any questions. We invite you to use this folder to keep this material and all your medical records safely in one convenient place.

The back panel could repeat your practice name and telephone number, along with office hours, special phone numbers for insurance, test results, and other designated calls, and the names and telephone numbers of physicians in the practice. (©1987 *The Doctor's Office*; 1858 Charter Lane; Lancaster, PA 17601. Reprinted with permission.)

Inside the Folder. You can mix and match a combination of the following items:

- The cover letter from the doctor, office manager, receptionist, or other staff member who made the initial contact with the patient or family member
- Your regular Patient Information Brochure
- A map that shows how to reach your office
- Biographical sketches for the doctor(s) and other key-staff members (the latter is a nice touch!)
- A copy of your most recent newsletter
- Information about the patient's insurance coverage if you know their carrier and have recent information
- Patient Information Sheet (Hx Form)
- An authorization for previous physicians or providers to release the patient's records
- If you're a specialist, you might also consider including:
  —educational pamphlets that address the patient's condition
  —information on fasting or other pre-visit instructions
  —and a preview of what their visit or treatment might include
- some practices now include charges for various services!

By using a folder instead of a printed booklet, you can select the right mix of items for the particular patient.

Information with a long life

To make the information you provide not just another piece of junk mail, include information that people will want to keep handy. A pediatric practice, for example, might include information parents would like to see at a glance in an emergency—who to call, their number, what to do if a temperature is above a certain threshold, do's and dont's, and so on. An obstetrical practice might include information on which problems you should call your doctor about during pregnancy. A general practitioner might offer information about bleeding and injury interventions. Family and internal medicine practices might convey information about risk factors for heart disease, cancer, hypertension, AIDS, stroke, and more.

These pamphlets are even more useful if you include the phone numbers of key community resources like the fire department, support groups, patient education providers, emergency services, and others.

The point is to package information about your practice along with resource information and facts compellingly relevant to your particular patient population. That way, they hang onto it and keep it in a prominent place where they, and others, see it.

HOSPITAL VISIT KIT

Some practices also distribute to their patients a hospital visit kit designed to make an impending hospital visit (for in-patients, out-patients, and lab patients) easier for the patient, for hospital personnel, and for the practice's own staff.

They provide a professional looking folder with contents written in plain people-talk, not obfuscated jargon. Enclosures describe the hospital location, the registration procedure, information about billing and insurance, and the patient's bill of rights, and a list of what to bring to ease the check-in process. These informative folders help your patients feel less intimidated and more comfortable as they ready themselves for their hospital visit. If you work with the hospital on the right contents for this kit, you can also include items that speed up, simplify, and demystify the check-in process. The ripple effect for you: fewer preadmission and post-discharge phone calls to you and your staff.

"Doctor's Office" newsletter (October 1986, pp. 8–9) makes these excellent suggestions about developing and implementing a visit kit system:

A. Use folders as covers for your visit kits.

This suggestion is being made for *marketing,* as well as for organizational purposes. You'll be able to present each patient with a professional looking *folio* that will guide him/her through every step of the hospital stay—and will project a strong image of your practice to the patient, the patient's family, and the patient's visitors.

We suggest you have two sizes of folders: an 8½" x 11" cover with one or two inside pockets, to hold all the information your long-stay or in-patient surgery patients will need; and a 9" x 4" side-entry envelope for the smaller amount of material your lab patients will need. Out-patient surgery patients can be given either folder, depending on the amount of information their visit and procedure call for.

Both kinds of folders should have your practice name and phone number tastefully printed on the outside. Both should be available through local printers and stationers—and we suggest you check out the various styles of folders and the varying costs of purchasing and imprinting them.

B. Gather as much basic information as you can.

Hospital forms that must be filled out prior to admission, insurance identification and information that the admissions office would like the patient to bring along, hospital rules and patients' rights, directional maps showing how to find the hospital, parking area, and proper entrance, floor plans showing where to go once you're inside the hospital, visiting hours, discharge procedures, etc.—This is the kind of information that will make an organized patient forever grateful to you for providing it. And for a disorganized patient— well, you and your hospital will be forever grateful if that patient's visit goes off without a hitch.

In addition to this basic material, there are also special folders or pamphlets that you can give to your patients: major operating room procedures, anesthesia, radiology, outpatient surgery, lab tests, hospital diet, physical therapy. Check with your hospital and other sources to find patient education materials that will be of help.

C. Provide the rest of the information your patients will need.

You should have a descriptive pamphlet of some kind for each of the major procedures your doctors do (in the office as well as at the hospital). These may be available from the hospital, from your professional society, or from a national association concerned with the particular condition. If pamphlets are not readily available from one of these sources, consider producing your own pamphlet(s), imprinted with your practice name and phone number, of course.

The appropriate descriptive pamphlet(s) can be added to each patient's folder, along with:

- the doctor's fasting and other preadmission orders
- postoperative instructions
- approximate (or, possibly, exact) fees that will be billed by your own office, and, possibly, the approximate amounts that may be billed by the hospital, anesthesiologist, lab(s), consulting and assisting surgeons, and whomever else.
- the patient's room number, when known in advance

D. Include a "highlights" cover sheet with each visit kit.

What are the most important things that each hospital patient must know prior to admission? Check-in time? Fasting orders? Insurance information the hospital must have? These are things that should be repeated on a "summary sheet" that goes on top of all the other material in each folder. This summary sheet can be a form printed on your letterhead on which certain items can be checked off or written in, or it may be a brief letter that follows a form and is individually typed for each patient on your letterhead. Whatever form it takes, put the summary where the patient can't miss it. If possible, call the patient's *attention* to the summary sheet, and, under ideal circumstances, *go over* the summary sheet word for word and point by point with the patient.

E. Set up a "library" of hospital visit information.

Preferably in a separate closet, store stacks of large and small folders, packets of basic information from your hospital, and descriptive pamphlets. Try to keep this material neatly organized, and make sure everyone on your staff knows what's there and how to present it to patients. Make a list of the pieces that are needed for each of your most common hospital procedures. Then, when a staff member isn't familiar with the procedure, he/she can simply go to the list and pull the necessary pieces for the folder.

F. When possible, hand out visit kits in person.

Usually, the best time to hand the patient a visit kit is when the decision is made to have the hospital procedure done. Go over the points on the summary sheet and then ask, "Do you understand everything we've talked about? Is there anything you'd like me to discuss? When you get home, will you read your visit kit and call me if there's something you'd like me to explain?" We realize this isn't always possible, but, when it is, you'll have a happier, more cooperative patient and a less-disrupted office day. ©1986 *The Doctor's Office*; 1858 Charter Lane; Lancaster, PA 17601. Reprinted with permission.

PATIENT EDUCATION READINGS AND PROGRAMS

To cater to many patients' emerging hunger for information as a basis for heightened involvement in their medical care, consider also providing patient education pamphlets, magazines or information cards or fliers (that you create or purchase) related to popular lifestyle and wellness concerns (smoking, nutrition, stress, etc.) and to the most typical conditions or illnesses relevant to your practice's patients. When you provide educational information, you not only cater to the patient's need for information but you might also save time by providing information in writing that you might otherwise need to supply during the office visit or in a follow-up phone call when the information you've communicated verbally recedes in the patient's memory.

Items provided by practices determined to be proactive in patient education include a mix of the following items:

- Information on how to reach your community's patient education hotline (e.g., Tele-Med)
- Brochures (often available free from organizations like pharmaceutical companies, the American Heart Association, the American Cancer Society, and other societies that focus on diabetes or hypertension or cancer, etc.)
- "Please ask me if I forget" cards: These cards educate the patient about questions they should be sure to ask the doctor during the visit in case their doctor doesn't think to discuss certain key issues, like follow-up care, appropriate time for next visit, medication instructions, etc.
- Articles written by your own doctors: Patients tend to be impressed by academic involvement of their physicians. They feel secure when they see that you write for the local newspaper or professional journals. Make available in your office "Please take one" copies of any printed materials you've developed on your specialty area. You can educate your patients about your views and at the same time build your credibility in their eyes. Some practices have a display area that spotlights their physicians' own work on a shelf under a bulletin board that reads "Hear it from our physicians," or some other attention getter that attracts people to the media or journal coverage achieved by you and your people.
- Newsletter with health update: Some commercially available newsletters are available on a subscription basis that you can purchase in quantity and imprint your practice's name on (e.g., "Women's Health Matters"). Or, do your own "Health Facts" newsletter.

A patient education strategy

Since patients today increasingly crave information about their health and their options, you can impress and educate your current patients and even attract new ones by going beyond the provision of pamphlets and developing a well conceived patient education strategy—a strategy that complements the patient education you already do one-on-one with patients who have individual needs. By making more than the usual few pamphlets available on a waiting area coffee table or rack, you can show a dedication to providing your patients with information and a desire to actively help them educate themselves about disease and prevention.

Options abound

A few pamphlets in the waiting area—that's getting increasingly common. But there are many more options that separate the sheepish practices from the goats! We'll describe here an integrated system for patient education, although if you don't want to install such a comprehensive, integrated approach, you might consider some of the individual components.

A Year-Long Agenda.   Divide the year into six patient education periods. Select one or two topics or education thrusts for each period. Depending on your specialty and target patient population, topics might include "Food for Your Heart," "Diabetes and You," "Diverticular Disease," "Childhood Infections," "Osteoarthritis," "Premenstrual Syndrome," "Reye's Syndrome," "Back Talk," "Healthy Aging," and more—in short, any topics that apply to many people and that you and perhaps your staff can address knowledgeably and authoritatively.

For each two-month period, prepare yourself and your staff by providing updates and materials on the topic, developing or locating handout materials, and lining up any promotional activities or events that you might want to sponsor.

By developing a year-long agenda of patient education topics, you convey the impression (and the fact) that you are a state-of-the-art, informed practice, dedicated to sharing facts and strategies with your patients whose health and wellness you are going the extra mile to promote.

Involve Everybody on Staff.   Prepare your whole staff and your office to educate your patients on the topic of the period. Make education available in short bits and through face-to-face and print vehicles like these:

- Post signs at strategic points (on bulletin boards, in waiting areas, in the bathroom, etc.) or have staff wear buttons that invite patients to ask staff about the topic of the period. The sign might read, "Ask our staff (or me) about ways to prevent backaches." Make sure everyone on staff can articulate two or three key points, warning signals, or tips in answer to the patient's question, and can refer the patient to further information sources if he or she wants to know more.

- Have staff hand patients a pamphlet (like those available from the AMA and medical suppliers). Or, better yet, prepare a letter or fact sheet or piece written by the doctor and tailored specially for your patients. Make sure staff know a good way to hand this information out, by saying, for instance, "Here's some more information about the subject. If you want to know more, Doctor _____ would be happy to talk with you."

- Have the doctor(s) speak to individuals and groups about the topic. Some practices hold two public education sessions per month on the subject, an evening session at a local public library or community center, and a daytime session within their own offices. This can attract new referrals too.

- Tell the public and your patients that they can call a certain number and hear a pre-taped message about the subject. Have the doctor tape this message, so it can sound personalized and create a feeling of a personal contact between the doctor and the caller, "Hello, my name is Dr. _____ and I specialize in pediatrics. I'm happy to talk with you about _____ *(the message)*. If you would like to know more or would like to consult with us about your concerns, please don't hesitate to call our office and ask for me personally at *(phone number)*." You can arrange for a special phone line to handle these calls at approximately $15/month, which is low, considering the educational value to your existing patients and the marketing value to future prospects. Some doctors do a variation on this theme by providing a tape recorder, tapes and earphones in their waiting rooms, and recently, some even have patient education videotapes that "educate while-you-wait."

How to Promote. To publicize your educational programs and resources, hang signs in your offices, announce in your newsletter, distribute fliers to patients, send fliers to community organizations, hang signs in the supermarket, and take advantage of the fact that community newspapers usually are willing to advertise educational programs free, even though the net effect is to promote you and your practice. If you plan for a year at a time, you can tell agencies, libraries, and senior centers your entire schedule which they will likely post in a visible place. Some practices even run paid ads and radio spots (although you might want to check with your local medical society about the norms for your area).

You Can't Lose. The patient learns. The patient often brings or tells others. New people get a glimpse of you and your colleagues before they have a problem. And you position your practice as dedicated to the health and wellness of the community and determined to promote knowledgeable consumers, whether the individual buys service or not.

Your Practice's Own Newsletter. Do you have a patient newsletter? Many practices, especially group practices, do. Filled with newsworthy features about patients, news about staff accomplishments and additions, descriptions about services, educational tidbits about illness prevention, surveys, pictures of staff, updated information about office hours and policies, and more. These are the typical contents of patient newsletters.

Sheldon Kress, M.D., of Internal Medicine Associates and the Greater Washington Preventive Medicine Center, describes the following contents of one issue of their excellent newsletter—"To Your Health":

- "In response to a recent patient survey, patients get three wishes"
- Announcement of expanded evening hours
- Introduction of new physician to their staff, highlighting how his presence will ease scheduling for patients

- Information about the incidence of breast cancer, the American Cancer Society's guidelines for breast screening, and how the reader can arrange a convenient appointment at her breast center
- Feature article on colo-rectal cancer (frequency, signs and symptoms, early detection, risk factors, prevention, and services available at Internal Medicine Associates)
- A reminder that patients can receive help with insurance and bookkeeping problems by calling a special number
- A thank you to people who have made referrals to their practice
- A survey inviting readers to rate their interest in several reasonably priced health education classes.

Other stand-out ideas

Also consider printed maps, compliance instructions, greeting cards, messages on the backs of bills, thank you letters, and more. When you seize opportunities for contact with patients—opportunities that other physicians miss—you stand out in the patient's mind as particularly patient-oriented.

Maps.   Before a first visit, send a "We're confirming your appointment" with a map showing exactly how to get to your office. And for patients referred by you to labs or other physicians or a hospital, provide a map that shows how to get from your office to there. And to demystify the maze-like hospital environment, show your patient the exact location of their destination, including the name of the office or department, the floor, the room, and the building name. Patients meander through hospital hallways in confused haze with a note in their physician's handwriting that says, "See Dr. Handley," or "Go to the lab," when people in the hallway and information desk don't know Dr. Handley and there are seven different labs throughout a campus of six buildings.

Compliance Instructions.   Patients appreciate *complete* written instructions when they leave your office. For the main conditions you treat, you can preprint these or make a checklist that you can quickly fill out. To excel in the instructions you provide, ask patients in a focus group or waiting room conversation to look at the forms you use and point to anything they consider vague or obscure. For instance, if you say to take a certain medication three times a day, how should the patient handle nighttime? Can they take the medication at mealtime, on an empty stomach, or exactly when and how? The practice that preempts feelings of insecurity and wondering on the part of their patients stands out as user-friendly and patient-centered.

Also regarding style, show a few patients the items you're planning to make available. Ask a few patients kept waiting to take a look while they're waiting. Get consumer input into color, type style, and layout.

Also, print big and bold. Especially for the sake of older patients, make sure the print isn't tiny. You want your patients to understand and remember their post-visit instructions—their medication doses and schedules. Your instruction sheets that show the current list of their medications with dosage and frequency can probably be enlarged on your copier, to make the print more readable. This tends to eliminate phone calls from some patients, and also shows consideration on your part.

Greeting Cards That Trigger Positive Associations.   Create a tickler system or special calendar that reminds your staff to send birthday cards to patients. And when you discharge a patient from the hospital, send a nice card wishing them a speedy recuperation and reminding them that you're there if they need you. Cards for all occasions—New Year, Valentine's Day, Thanksgiving, etc.—make people smile at your thoughtfulness. And how about a reminder card sent to patients you haven't seen in a while? They might say, "It's been a year, hope you're well."

Bill-backs.   On the bottom or back of invoices to the patient, include a cartoon, news item, or tidbit of medical memorabilia. The extra attention this attracts not only speeds up payment, it also sweetens the otherwise sour taste of a bill or payment reminder.

Thank You Letters.   Again, you have so many *good* excuses to connect to patients in writing. Thank them for a referral, share a low-salt recipe, remind them about a forthcoming appointment in a welcoming manner. And, if you want them to tell their neighbors about you, send their *kids* a letter with a sticker, a cartoon, a pen, or something else. Kids love mail and get very excited about it.

"Many Happy Returns" Card to New Patients.   Encourage new patients to return by sending them a follow-up mailing that includes:

- Key names and phone numbers for people who can answer different kinds of healthcare questions
- A survey or response card that invites their reactions to their first visit to your practice
- A business card with your name, address, and hours
- And *if* your practice competes with other practices on affordability, include also a discount coupon worth 15 percent off the next visit's fees. (Try out this

concept on a few patients before you do it, to make sure it doesn't offend or make your practice seem like the low-priced and, therefore, low-quality option.)

An Apology Letter.   Doctors with the humility and interpersonal sensitivity to apologize to patients who have been inconvenienced by them inevitably come out winning. An emergency arises, or you keep people waiting. In situations where you're in the wrong—when you keep patients waiting, when you forget to call the pharmacy, when you are late in responding to their phone call—apologize not only in person but also in writing. A gesture of apology goes a long way with patients to right a wrong and make the patient perceive you as considerate after all. Simply defuse their annoyance or anger with the facts and a sincere apology. Recognize that you've inconvenienced them and express your regret. Here's an example:

> Dear Mrs. Fantz,
>
> I want to personally apologize for the fact that you had to wait so long in our office on July 18th.
>
> I'm very sorry to say that another of our patients had an emergency that I felt had to become our first priority. We could not anticipate this in time to alert you to the fact that your appointment would be delayed.
>
> I respect the value of your time and when we schedule an appointment with you, I consider it a promise to provide the service you expect and deserve. I'm very sorry that the emergency on July 18th caused me to break that promise.
>
> Again, I'm very sorry we caused you this inconvenience. I want to assure you that in the future, we will do all we can, within our control, to fulfill our commitment to you.
>
> Thank you for your continuing trust and confidence.
>
> > Sincerely,
> > *(signature)*
> > Margaret Harris, M.D.

Patients don't expect you to be perfect, but they do believe they deserve honesty and an explanation when you're not.

WORDS TAKE WORK

We've presented a few examples of ways you can heighten patient satisfaction through increased written communication with your patients. But communicating takes time, and who has it?

Some medical practices find that, within their own staffs, they have a closeted writer who would find it enhancing to their job to develop or adapt the kinds of written materials described. Other practices hire a free-lance writer or public relations firm to develop boilerplate letters and notes that your staff can then adapt and generate in a quick and easy fashion.

Is the expense and effort worth it? You'll know if "Out of sight, out of mind" is interfering with your patients' loyalty to your practice. If so, carefully designed, positive, patient-centered communications extend your reach and give continuity to your relationship with your patients even when they're out of sight.

9

Telephone Tact and Tactics

Telephone, *n*. An invention of the devil which abrogates some of the advantages of making a disagreeable person keep his (or her) distance. (Ambrose Bierce, *The Devil's Dictionary*)

If your phone service has ever gone dead, then you've probably had the occasion to appreciate the massive amount of business you and your staff handle via phone. It's hard to imagine how the old-time doctor even functioned without utter dependency on telephone lines, hold buttons, call transfer, call-forwarding, ring-again, and other features that we and our patients have come to depend on as nothing less than a lifeline.

That's why your telephone systems and practices are so powerfully important to patient satisfaction. The telephone is your lifeline. A ringing phone is liable to be a patient, a patient's loved one, a prospective patient, a referring doctor, another referrer—in other words, a customer or someone who attracts or repels customers.

PATIENTS EXPECT SO MUCH

The general public relies on phones for so much everyday activity that, to many people, a phone feels almost like an appendage. While people understand that your busy schedule might make it impossible for you to see them in person at a moment's notice, people are far less understanding of frustrations they suffer when they seek information or access by way of "a quick call." And that's what people primarily want: information and access—delivered with courtesy and a quick willingness on the part of the voices who answer. They want timely attention to their needs. They want to be treated with respect. They want their requests to be taken seriously and considered important, not regarded as an interruption. And they want answers to their questions, not buckpassing or a runaround. That's what patients want—plenty!

WHAT DO YOU WANT?

Meanwhile, you have your needs to fulfill. You undoubtedly want to handle calls efficiently and courteously, but without placing stress and strain on the energy of you or your staff. You want to handle as much as possible by phone to alleviate unnecessary appointments that demand even more of your time. And you want people to perceive their phone interactions with you and your staff to be satisfying to the point of increasing loyalty to your practice and encouraging repeat business.

Patients want:
- courtesy
- answers
- now

You want:
- efficiency
- information
- satisfied, not harried, staff
- satisfied callers

To achieve these result for you and your patients, you need to manage your telephone service, ensuring that you establish, monitor, and fine-tune three aspects:

- The technology
- Access
- People skills

THE TECHNOLOGY

Patients care first of all about whether your phones are answered without delay. Here is a list of patient frustrations with their physicians' phones—rank-ordered from most frustrating to least frustrating:

- You get a busy signal and have to call back.
- You get a machine that asks for your name and number and promises a return call who knows when.
- A human being answers and puts you on hold before you can get a word out.
- You get a machine response, saying, "All lines are busy. Please hold."
- You get a human being who asks you if you would mind holding.
- You get through immediately.

To reduce caller frustration, your phone technology (and of course, your people) must be adequate to the task. You need enough phone lines and an answering system that prevents callers from ever getting a busy signal and thus shouldering the burden of calling back. Ideally, you would have enough reception staff to handle the volume of calls you tend to get simultaneously. But knowing that the cost of that might be prohibitive, you need back-up systems that help patients wait their turn without climbing the walls with impatience and resentment.

Consider a branching system made possible easily by new technology. Think of the volume of calls related to appointments and bills. These never have to reach the doctor's ears. Ideally, if your practice is large enough, you might have a direct line to billing or appointments, so that not all callers have to go through a central receptionist. This cuts down on call volume to the receptionist, and it also reduces the time it takes for the patient to reach the appropriate person. With new telephone technology, you can have a machine triage calls by category and direct them to the right extension. For instance, the machine says, "Hello, Redwood Pediatrics. If you want to talk with someone about a medical question or problem, press '1' on your telephone and wait for an answer. If you want to make an appointment, press '2'. If you have a question about your bill, press '3'. If you don't have a push-button phone or you want to reach our receptionist for help, just hang on please and someone will be right with you"

Ironically, patients tend not to mind this kind of branching system. What they mind most is *people* giving them the runaround. So, if you must forward calls from person to person, consider a mechanized way to do this that might make the first forwarding move quick and mechanical, so that the people who then receive the call are receptive, welcoming, serving, and the place where the buck stops for the kind of call they receive.

Your technology also needs to be easy to use by staff. Some newfangled phone systems have wonderful features, but, without adequate training of all staff, those feature obstruct excellent service to patients rather than providing it.

And how about your staff and patients within earshot of your phones? Are they driven crazy by an abrasive, buzzer-like sound, instead of the more soothing, less intrusive tones now available?

Some physicians jump at the new customer-friendly phone features available. Others feel that their old systems are adequate and changes are not worth the investment. But since customers are so concerned about telephone service, the attitude of "We can get along without improvements" may be short-sighted. A simple survey of your patients' perceptions can help you decide whether improvements are, in your practice, worth the investment.

Ask your patients:

1. How would you rate the service you get from our office over the phone?
2. How would you rate the service you get from your physician over the phone?
3. Are you able to get through to us when you need to?
4. How do you rate the courtesy with which your calls are handled?
5. If this were your office, how would you improve our phone system or methods?

To find out the facts about how long your callers are waiting, try a mini-audit of telephone wait time. Specifically, monitor calls for three days. You may be able to find a volunteer, a telecommunications graduate student, or a staff member whose duties you can delay for these three days. Have this person monitor the number of calls into your office, the length via stopwatch of every third or fifth call (you can extrapolate to all calls from that), and the time on hold.

Based on these service audits, you can determine how big a problem your phone system is and know whether to make it a priority worth tackling in your practice enhancement strategy.

REGARDING ACCESS

When patients or concerned family members want to reach the doctor's office, they want to reach the doctor's office! They want ready access. Since no physician can be instantly available 24 hours a day, that access is rarely possible. But patients still want it. To cater to this need, you have to rely on other people, covering physicians, answering services, answering machines, and beeper systems. Fortunately, telephone technology has advanced to a point where you can purchase access tools that make your life and the patient's life easier. In fact, with beepers and answering services, and mobile phones, you can, if you want, have nationwide mobility while your staff and patients continue to have access to you.

All of these phone options have their place. Once you decide which options best serve your needs, the key to their effective use by patients is patient education. You need to make sure that your patients understand thoroughly how to have access to you or a trusted backup person in what they consider an emergency. On the following patient information card, consider the clarity by which one practice communicates all about phone access to its patients.

How You Can Reach Me When You Need Me

When it comes to health and illness, you never know when you'll need attention or advice. As a result, you might want access to me or others in our office at times when our office is closed—at night, on weekends, and during vacations.

I realize how important it is for you to reach me or a trusted back-up physician when you need to, so I want you to know exactly how to gain access to me or others in our practice any time of the day or night. I want you to know that when I am not available, I always have another physician I trust on call to respond to your needs. I can assure you that I stay in close contact with this back-up physician, since I'll want to know what's happening with you in case I am needed to help.

During regular office hours: call our office at 000-0000 between 8:00 AM and 5:00 PM Mondays thru Friday, and between 9:00 AM and 1:00 PM on Saturday. That's when we're open, and our staff can take your call. I'll try to speak with you when you call, but usually, if I'm with a patient, involved with an emergency or out for a period in order to make my hospital rounds, I won't be able to speak to you right at that moment. Please explain your situation to whomever answers and he or she will help you or will see to it that I or another appropriate person does as soon as possible.

Outside of Office Hours: Before 8:00 AM and after 5:00 PM, I am generally not available to take calls in my office. But if you call my office, our answering service will take your call and make sure I get the message within the hour. I make sure I call my answering service every hour that I'm otherwise unavailable. I make sure to keep our answering service people informed of my whereabouts and also they always know how to reach an on-call physician at all times.

I place a high value on returning your phone calls as soon as I possibly can. However, sometimes I have literally dozens of calls to return and it might take me some time to get to yours. I want you to know that I'm trying to reach you and every other one of my patients as fast as I can without sacrificing the quality of attention and help I give to each. I apologize in advance for any uncomfortably long waits for a phone call back from me.

Again, I want to assure you that by following these guidelines, you can have access to me or a trusted back-up physician with whom I'll keep in close contact—any time of the day or night, because I want to be there for you and your family.

REGARDING ANSWERING SERVICES

Some of the patient complaints about telephone handling would disappear if medical practices shopped carefully for service-oriented answering services that employ people who both understand medical practices and are willing to work closely with the physicians to expedite appropriate communication between physician and patient. You have to demand knowledgeable answering service staff, you have to train them to handle your patients knowledgeably, and you have to monitor their compliance with your preferred phone management practices. Some practices require quarterly full-day training for their answering service providers. They make this training a condition of a long-term contract with the answering service. Such sessions include training and orientation to your specific ways of doing things:

Training and Orientation Agenda for Answering Service Staff

- Our practice's size, scope, and specialty
- Our practice's patient-centered philosophy
- Getting acquainted with our physicians and their ways of doing things
- How to screen calls in order to judge appropriate followup
  —when to call an ambulance
  —when to call the doctor on call
  —when to wait until the doctor on call calls
  —when to call certain other staff members
  —when to take a message and promise a call-back as soon as the office opens
- How we like messages to be taken

PATIENT-FRIENDLY STAFF

Technology and access are important, but according to consumers, not as important to your telephone reputation as your own staff's behavior on the phone.

How capable are your staff when it comes to handling the phone? Have them take this quiz (See Table 9–1) and examine the skills they have versus the skills they need in order to excel at telephone tact and tactics.

Table 9-1. Quick Telephone Self-Quiz.

Do you come across on the phone like "Oscar the Grouch"?
Does your TONE OF VOICE say, "Get off my case"?
This quiz is designed to give you insight into your phone skills.

1. When a caller refuses to give their name, do you:
   a. Hang up on them
   b. State: "I need your name in order to help you"
   c. State: "I can't put you through unless you give me your name"
2. If a second call rings on your line and no one else is around to pick it up, do you:
   a. Continue to let it ring
   b. say to the first caller: "Will you please excuse me. I must answer another phone."
   c. You say to the first caller—"hold on a minute".
3. When returning to a caller after putting them on hold, do you say:
   a. "Sorry, it's been a crazy day today"
   b. "Hello"
   c. "Thank you for waiting, Mrs. _____. I can help you now."
4. When a person calls with a complaint, do you:
   a. Listen to the whole complaint and show you understand.
   b. For efficiency, try to change the caller's point of view.
   c. Interrupt the caller and say, "You're talking with the wrong person"
5. If you can't understand what the caller is saying, do you say:
   a. "What did you say? Talk a little louder"
   b. "I can't understand what you're trying to say"
   c. "I'm having difficulty in hearing (or understanding) what you're saying. Would you please repeat your last statement?"
6. When you answer the phone for someone who is not in the office, are you likely to say:
   a. "She/he hasn't come in yet"
   b. "She/he has a doctor's appointment"
   c. "She/he's not in the office at the moment"
7. When you receive a call and the person is in a meeting or on another line, do you say:
   a. "She/he's busy right now. Will you please call back later?"
   b. "She/he's unavailable right now. May I take a message and have him/her call

you back?"
   c. "She/he cannot be disturbed. You might be able to reach her at 3 P.M."
8. How long do you think it's okay to leave someone on hold?
   a. 3 minutes
   b. 1 minute
   c. 2 minutes
9. When you are rushed or under stress, do you tend to:
   a. Keep it to yourself and handle people calmly
   b. Apologize for your mood and hope they don't take it personally
   c. Let it show. After all, no one's perfect.
10. How many times do you usually allow the phone to ring before answering it?
    a. 1-2 rings
    b. 3-4 rings
    c. 5 rings or more
11. When you want to ask someone else in the office for information for a caller, do you:
    a. put the phone on hold
    b. place your hand over the receiver
    c. put the phone down on the desk.
12. When putting someone on hold, do you say:
    a. "Please hold!" and put the person on hold
    b. "May I put you on hold for a minute?" and wait for a response
    c. Nothing ... just put the person on hold.
13. When you get a call that should really be handled by another person or department, do you:
    a. Apologize nicely that you can't help and wish the person luck in finding who they need?
    b. Find out who the right person is and let the caller know?
    c. Find out who the right person is, locate their number and transfer the call?
14. When you call someone and realize you have the wrong number, do you:
    a. Hang up immediately, saving your breath and theirs
    b. Apologize and tell them you have the wrong number
    c. Say, "What's your number?" or "Who are you?"

SCORING KEY

1. **The best answer is (b). It's assertive and cooperative.**
   (a) is rude
   (c) shows a lack of consumer orientation
2. **The correct answer is (b). It shows courtesy and acknowledges the caller.**
   (a) is annoying and no one likes to wait.
   (c) is abrupt and leaves the caller confused and irritated.
3. **No question about it, (c) is the answer. It makes the caller feel important. Addressing people by name scores big points.**
   (a) the caller really doesn't want to hear about how frustrating your day has been. They have problems of their own.
   (b) "Hello" is not enough after they've been waiting for you.
4. **Of course, (a) is the answer. It allows the caller to express their complaint and shows them you're concerned.**
   (b) frustrates the caller and often leads to an argument.
   (c) alone angers the caller. Add a little concern and help them find the right person. That makes it okay.
5. **Yes, (c) is definitely the correct answer. It acknowledges the fact that you are having a problem hearing the person and are concerned about getting the full message.**
   (a) sounds bossy.
   (b) blames the person and makes them feel defensive.
6. **You guessed it! (c) is the correct answer. It gives the caller the impression that the person is engaged in a business matter.**
   (a) suggests that the person is late getting to work
   (b) the party shouldn't be told anyone's personal business.
7. **The correct answer is (b). This statement indicates your willingness to be of service to the caller.**
   (a) and (c) irritate the caller. You should offer to take a message.
8. **Telephone etiquette states that (b) is the correct answer. Responding quickly, even though you have to ask the party to hold for a minute, makes people feel that you want to assist them.**
   (a) and (c)—A minute goes fast when you're talking, but it's long and agonizing when you're waiting.

9. **The best answer is (a). It shows a professional demeanor.**
   (b)—If you slip, this isn't a bad idea. It's best, though, not to let it happen in the first place.
   (c)—The caller is innocent. Your ill will makes you and the hospital look bad.
10. **The correct answer is (a)—1–2 rings. It's common courtesy.**
    (b) and (c)—People become impatient when they have to wait for an answer.
11. **(a) is the answer. This is professional.**
    (b) and (c)—The caller should not be subjected to background noise and office conversation.
12. **The correct answer is (b). Asking permission to put someone on hold shows good manners. The person may be unable to wait.**
    (a) doesn't give the person a chance to respond. They may not want to hold on.
    (c) is rude and angers the caller.
13. **The best answer is (c). It eliminates the caller having to play a guessing game.**
    (a) doesn't help the caller in finding the correct person, and shows a lack of concern on your part.
    (b) You stopped one step too soon. This transaction is complete when the call is transferred.
14. **The best way to handle this is (b). An error has been made and expressing your regrets is proper telephone etiquette.**
    (a) is inexcusably rude!
    (c) is rude and an invasion of privacy

If you scored . . .

10–14   You're a Ringer! You get the Merit Award for Outstanding Phoning.
5–10   You're getting there! Call forward and transfer your skills to handle the situations you missed.
1–5   Sorry . . . wrong number! Hang up and try again!

Source: HOSPITALity News, Albert Einstein Medical Center, Philadelphia, PA 19141; © 1983 and reprinted with permission

Given the importance of the phone to your reputation, phone answering behavior should not be left up to the individual judgment of your staff members. You need telephone protocol. You need to set clear expectations about how phones are to be answered in your practice, in a way that reflects your patient-centered practice philosophy. You need to define excellent telephone skills and help staff enact them in the variety of situations that typically arise in your practice. You then need to declare that excellence is required, not optional.

The telephone calls for tact

Consider the following tips to help establish guidelines with your frontline people for using the phone. These points help your key people use the phone to not only communicate information but also to demonstrate the professionalism and excellence you want to characterize your practice.

1. *Greeting*. Take a breath and smile before you pick up the phone. Introduce your practice and yourself ("Parkland Medical Associates, Pat Cather speaking"). A "Good morning" or a "May I help you?" helps.

2. *Tone*. In general, be careful to speak clearly and succinctly. Be neither casual ("Who's this") nor too formal ("May I ask to whom I am speaking"). Strive to sound professional ("May I ask who's calling").

3. *I'm sorry but*. If the caller asks for someone who is not in, say, "He's not available right now. May I take a message?" or "She's out of the office now. I expect her back at four o'clock. May I take a message?" If the person is out of town, ask the caller if he would like to speak with someone else.

4. *Messages*. Always find out and write down the caller's name and telephone number. If possible, record the subject of the call. This will help the person called to determine the best call-back order.

5. *Transferring calls*. Never say, "You've got the wrong office." If a caller isn't where she wants to be, tell her where she is and help her get where she's going. "This is Reception, not Billing. Would you like me to transfer your call for you? I'd be glad to. But in case something happens or you get a busy signal, the number for Billing is 555-5555"

6. *Closing*. At the end of a call, say something that leaves a cordial last—and lasting—impression, like, "Thank you for calling." Let the other person hang up first.

7. *Phrases to avoid.*

"She's impossible to find or reach, but as soon as I can, I'll give her your message."

"She's working at home."

"I really don't know where he is, but I'll tell him you called."

"She's always away. It's a real challenge to get her."

"He'll be back on Monday. Would you try again then."

"I'm sorry, but he's at the proctologist. Can I take a message?"

(The Einstein Consulting Group, York and Tabor Roads, Philadelphia, PA 19141. ©1986, and reprinted with permission.)

When you set guidelines, make sure you identify appropriate behavior for handling the critical times or "moments of truth" when patient satisfaction is at stake over the phone. For example:

- When the patient calls for an appointment
- If you must reschedule a patient's appointment
- When the patient wants to speak with the doctor
- When the patient needs to be reminded to schedule a follow-up appointment
- When the caller is kept waiting longer than he or she thinks is tolerable
- When the caller thinks he or she has been given the runaround
- When the caller has waited for a doctor to call back, with no result
- When people have who-knows-what complaint

Each of these situations can be handled with either skill and finesse, or the kind of awkwardness or disregard that leads to an escalation of anger. You need to develop protocol for these recurring and inevitable situations and train your people to handle them with aplomb.

The "Doctor's Office" newsletter included a rich variety of typical telephone situations along with possible responses. Use these with your staff as a springboard for developing a protocol that best fits your office practice and personal preferences. Once you have a protocol developed with staff and physician understanding, incorporate it into your personnel management practices and office procedure manual. And until these responses become second nature to staff, encourage them to keep a copy nearby as they handle the phone (see Table 9–2).

Watch your language

Also, make sure you help staff become careful about their telephone language. Since the phone prohibits warm, caring looks and gestures, you have to rely on

Table 9–2. Typical Telephone Situations.

SITUATIONS THAT COME UP WHEN THE PHONE RINGS	RESPONSES
The phone rings, beeps, chirps, or otherwise signals.	Answer by the third ring. Identify yourself immediately, "Dr. Eberly's office, this is Barbara, how may I help you?"
The caller asks for information without identifying him- or herself.	"O.K., and your name is . . . ?
The caller's name is hard to understand, either because it's unfamiliar or not pronounced clearly.	"Would you please spell your last name?"
You're not sure if it's a new or an established patient.	"When did our doctor see you last?" (Better than asking a long-time friend of the practice, "Have you been here before?"!)

APPOINTMENT REQUESTS	RESPONSES
Emergency	"What symptoms are you having?" (Consult 'Emergency' chart, or refer the call directly to your nurse or doctor.)
Same-day request (when your schedule is full) . . .	Ask: "How long have you been having these symptoms? Have they gotten worse today?" Then ask the nurse if the patient must be seen today . . . should be referred to another physician . . . or scheduled for a later day.
If the patient *must* be seen today . . .	"I see this is urgent, so we'll work you in at 00:00 today. Since our schedule is so full, you may have to wait a bit. Is that O.K.?"
The patient's "regular" doctor is booked solid . . . but another doctor in your practice has an opening.	"Dr. Mead's schedule is completely filled today, but at his request we're scheduling patients with Dr. Ash. She can see you at 00:00."

The patient asks to see a doctor in your practice who is not taking new patients. You want to convey the point that the *practice* IS welcoming new patients with open arms.

"Dr. Mead is pretty heavily scheduled, and he's asked us to schedule new patients with Dr. Ash or Dr. Hampshire. Would that be O.K. with you?

A new patient has just been scheduled.

"Mrs. Stone, we do request payment at time of service, and our initial office visit fee is $00.00. If additional services are necessary, we can discuss those fees with you at that time. Now, may I have your home and business telephone numbers? And (if the appointment is three or more days away), if I can have your home address, I'll mail you a copy of our Patient Information Brochure."

A new patient tells you he's been referred by an established patient.

"Oh, I'm happy to hear that! We appreciate it when patients recommend us to their friends."

A patient asks for directions to your office.

"Are you close to _____?" "Let me tell you the best way to get here from there." (Have the receptionist read written directions to your office.)

A patient calls to cancel . . . at the last minute!

We're disappointed you can't make it. When would you like us to reschedule your appointment?"

A patient calls to cancel and gives reasonable notice.

"Thanks for your consideration in letting us know in advance. Now, when's a good time for us to reschedule your appointment?"

A patient calls to let you know, "I'm going to be 'a little' late."	"Thanks for calling . . . when do you think you'll be here?" Check the day's schedule and go on to either: (a) "We should be able to work you in at that time—but you may have to wait a few minutes." (b) "We've reserved that time for other patients . . . could you come in at 00:00? We should be able to see you then."

CALLS FOR THE DOCTOR	RESPONSES
A colleague calls.	"I'll get him for you . . . hold on just a moment." Or: "She's out of the office right now. We expect her back at 00:00. Should I have her call you when she returns, or try to contact her immediately?"
Bona fide emergency (patient, hospital, nurse, whoever).	"I'll interrupt him . . . may I have your phone number? I'll call him to the phone. Please hold on!"
Nonemergency illness, treatment, or diagnostic calls from patients, hospital, nurse, corporate clients, etc.	Determine the *exact* question the caller wants answered; jot it down on a memo pad, along with the caller's name and phone number, and promise that someone will call back by a designated call-back time.
Salesperson calls.	"The doctor is with a patient now. Ms. Merly makes all purchase decisions in that area—please hold a moment and I'll put your call through."

PATIENT CALLS FOR INFORMATION ABOUT YOUR PRACTICE	RESPONSES
A new patient asks, "Does your doctor treat _____?"	"If you're having those symptoms, our doctor can examine you, determine the exact nature of your condition, and then discuss the various treatment options with you."

A patient asks, "Can you send me somewhere for an x-ray?"

"The doctor will examine you first, to see if an x-ray is necessary. We don't like to expose our patients to unnecessary x-rays."

A patients asks, "Can I get a prescription for _____; I've used it before when I felt this way."

"Our doctors *never* prescribe medications without diagnosing the patient's condition. If you'd like, I can give you an appointment for an examination . . . ."

"What insurance plans do you accept?"

"We participate in Medicare, Blue Shield, and a number of private plans, and an HMO. If you tell me what kind of coverage you have, I can connect you with someone who can answer your specific questions."

Clinically related questions, such as medication dosages, from current patients.

"I'll get your chart, and then I'll ask the nurse to speak with you. Can you hold, please?" (Wait for a reply; if you must keep the patient "on hold" for more than a few moments, get back to him or her, and ask if he or she can hold a moment longer or if someone can return the call.)

An established patient calls to request a prescription refill.

"Do you have the prescription label in front of you? O.K. Please give me your name; the pharmacy name; prescription number; name of the medication; and the directions listed on the label. If you don't hear from us by noon, it will be at _____ pharmacy."

EMPLOYMENT-RELATED CALLS	RESPONSES
A job applicant calls.	"We don't have an opening right now, but we would be interested in seeing your resumé . . . could you send us a copy, along with a handwritten letter telling us a little about yourself? We'll keep your resumé on file for a year, and if anything comes up, we'll call you."
An employee calls to let you know he or she won't be able to make it to work that day.	"Are you all right? I'll let Dr. Dover know you'll be out."
A bank or other credit granter wants to confirm a staff member's employment.	"Could I please have your name, company name, and firm number? Our Office Manager will be happy to return your call."
A prospective employer asks for a reference for a former coworker.	"Could I have your name, company name, and phone number? I'll ask our Office Manager to call you back."

MISCELLANEOUS CALLS	RESPONSES
An attorney or insurance company asks for patient's diagnosis, dates of service, or other information.	"I'm sorry, we do not provide any type of patient information over the phone. I'll need a written authorization from our patient allowing us to release specific information to you. Please send a request outlining the information you need to our Office Manager, Marcia Prudence."

Source: "The Doctor's Office," 1858 Charter Lane; Lancaster, PA 17601. ©1988, and reprinted with permission.

tone and words. And words mean different things to different people. Careful scrutiny of the words and phrases people use is important in order to eliminate the ones that alienate people.

If you tune into the phone line from the patient's perspective, you will most certainly prefer the phraseology in column B over the unintentional atrocities in column A:

A	B
I'm sorry he's all booked up today. He can't see you until tomorrow.	May I have an idea of the problem? The doctor has an opening at _____ tomorrow. He is scheduled this afternoon.
I'm sorry I can't fit you in today.	Could you come at _____ tomorrow?
We are running late.	The doctor's schedule was interrupted—or The doctor's schedule was interrupted by an emergency.
I'm calling to remind you of your appointment.	I'm calling to confirm (or verify) your appointment.
We've had a cancellation.	We've had a change in schedule.
The doctor is recalling you.	It's time for your regular examination.
Are you an old patient? *or* Mr. Thorson is an old patient.	When were you last seen? *or* Mr. Thorson is one of our regular patients.
The doctor's at a convention.	The doctor is attending an educational seminar.
You misunderstood me.	There must have been a misunderstanding.
Are you a patient here?	When were you last in our office?
Hold on.	Can you hold while I get that information?
Okay, goodbye.	Thank you for calling, Ms. Smith.
Doctor's Office	Dr. Hershey's Office, Mary Mint speaking. May I help you?
Dr. Beck isn't in today.	Dr. Hershey is seeing patients in the office today. May I give you an appointment with her or would you pre-

fer to see Dr. Beck tomorrow at
_____ ?

Yes, we are taking new patients.

Yes, may I schedule something with
Dr. Beck for you?

(The Doctor's Office, 1858 Charter Lane; Lancaster, PA 17601. ©1988, reprinted with permission.)

The words and phrases in column A are used without thought as to how they fall on patient ears. That's the point. Telephone behavior, like other staff and physician behavior, needs to be examined and reshaped, so that patients feel they're in the hands of professional and caring people.

Counter staff forgetfulness

Occasionally, reinforce the importance of telephone effectiveness and the requisite skills in communications with your staff. In other words, remind them of the importance of their telephone presence. Here's an example of such a communication:

To: Staff
From: Herb
Subject: The Power of the Phone

   In talking with patients recently about what they like and don't like about our practice, I've heard several emphasize the importance of how we handle the phone. The fact is, and patients reinforce this point, when we're on the phone, our reputation is on the line! Our styles for handling calls reflect not only on every one of us but also on our total practice.

   Given this fact, I would like to draw your attention to several telephone guidelines that, when followed, make a positive impression on our callers:

- Before you pick up the phone, finish your other office conversations.
- Put a smile on your face, even before you say "hello."
- Answer promptly—preferably on the first or second ring—and identify yourself as you do.
- Listen attentively to the caller. Concentrate on what he or she is saying. If you can't understand what is being said, tactfully interrupt and say, "I'm having difficulty hearing you. Would you mind repeating that?"
- To secure the attention of someone in the office who is on the phone, place a written note in front of that person explaining that

you need to talk with him or her. And be sure to wait for a response.

In our next staff meeting, I would like to discuss other ways we can be *phonetastic* and achieve the reputation for responsiveness and courtesy that we deserve.

SPECIAL AND SOMETIMES STICKY SITUATIONS

Beyond the basic skills you advocate and expectations you set for staff phone behavior, sticky situations still arise. Ideally, you will foster an atmosphere and a periodic staff meeting in which staff will discuss how best to handle the more challenging phone procedures.

Here are a few questions likely to arise in such discussions, and a few thoughts in response to each.

Q: First impressions matter so much, is there anything different about the way you would handle the call from a first-time patient?

A: For most patients, their introduction to a medical practice is the person who answers their initial telephone inquiry. The secretary, receptionist, or whoever answers the phone must convey a sense of competence, caring, and professionalism. First-time patients are apt to be concerned and frightened about their symptoms. *You* must be reassuring and confident. First-time patients are apt to be nervous about seeing a new doctor for the first time. *You* must convey sincere trust in the doctor. First-time patients may be worried about how long they'll have to wait to see the doctor. *You* must be optimistic, but honest in your assessment of the time delay. And no matter what, try to end the call on a positive note like, "I'll look forward to meeting you."

Q: You never know when several people are going to call at once. How do you juggle many calls simultaneously without turning off at least some of your callers?

A: Answering telephones in a busy office can often seem like a circus juggling act. People who have to do this become alarmed—even confused—when more than one call comes in at a time. The task requires a cool head, manual coordination, and a few points of telephone etiquette. Here are a few tips to help your staff juggle phone calls with poise.

- When putting someone on hold to answer another call, ask the caller's permission: "Would you mind waiting a moment while I answer another line?" And if the caller is willing to wait, when he or she comes back on the line, resume the conversation using the caller's name: "Mr. Jones, thank you for waiting. You were saying that . . . ."

- If the second call can't be taken care of briefly, ask the caller if he or she will wait until the first call is completed, or whether he or she would rather be called back later.
- If the second caller prefers to be called back, take the appropriate information and call back promptly.
- If the caller prefers to wait on hold until the first call is completed, be sure to check in periodically to indicate you haven't forgotten him or her, and to ask if he or she wishes to continue to wait.

Q: The phones are ringing, and patients are standing in front of you waiting to talk with you. How should we handle this conflict without slighting either the patient with you or those on the phone?

A: If you're speaking with someone face-to-face and the phone rings, finish your statement, say "Excuse me a moment please," and then answer the phone. Or, if the initial conversation is on the phone, finish your statement and ask the person to hold. Use your judgment to assess the priority of either conversation. Ask callers if they want to remain on hold or be called back, or apologize to the person before you for having to wait, and finish the phone call. Such conflicting demands can be unnerving; try to remain calm and show that you're trying hard to meet both people's needs.

Q: What if the caller has a serious complaint?

A: Although you and your staff might do all you can to prevent complaints, they are inevitable. And although nobody really *likes* to handle them, somebody has to.

Here are a few tips that can help all staff associated with your practice to better handle complaints—and help keep your practice's reputation intact at the same time.

1. Allow the speaker to express their complete thoughts. Don't interrupt. *Listen.*

2. Write down all important details, including short phrases and major facts.

3. Repeat these facts back to the caller to be sure you have them right.

4. Be sympathetic. It helps to calm the caller.

5. Maintain a pleasant tone. Don't lose your cool!

6. Tell the caller exactly what you plan to do with the complaint, to whose attention you will bring it, and if and when they can expect a response.

7. Apologize to the caller for the inconvenience or difficulty, even if it's not your fault or the fault of anyone in the office. This is an important gesture of goodwill toward the public.

8. Then, be sure to follow through. How complaints are handled dramatically affects how your patient following feels about your practice.

Volume control and time-saving

If your practice is besieged with calls and you can't afford to or don't want to expand your reception staff, you can control the number and length of incoming calls by instituting efficiency measures. First of all, analyze your incoming calls and have the analyst record the reasons why people are calling. Sort out the calls that are necessary from those that might have been avoided had you communicated with patients more effectively.

For instance, upon analysis, many practices discover that in well over half of their incoming calls, people merely have a nonpersonal question, like "Where do I park?" or "How late are you open on Thursday evenings?" or "How often do I have to change my dressing?" These are the kinds of calls that tend to drive staff crazy especially if they hear these kinds of questions day after day.

If they do, it means that earlier communication that should have happened did not happen or was not effective. You should take a new look at your Patient Information Brochure and New Patient Kit to make sure that the major call-evoking questions are addressed. And if they already are, you probably need to position them more prominently in your printed materials.

Also, consider revamping your office forms to make them truly informative and self-instructional, using plain talk. Rule of thumb: communicate facts like these at the first opportunity in order to ease the patient's mind and also prevent an onslaught of unnecessary phone calls that flood your office arteries. For instance, some recurrent questions should be addressed in your New Patient Information Kit or in an appointment confirmation call or note, or in a prior visit with the doctor, or on an individualized "Follow-Up Instructions" summary given by the doctor to each patient to explain their pills, when to change their dressings, and so on.

The point: pre-answer questions that otherwise result in a deluge of phone calls that could have, at least in many cases, been avoided.

Another challenge: absorbing and recording "quality" information when the phone is ringing off the hook. With many incoming calls, the receptionist walks the tightrope between handling a volume of calls and at the same time gathering quality information that saves time for the physician and other staff. Some practices analyze the quantity and purpose of their incoming calls and develop a message form that helps them gather complete information and record it quickly. An example is shown in Table 9–3.

The type of form shown in Table 9–3, which you can tailor to better suit your type of practice, can consume less of the receptionist's energy in having to think of what to ask, and can leave this person free to concentrate on listening to and

Table 9–3. Telephone Message Form.

Patient name _____ Time of call _____

Caller (if different) _____ Adult? _____ Child? _____

Phone: (H) _____ (W) _____

Referred by _____

Regarding: _____

Purpose of appointment:

☐ wants to see you because _____

☐ for second opinion because _____

☐ new symptoms _____

☐ routine follow-up on _____

☐ Wonders if it's ok to _____

☐ Has questions about _____

☐ Wants referral for _____

☐ Other _____

Insurance _____

Remarks _____

Appointment with _____

Receptionist's initials _____   Call Date _____

Source: "The Doctor's Office, 1858 Charter Lane, Lancaster, PA 17601; [1988, and adapted with permission.

absorbing the caller's concern. Practices that use forms like this then file them in a dated tickler file, so that this form is available to brief the physician on the day the person arrives for his or her appointment. At that point, the physician can tell how long the patient had to wait when they scheduled their appointment, and they can notice nuances of the original call that they can follow up on with the patient, thus showing the patient how good the communication is within their office.

THE NEED FOR SKILLED BACK-UP

When your receptionist can't answer, the others in your office who might be in the best position to pick up that call should be equally well trained. The patient calling deserves courteous, competent treatment on 100 percent of their calls, whether the right receptionist is available or not. Everyone should be ready to answer the phone if the receptionist can't—and quickly. But that doesn't mean that whoever answers must handle the concern. It usually takes an inordinate amount of time for someone not equipped to find an answer to try, with all best intentions, to do so. It's better to route the question to the right person (billing, Rx information, a review of chart instructions, an insurance question, etc.) or if they aren't available, say "Let me find Sally. She's best qualified to give you the thorough and accurate answer to your question."

THE POWER OF THE CALLBACK

It's painfully true that phone calls can consume large chunks of time. But carefully timed phone calls that you initiate to your patients are as powerful a patient-pleaser as you can expect to find. After a visit, for instance, calling to find out how a patient is doing—a clearly human and unexpected gesture—is an awesome differentiator among physicians and their degree of patient concern. Most patients are thunderstruck. They feel you wouldn't have taken the time if you didn't care. Ideally, the physician makes these calls, even to a few selected patients each day, and/or another staff member can extend that reach by making calls on behalf of the physician.

Around a hospital admission

When you've admitted a patient to the hospital, consider calling his or her family the first or second night to see if they have any questions. You can empathize with their apprehension around their loved one's hospital visit, and you can help to alleviate it.

And after your vacation

The callback is especially important after your vacations, at the annual golf tournament, off-hours, or in some other way off-duty—at the very time when you are probably most inundated by a backlog of appointments and pressures and catching up. While away, you had a back-up system that directed your patients to a covering physician or group. More often than not, patients don't like this situation any better than you do.

If patients identify you as their doctor, they are typically unhappy about having to see a covering physician in your absence. Some irrationally feel angry that you weren't there for them when they needed you. Others just hesitate to see a stranger, a physician they didn't choose at a time when they need a doctor and don't have the luxury of time to go doctor-shopping.

From your point of view, when your patients see a covering physician, you are inevitably being compared to that covering physician. You want to have a wonderful physician cover your patients, but if that physician is really wonderful, your patients might in some cases prefer this new person. Fact is, many patients switch doctors after seeing a covering physician that they perceive to be a cut above their own doctor.

Instead of being passive in this situation, you can make it your business practice to touch base with your patients. Probably the physicians covering for you provide you with a list of patients seen and reports on their visits. If they don't provide you with this information, make sure you ask for it.

Then, once you know which of your patients were seen by Doctor Alternative, reestablish contact with your patients by calling them, especially if notes on their condition suggest a serious problem or one that is likely to need follow-up. If you can't call everyone, have your staff help out. In these calls, let your patient know you're back, available, and concerned about how they're feeling. See if they want or need to set up a follow-up appointment with you.

It takes time, yes. But patients are impressed. They feel more secure in your hands; they stop wondering if you know about what's been happening to them. They feel personally attended to. And, in many cases, you prevent patient drain.

YOUR REPUTATION'S ON THE LINE

Your patients consider the telephone their lifeline to you. Every time your patient calls you, the reputation of you and your practice is on the line. Patients frustrated in their efforts to gain access, information and appointments consider your practice with reservations. They resent obstacles to receiving the service they feel they are more than paying for. In knowing the power of the phone, impediments to smooth phone service should become a top priority. Otherwise, you are perpetuating what seems to patients to be an insurmountable barrier to healthcare and a barrier that they will avoid by considering the practice down the street.

10

Time, Access, and Availability

Healthcare consumers care deeply about respect for their time and access to their doctors when they need it. The amount of time their doctors spend with patients, how easy it is to make an appointment, how often their doctors keep these appointments, and finally how easy it is to gain access to physicians are criteria people use to judge the responsiveness and consumer orientation of medical practices. In this chapter, we examine these sensitive, even delicate, issues by focusing on these specific areas:

- Scheduling appointments
- Managing time
- Access and availability

BEGINNING WITH APPOINTMENTS

What is a good appointment system? If you ask patients to define it, they cite three desired characteristics:

- The patient can be seen on the day desired
- The patient's waiting time is kept to a minimum
- Enough time is allotted to each patient for their particular type of visit or consultation

When designing or improving your appointment system, consider especially these three factors:

1. *Type of patient visits and how much time to allocate to each.* Different practices allocate different lengths of time for patient visits. Obviously, a general practice—which handles everything from allergy shots to full physical exams— needs a flexible scheduling system that allows for shorter and longer visits. It also requires that the person making the appointments understands these distinctions and, based on the patient's information, whether to allocate a short or long visit.

2. *Who can come when?* Different patients also find certain times of day more convenient and practical than others. Your system should encourage reserving specific times for certain groups of patients, times especially convenient to them.

- *Employed People.* Typically, people who work appreciate early morning, evening, or lunch-hour appointments. These interfere least with their work.
- *Unemployed parents of young children.* They often prefer midmorning appointments. They can handle their family responsibilities in the morning, take Billy to your office, and get him home for his nap on time.
- *Older people.* Seniors usually choose appointments between noon and 3:00 PM. They can visit you in your office while the business world is filling restaurants, then have lunch later when working people fill your office.
- *School-age children and their parents.* Kids tend to prefer appointments during school hours, but their parents usually prefer after hours appointments. It's probably best to cater to parents!

3. *When you need to be in and out of the office.* Your office hours need to allow you adequate time to see patients and to make hospital visits and consultations. You need to plan an appropriate allocation of your time to this mix of activities.

Dr. Jones, for example, sees patients in the office every day after 1 PM. and visits patients in the hospital every morning. Dr. Smith does the reverse. Dr. Brown is in surgery from 6:30 AM until 11:00 AM every Monday, Tuesday and Thursday and sees patients in the office every afternoon. Dr. White visits patients in the hospital three evenings a week. Dr. Alert visits patients in the hospital after evening hours often until 11 PM. Who is correct?

Obviously, there are no hard and fast rules. The Super Docs we consulted agree that the key is to pay attention to the needs and preferences of your patients.

ASK YOUR PATIENTS

One approach is to consult your customers. Patient questionnaires or surveys can help you determine whether your office is open at the best times for the patients *you* see.

Questionnaire items

1. What are the times you generally use our office? (list alternatives)

2. Check off below all the appointment times that are possible for you. (list alternative)

3. Which two time slots do you like best? (list alternatives)

4. Which two time slots do you most dislike? (list alternatives)

Once satisfied that your hours are the best for you and your patients, the next step is to use this time sensibly. The following (from "The Doctor's Office") is a good guide for your appointment scheduler to follow:

- Block out "reserved" emergency time and use a highlighter to indicate your emergency blocks. This lets you schedule same-day calls without disrupting your entire schedule.

- Show the doctor's out-of-office schedule in the appointment book. This lets you know the doctor's whereabouts, and helps you predict his or her arrival time more accurately.

- Block out one or more telephone callback period(s) each day, so your doctor can return calls at a convenient time. And, you can do much for patient relations by letting the patient know the approximate time the doctor will call.

- Have a good idea of how many minutes are required for each procedure. This helps you schedule the right amount of time for each patient in particular and for the practice in general.

- Write in the reason for each scheduled office visit. This lets your doctor and/or nurse prepare for the visit more appropriately. It also assures that you allow enough time for patients scheduled around that appointment.

- Write in each patient's phone number. This gives you faster access to the patient if you have to reschedule the appointment.

- To cut down on no-shows, call new patients to confirm their appointments.
- Update your patient information forms at least once a year. Phone numbers, addresses, and employers are constantly changing.
- Keep quick-reference lists of patients you have been forced to discharge from the practice because of their "difficult" behavior and whom you do not want to see unless it's an absolute emergency. You may want to keep some other lists available, also. These include patients who should be reminded that they have a balance outstanding and patients who can be seen on short notice. Of course, be sure to keep these lists confidential.
- Keep track of the total numbers of patients you see each month, plus the number of new patients you see each month. You'll be able to see how quickly your practice is growing, so you can add extra hours or make other plans to accommodate this growth.

Think about your scheduling. Is there a system to it? If so, does that system help your practice reach specific objectives? Maybe now's the time to think through a new system, and these tips could very well make that system more helpful to your practice. (*"The Doctor's Office,"* 1858 Charter Lane; Lancaster, PA 17601; ©1988 and reprinted with permission.)

Long appointments

Most people don't know how long a forthcoming appointment will take unless you tell them. Some people call at 3:00 in the afternoon and hope you'll "squeeze them in" between 4:00 and 4:15 PM, not knowing that what they need might require a long appointment. Others arrive to undergo a certain hour-long procedure at 4:00 and announce, "I hope you can get me in and out quickly because my three-year old will be standing alone on a street-corner outside of day care at 5:00."

People won't know how long they can expect to be with you unless you tell them in advance:

> Mr. Perkins, removal of that toenail takes approximately 30 minutes. Dr. Stein has a 30-minute appointment available, let's see, on March 4, from 9:00 AM to 9:30 AM. Will that time be convenient for you? Great, Mr. Perkins; then we'll see you at 9:00 on March 4th and you can expect your appointment to take 30 minutes.

If you alert patients to the length of their appointment, you save yourself time and angst later, because your patients are more likely to allocate their own time accordingly—and even be on time in the process.

OTHER CREATIVE, HIGH-PAYOFF APPROACHES TO TIME

1. Open One Hour Earlier.   Do you already open your office, or rather staff your office, at least an hour before office hours begin? Many physicians have found that it pays to do so. Although, of course, you need to pay your staff for these extra hours, the returns justify the expense.

First of all, *you'll be ready for the onslaught.* If you have a busy practice, then you're used to the day beginning with a barrage of phone calls from people who've probably been watching their watches until the start of the business day. People are concerned about something they consider urgent or they're trying to squeeze in their call to you before the start of their own work day, or they need to plan their day around their appointment time. If these calls and your patients arrive at the same time, havoc can ensue. Your staff can go crazy and your patients, many of whom have already had their answering machine messages seemingly ignored, are feeling impatient, even demanding. If you're staffed to handle the first onslaught in a calm manner, that onslaught slows down and your staff can handle ensuing calls with more thoroughness and finesse as your first patients begin to arrive.

Another advantage of staffing before appointments begin is *the marketing advantage.* Many practices will not open early. So, if you do, you have the advantage of giving people better access to your office and prompter service than other practices provide. And you can publicize this extra convenience in your Patient Information Brochure, practice promotions, and newsletter if you have one.

> We offer you early morning access! Every day, we begin answering your calls an hour before our practice sees its first patient. And, our own staff answer the phone, not an answering service! That's because we know you want your questions answered before you have to face your own busy day.

2. Open Time.   Many offices like to keep certain times open every day or every other day for walk-ins and call-ins. There is a growing tendency for patients to expect this practice. This may be due to the increase in walk-in centers, or Docs in the Box. If you don't have this type of option, you may be losing business to convenience centers. Many patients with established relationships with an office-based doctor are choosing or feel forced to go to a convenience center because:

- Their doctors were too busy to see them
- The patient didn't want to wait as long as they would have to at their regular doctor's office.

If you can't offer your patients convenience, someone else will. By maintaining certain open hours, you have the flexibility to accommodate people who have unanticipated needs for attention and service.

3. Flexibility for Short Appointments.   How about the "quickie" appointment? Do patients really need appointments for allergy shots, doctor's notes, etc., and worse, can these patients be kept waiting hours for a one-minute need?   The creative, consumer-oriented practice develops creative approaches to these types of situations. Some offices have regular times when they take quickie needs on a first come, first served basis. For instance, 7–7:30 AM, 11 AM to 12 PM, 4:30 to 5:00 PM are set aside for visits that do not involve the doctor but take up staff time. Others set a time limit and fit you in with a fixed number of these quickies per hour. Four to six quickie visits can then be accommodated each hour, and each person will wait no more than five or ten minutes. The key here is for the patient to know your system—why you've created this system and that you have the patient's best interest in mind.

REMEMBER THE GOOD OL' DAYS

It wasn't that long ago that many doctors had "open" office hours. Patients would just show up for shots, exams, and medications. They knew what to expect, including long waits, since patients were generally taken on a first-come basis and long waits were expected. The move toward a "system" for scheduling was sparked by a desire to increase efficiency and decrease waiting time. The promise of a "time" when you could see the doctor consequently raised expectations and led to unprecedented patient frustration since their expectations were violated.

It is interesting to note the popularity, however, of the MediQuik, Doc in the Box operations that promise and deliver access to a doctor when you need one. It raises the question of what patients want most. In reviewing your scheduling system, make sure you've included some slack in your rope for accommodating at least some emergencies and "Service now!" patients.

ACCESSIBILITY

A clear scheduling system mutually beneficial for the doctor and the patient will certainly improve patient satisfaction. But scheduling appointments is only half the battle. The other half has to do with the patient's need to gain access to the physician for questions, concerns, and information—by phone. Although this subject sends shivers down the spines of most doctors, it is possible, with careful planning and patient education, to create ways that afford ease for the patients and protection for the physician.

What do patients need?

- An understanding of when the best times are to reach the doctor by phone for nonemergency concerns
- An understanding of how to reach the doctor for real emergencies
- An understanding of what constitutes an emergency

Access for nonemergency phone calls

By educating the patient, you can avoid premature phone calls. For instance, some patients call for test results before the results are ready. Then, they call again. You should be careful to tell patients when their results will be ready and whom to ask for when they call. Otherwise, they might call often and ask for you unnecessarily.

> Your test results will be back on Tuesday. I suggest that you call on Tuesday afternoon for the results. If the test comes back negative, I will not need to speak to you. If it is positive, my secretary will be instructed to make an appointment.

The point here is to let the patient know, when leaving the office, what to do next, whom to call for results, and what your next steps will be.

Progress reports

"Take two aspirins and call me in the morning" could mean many things. Does it mean, "Call me personally" or "Call to make an appointment"? These instructions are still unclear and incomplete, even if you mean "Call and ask to speak with me during office hours tomorrow." So, give direct, complete instructions:

> 1. "Call me between 9–10 AM and ask to speak with me. If I'm not available, I will call you back."
>
> 2. "Call the office and let my secretary know how you are so it can go on your record. If your fever doesn't go down, I want to see you right away, and it will be fine for you to drop in without an appointment."

Emergency calls

In many cases, patients will either underestimate or overestimate the seriousness of a condition unless you clarify it for them. It helps to spell out the following:

1. What is "normal" and needs no follow-up
2. What is "not normal" and should trigger a call to the doctor during (or, if necessary, after) office hours.
3. What is an emergency case that warrants immediate notification of the doctor.

Most patients want to know that their doctor is there for them, available to help them when they need it. Most patients don't *like* to call their physicians at 4 AM, but often they don't know what to look for or when to be alarmed enough to make that intimidating call.

Here's an example. A young mother took her baby, who had a high fever, to see the pediatrician. Medication was prescribed and the doctor said, "Call me in a few days to let me know how the baby is doing." Mom called late that night, in a panic, when the fever was still high. Had the physician said, "Often young children get higher fevers and keep them longer than adults. The baby's fever might not break tonight, and may, in fact, still be high for several days. Here's what to do . . . . And, here's what I want to know about right away. . . ."

Screening calls

Most doctors rely on an answering service to screen emergency calls. These services can be a curse or a blessing depending on how competent they are. The key is to let these services know exactly what you need to know and what they should ask the callers.

One physician we interviewed gives her beeper number to patients, in addition to giving them her office and answering service numbers. This sounds extreme, but her rationale is that if she is clear about how and when to use the beeper, it makes her patients feel so secure that they are *less* likely to call her. In fact, she reports that very few patients actually use the beeper. Most call the office or service. And the few patients who do use the beeper do so appropriately. In other words, when people feel that they have access, they are less nervous and panicky and less likely to make the call, because they know that if things get worse, they can always call.

WAITING

The Keckley Report (Paul Keckley, Nashville, TN; May 18, 1987), reports a study in which, when patients were asked, "What do you most dislike about visiting your doctor?" the largest percentage (49 percent) of the respondents answered, "The office wait."

Healthcare Marketing Trends (Delphi Forecasts, Nashville, TN, January 12, 1987) says that, according to patients, 15 minutes is the longest acceptable time to be kept waiting. If the wait is expected to be longer, patients want an explanation. If the wait is to be very long—more than 30 minutes—patients would like the option of rescheduling the appointment.

Handling waits

Unfortunately, there will still be the inevitable wait, even if you employ the most creative and flexible scheduling system. The key is what to do about them. At times like these, extending goodwill to anxious patients can pay big dividends in return visits and patient loyalty. Here are a few thoughts to share with your staff to help promote empathy and responsiveness around delays, and to help patients wait patiently.

- If the caregiver is detained, explain the reason simply and briefly, and tell the waiting patients approximately how long the wait will be.
- Be sure patients are as comfortable as possible during this time.
- If the wait will be considerably longer, give the patients the option to go out and run a few small errands without losing their place in line.
- Arrange with a local delicatessen, ice cream parlor or hospital coffee shop to provide coupons for patients to have a small snack while they're waiting.
- A delay on the part of the caregiver may mean patients will be late for other appointments and meetings. Make a telephone available to patients to let others know they're running late.
- Remind the caregiver how long a patient has been waiting, so the caregiver can apologize and offer an explanation.
- A written note of apology for a long wait—or a 10 percent to 25 percent discount on the bill—will go a long way toward establishing goodwill; it identifies the organization as time-conscientious and its people as considerate and respectful of patients' time.
- Time is valuable not only to healthcare professionals but to patients as well. It's good practice to help patients focus on your consideration and thoughtfulness rather than on the length of time they're being kept waiting.

The waiting environment

In Chapter 6 on the environment, you'll find suggestions about waiting room ambience and amenities that help alleviate the discomfort of waiting. The more you can help people pass the time quickly, the shorter every tedious minute feels. Some offices have children's play areas, jigsaw puzzles, personal computers, hand-puzzles, drawing materials, up-to-date and offbeat magazines, and more.

Draw attention to time or away from it

Some doctors have eliminated clocks from the waiting rooms so patients won't be so clock conscious. Does this help? We think not much. It's better to work on eliminating, easing and explaining waits rather than ignore them or hope the patient won't realize the time.

Patient perceptions of time with the doctor

"My doctor doesn't spend time with me," or "My doctor appears to be in a rush," or "I never get the kind of answers I want from the doctor." These are all comments from patients. Where does this come from? Patients' perceptions of how much actual time the doctor spent with them is colored by many things.

1. *Friendliness.* Does the physician appear relaxed, concerned? Is there eye contact sustained?

2. *Questions asked.* Does the physician enable me to ask the questions I want to ask?

3. *Questions answered.* Do I get the answers I need and want?

4. Once in an exam room, how much time do I wait to see the doctor?

5. Does the doctor show a desire to get rid of me (by putting hand on door knob, looking at watch, etc.)?

If two doctors each spend ten minutes with a patient and one of these doctors, from the patient's point of view, appears helpful and friendly, and the other curt and disinterested, the patient *actually* perceives the caring doctor as having *spent more time* with him or her. This suggests the need to focus on *quality time*, not just an increase in *time spent* with patients. Actual time may have little or no relationship with patients' perceptions.

A CREATIVE ALTERNATIVE INVOLVING COORDINATED USE OF STAFF

A *very* busy orthopod maximizes the amount of time spent with patients by utilizing other staff and office systems. This high-volume office schedules ten minutes with the physician per patient, yet the patient is in the office and seen by staff for at least 20 to 30 minutes. The patient is first seen by a physician's assistant who asks pertinent questions and fills in questions on the chart. The physician's assistant escorts the patient to the exam room and lets the patient know what to expect from the rest of the visit. The physician reviews the chart briefly and then examines or speaks with the patient. The physician outlines the treatment plan and answers questions. The physician's assistant returns to the patient once again to go over the treatment plan, medications and answer any follow-up questions.

This approach may seem like an assembly line—very structured and impersonal. Actually, patients feel that it is thorough and highly professional.

In conclusion, patients cannot be left stranded. Often five or ten minutes is just not enough time, and the alternative may be to employ other personnel to spend *additional* time with patients.

But what if the patient needs *me?*

Some doctors have stated that they suggest an additional appointment for further discussion or ask the patient to wait in the office for a bit until they can see clear to taking a larger, uninterrupted period of time.

Other alternatives

Focus on One Problem at a Time.   Some physicians do feel under pressure to solve every problem that a patient brings up. This can only lead to frustration on both parties, and a better alternative is to try to focus the patient and give "quality time" toward one problem.

Questions like, "What would you like help with today" may direct the patient. Sometimes, you may need to be clearer: "I don't think we can cover everything in this one visit." Often, you may need to separate the major issue for the patient. "I'm concerned with _____ problem right now. I'd like to spend time talking about what to do with that. We can, at another time, talk about some of your other concerns."

First Time Patients.   Many doctors like to spend up to one hour with a first-time patient, knowing that this investment in the beginning will pay off in many ways in the future. Therefore, they like to schedule a finite number of these visits during each week. It also helps to schedule these appointments before lunch or toward the end of the day so other patients aren't kept waiting. This schedule also allows doctors to focus on that particular patient.

FROM THE DOCTOR'S POINT OF VIEW

Generally, physicians view the issue of time as a problem. Physicians feel that:

1. There are not enough hours in the day to do it all well.

2. They are pressured to see a high volume of patients to support the practice, which means less time per patient visit.

3. Patients' expectations of them have become unreasonable regarding time.

4. Visiting patients in the hospital is becoming more difficult and time-consuming.

5. More emphasis needs to be placed on making things easier for the doctor, since ease-of-practice ends up helping patients.

IT'S ALL IN YOUR EXPECTATION!

It is curious that two offices can have similar systems and experiences and yet get very different results and feedback from patients. Part of this is due to the discrepancy between our expectations and our experience. When the experience matches our expectations, good or bad, we seem to have a higher degree of satisfaction. So, it seems that, in addition to raising satisfaction by improving systems and practices, we should also be meticulous about letting our patients know what to expect—especially regarding time.

Questions to consider

In your office:

- How easy is it to get an appointment?
- How convenient are your office hours for your patients?
- How long do patients generally have to wait?
- Is the environment pleasant so people don't mind a short wait?
- Do you explain waits when they occur?
- Do you offer alternatives?
- Do patients appear satisfied with the length of their appointments?
- Do patients know how to reach the physicians?

Time is a sore spot for people. People draw conclusions about you based on their perceptions of your respect for them. And they draw conclusions about your generalized respect for them as a person based on your treatment of their time. If you haven't yet received a bill from a busy attorney for $125/hour of waiting in your office, you probably will.

Knowing people's sensitivity to time issues and knowing how much respect for the patient's time means respect for the person, energy and expense channeled into more effective time management pays off in patient satisfaction and patient loyalty.

III
Managing Staff for Patient Satisfaction

If you ask patients, they're quick to point out the powerful impact of your staff's behavior on their perceptions of your practice. Rude words, a few extra minutes of neglect, raised eyebrows when a patient asks a question, all repel people from your practice. On the other side, a few extra words of concern, calling people by name, apologizing for an uncomfortable wait, patience in the face of a string of questions and confusion about billing all make patients feel you and your employees care. And they don't think you take them for granted. Patients expect and deserve courtesy, care, attention and concern in their interactions with physicians and staff. Dissatisfaction with staff behavior turns patients and their families away, hurting the ability of your practice to attract and retain patients. Given the increasing competition for patients, many physicians are instituting programs to assure that their practices are consistently positive in the most important aspect of assuring patient loyalty ... employee interactions with patients.

YOU SET THE STANDARDS FOR STAFF BEHAVIOR

No matter how small or large your staff, you can enhance your practice by devoting explicit attention to building among your staff a strong service philosophy, establishing clear expectations for staff behavior, holding people accountable, and providing support, encouragement and reward for performance that pleases patients.

The challenge is to create a "service culture"—a climate and way of doing things that screams to patients, "We care about you as a person; we respect you and your time; and we do all we can to act in your best interests."

This section is designed to help you examine your current "culture" among staff and bolster your management practices so that your staff are powerful patient-pleasers.

11

How To Build a Patient-Oriented Culture

Staff behavior can be elusive. After all, you're busy doctoring and your staff are (or should be) busy supporting your efforts. It is frankly impossible to witness or police interactions between employees and patients (see Figure 11–1).

In this chapter, we identify the essential components in a successful strategy to achieve excellence among your staff in the human ingredient of your practice.

"SYSTEMS" APPROACH NEEDED

> For every complex problem, there's a simple solution, and it's wrong. (H.L. Mencken)

For your staff to feel and act truly service-oriented, you need a "systems approach," not just training. A systems approach is in contrast to a "training" approach. Some medical practices want improved staff behavior toward patients, so they institute a training program that focuses on refining the staff's "customer

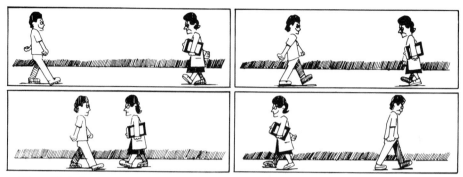

Figure 11–1. Cartoon from *Guest Relations in Practice.*

relations" skills. But, usually, training alone does not move staff toward excellent interactions with patients on service dimensions.

Example: In one practice, the front-desk receptionist was reported to be unfriendly and curt with patients. The physician sent her to a training program on customer relations skills. Upon her return to work, motivated by the training she received, she sat down in the waiting room for a few minutes to comfort an elderly patient. The physician entered the scene and asked her to step back into his office for a moment. He then confronted her for being away from her desk and "making chit-chit" with patients when she was supposed to be working. The receptionist was upset, because she had been inspired by her foray into customer relations training to pay special attention to patients who seemed particularly distraught, to take a bit of extra time to comfort them and make the kind of attentive small talk that eases anxiety. Full of energy for reaching out to this patient, the receptionist had later been berated by the very same physician who had paid her way to customer relations school. His grounds: that her behavior interfered with her and his office's productivity.

Most people know how to be wonderful to other people if they bring the best of what they know and apply it at work. But if they do that and their behavior is discouraged, they stop doing it.

This means that step one involves getting clear on what you really want from your receptionist and other staff and instituting policies, strategies, expectations, rewards, and opportunities—all with the goal of raising standards of employee behavior to the level of excellence, and holding people accountable to those standards.

Literally every component of your practice that shapes employee behavior needs to be examined and, where necessary, modified to achieve, sustain, and support excellent staff behavior toward your patients.

The practice manager or physician who wants to improve staff behavior toward patients must take a fresh look at your practice's policies and procedures that influence employee behavior toward your patients, and make sure that these policies and procedures support, and do not impede, patient satisfaction.

The challenge: to align or adjust your practice so that all forces that shape employee behavior push for staff behavior consistent with your patient satisfaction objectives. These forces we call the Six Pillars of Staff Behavior, because they must be strong to support patient satisfaction:

1. Your practice philosophy and power as role model
2. Clear expectations and accountability, including job descriptions, performance appraisal, feedback and discipline
3. Hiring and new employee orientation
4. Training and development on key interpersonal skills
5. Reward and recognition
6. Employee involvement and employee as customer

Strategically, you can enhance your practice by determining the degree to which these six pillars are in place, and then taking action as needed so that you establish standards, support, reward, and hold staff accountable for the behavior that gratifies patients.

THE ROLE OF THE "MANAGEMENT"

Clearly, to pursue the model presented, you need active, deliberate practice management and a person or two who take responsibility for spearheading your effort to create a patient-oriented, service culture. The most likely people to adopt this leadership role are the managing physician or an office manager, who need to build the pillars that support excellent behavior on the part of staff. To manage staff to achieve enduring patient satisfaction, key responsibilities include:

- Be first and foremost a role model.
- Hire service-oriented people with polished interpersonal and communication skills.
- Orient new staff to the philosophy and expectations that support excellent customer relations.
- Set and communicate clear behavioral expectations to staff.
- Train staff in skills needed to meet expectations, or find people who can.
- Uphold high standards by monitoring performance and confronting, disciplining, and terminating when necessary.

- Recognize and reward excellent behavior that satisfies patients; make examples of exemplary people.
- Hold staff meetings that refresh awareness of the importance of staff in achieving patient satisfaction and explore new ways people can heighten their effectiveness.
- Engage staff ideas and energy in solving problems that impede patient satisfaction; invite staff involvement in making the practice one they're proud of.
- Solve systems problems and make procedural decisions that enable staff to work efficiently and gain satisfaction from the job.

In short, managing for patient satisfaction is a multifaceted job and requires dedicated attention.

AUDIT YOUR STAFF MANAGEMENT PRACTICES

If you want to audit your current practices regarding staff behavior and identify practices that need strengthening, try this audit. Have at least two people from your practice complete it and compare responses:

Staff Management Audit

As long as your practice has patients and employees, it has an ongoing need for attention to patient satisfaction and an ongoing need to build, maintain, expand, trouble-shoot, and improve your practice enhancement strategy.

This audit helps you diagnose strengths and weaknesses in your efforts to manage staff for optimal patient satisfaction and suggests alternative directions for practice enhancement.

Directions

Think about your practice. Consider each statement on this survey and check *true* or *false* for each as it applies to your practice. *Answer all questions*—force yourself to choose the best answer, even if you prefer a middle-of-the-road answer.

	True	False
A. SUCCESS SIGNS		
1. Patients hardly every complain about employee attitudes and behavior.		
2. Our practice's atmosphere is generally seen as very friendly.		
3. Physicians are generally satisfied with the co-operation they get from staff.		

	True	False

4. Physicians are generally satisfied with staff behavior toward their patients.

5. Our employees speak positively about our practice to outsiders.

6. Staff generally see our physicians as hospitable toward them.

7. Our physicians are generally seen as hospitable toward patients and their companions.

8. If someone accompanies a patient to our practice, our employees typically help these friends and family get as comfortable as possible.

9. Our employees are friendly toward patients and their family and friends in hallways and waiting areas.

10. Our practice has a reputation in the community for being a friendly place.

11. Generally, we have a spirit of team work and cooperation among our employees.

12. Our organization is not faced with much competition.

A.   TOTAL # TRUE

B.   *AWARENESS HIGH?*

1. Most of our employees can explain the importance of patient satisfaction to our practice's health and to their own job security.

2. Most of our employees can explain the importance of *physician* satisfaction to our practice's health and to their own job security.

3. Most of our employees can explain the importance of coworker cooperation to our practice's health and to their own job security.

4. Our employees at all levels are generally aware of the new economic challenges that practices like ours face and strategies for tackling these challenges.

5. Our employees are generally aware of their importance in attracting and retaining patients.

6. In our written materials, our high priority on patient satisfaction is stated and restated . . . to

True | False

reinforce its importance in our practice.

7. We circulate written materials that feature patient relations concerns, events, and accomplishments.

8. Our management frequently refers to patient satisfaction as the driving force in our organization.

9. We have systems for updating our employees on the economic challenges ahead for our practice, so they know how we're doing and what we're doing to succeed.

B. TOTAL # TRUE

C. *ARE STAFF HELD ACCOUNTABLE?*

1. Courteous, respectful, and compassionate behavior toward patients and their companions is a *requirement* in our practice, not an option.

2. For our employees, we've instituted clear, written behavioral expectations that describe customer relations behavior in specific terms.

3. Managers and supervisors hold employees accountable for their behavior toward our patients and companions, confronting problem employees when such employees darken our practice's image.

4. In our practice, we are encouraged to coach, discipline and eventually terminate employees who persist in their failure to meet high patient relations standards.

5. Generally, our management shows courtesy, friendliness and a caring attitude toward patients and their companions.

6. Management here is/are under pressure to be role models of positive behavior toward our patients and one another.

7. The atmosphere in this practice makes it impossible any longer for rude and belligerent employees to remain secure and accepted year after year.

8. Our management has established and communi-

		True	False

cated clear, *job-specific* expectations to staff.

9. Our management has communicated clear expectations to staff they supervise.
10. Specific patient relations responsibilities are built into job descriptions.
11. Our hiring practices include specific techniques for screening applicants for interpersonal instincts and skills.
12. Patient satisfaction behavior has a prominent place in our performance appraisal process.
13. Employees who show excellent patient relations receive appreciation and praise for their efforts.
14. The quality of one's behavior toward our patients affects employee pay increases.
15. Our New Employee Orientation emphasizes the importance we place on patient satisfaction and communicates the specific behavior expected of every employee to achieve this satisfaction.
16. Our practice has systems for recognizing employees who are wonderful to patients.
17. The quality of one's behavior toward our patients affects promotions.
18. Employees can't take out their frustrations on each other here without being confronted.

C.   TOTAL # TRUE

D. *DO YOU HAVE SYSTEMS FOR EVALUATION, PROBLEM-SOLVING AND COMMUNICATION?*

1. We have systems in place to assess patient satisfaction with our staff and services.
2. We have strategies in place to tap physician satisfaction with our staff and services.
3. Generally, our staff welcome and invite patient complaints, since complaints give us a chance to show our concern and responsiveness.
4. Generally, people here are apologetic and concerned when patients are not satisfied; staff bends over backwards to resolve complaints.
5. When patients have a complaint or concern,

	True	False

they know who to contact.

6. We have a clear system for following up on patient complaints and requests.
7. When employees have complaints or suggestions, they know specific channels for expressing them.
8. Our management generally responds to employee concerns, even if they don't solve them.
9. Our management is generally perceived as open to employee complaints and suggestions.

D.   TOTAL # TRUE

E.   *ARE SYSTEMS AND AMENITIES COMFORTING, EASY-TO-USE AND CONVENIENT?*

1. We examine our systems periodically to see if we can make them more "user-friendly."
2. Generally, evaluations of cleanliness are positive in our practice.
3. Generally, people can get from place to place in our practice without getting too frustrated or confused.
4. Generally, the registration process runs smoothly without long waits.
5. Generally, a patient's experience here runs smoothly without undue confusion or long waits.
6. Our employees generally are tolerant of problems in our organization because they're aware of management's commitment to making things run smoothly.
7. Generally, systems in our organization work smoothly enough that employees don't have to apologize endlessly for problems and breakdowns.
8. We periodically examine those services with the greatest effect on patient satisfaction, to see if we can improve them.
9. We look at the amenities or extras we offer pe-

	True	False

riodically to see if we can increase patient comfort and satisfaction.

E.   TOTAL # TRUE

F.   *DO YOU HAVE SYSTEMS FOR IMPROVING EMPLOYEE SKILLS?*
1. Our practice offers or subsidizes attendance at training programs periodically to upgrade the patient relations skills of employees.
2. We train our people in telephone skills.
3. We offer or subsidize attendance at training in handling complaints, so that complaints are seen as giving us another chance to satisfy our patients.
4. We offer or subsidize attendance at professional renewal programs to help our staff and others handle the stress, pressure and burnout felt by many these days.
5. We have strategies for team-building, so that problems within our staff are not ignored.
6. We have a method for identifying individuals with mediocre skills and developing training that upgrades their skills.

F.   TOTAL # TRUE

G.   *ARE YOUR PHYSICIANS INVOLVED?*
   (for larger practices)
1. Physicians are aware of our practice's priority on patient satisfaction.
2. Physicians see themselves as an important part of our practice enhancement strategy.
3. We've made physicians aware of the specific behaviors that satisfy patients.
4. When a physician violates our patient relations standards, that physician is confronted in a constructive way.
5. When doctors have a complaint, they know who to contact.
6. We have a clear system for responding to physi

	True	False
cian complaints and needs.		
G. TOTAL # TRUE		

How To Score

1. Make sure you respond to every item.
2. For each section, count the number of *True* answers and write the total at the end of that section.
3. Now, transfer the totals for each section to the column below that reads *Total*.

	Section	Total	×	Factor	=	Score 0 to 36
Success Signs	A		×	3	=	
Awareness	B		×	4	=	
Accountability	C		×	2	=	
Systems for Evaluation, Problem-solving, and Communication	D		×	4	=	
Systems and Amenities	E		×	4	=	
Skill Development Strategies	F		×	6	=	
Physician Involvement	G		×	6	=	

4. Now multiply each *total* above by the factor next to it, and write the answer in the box in the score column.

How To Interpret Your Score

The highest score possible for each category is 36. Higher numbers are positive. Lower numbers reflect problem areas that interfere with customer satisfaction. To learn from these, go back and analyze the items that deflated your score, since these reveal promising directions for action.

A. *Success Signs*: This score reveals how successful your practice already is in achieving customer satisfaction. Practices with higher scores here should feel accomplished! In the future, the challenge to you is to maintain and even strengthen your successes.

B. *Awareness:* The lower the score, the more you need to consider strategies for raising employee awareness of patient needs and expectations, what your practice stands to gain from excellence and what every employee can do (and must do) to help.

C. *Accountability:* Do your staff behavior standards have "teeth"? Lower scores here indicate a weak foundation. Employees might know all about the value your practice places on patient satisfaction, but without accountability mechanisms, you can't expect lasting results.

D. *Systems for Evaluation, Problem-solving and Communication:* To sustain employee motivation and energy for practice enhancement, your practice has to have underlying systems for *ongoing* evaluation, problem-solving, and communication. Otherwise, employees get disillusioned and frustrated. Lower scores here need to be taken very seriously, since they indicate an undercurrent of employee feelings that interfere with people's ability to extend themselves to patients and coworkers.

E. *Systems and Amenities:* People skills aren't enough! Employees can only apologize so many times for patient discomfort, inconvenience, and cumbersome systems. Lower scores in this area suggest that systems problems and insufficient amenities or extras for your patients interfere with your achieving high levels of patient satisfaction.

F. *Skill Development Strategies:* The interpersonal skills among staff that impress patients are not easy. It's not hard to be good, but it's hard to be excellent, to impress your patients with your compassionate, responsive and respectful treatment. This takes skill! Lower scores in this area suggest the need for skill-building programs and other employee development strategies.

G. *Physician Involvement:* If physicians are not involved in your practice enhancement strategy, then your employees are probably angry! Also, physicians are caregivers and part of the team, so how can you exempt them?! Lower scores in this area indicate a need to develop or strengthen physician involvement.

This inventory suggests possible directions that your practice might pursue. In the following chapters, we will present nut-and-bolt strategies for building on your practice's identified strengths and bolstering weaknesses so that your staff do all they can to satisfy and even impress patients.

CONCLUSION

The pillars that support effective staff behavior can serve as a checklist of specifications for the design or improvement of your approach or as an analytical device for identifying gaps in your current practices.

Achieving excellence in staff behavior toward patients calls for a long-term and substantial commitment. Your practice should not allow its commitment to fade, nor should it slacken in its strategic efforts to bring about continued improvements. In short, this requires dedicated management. You need to manage staff in a way that creates a service-oriented culture where everyone strives to meet patient needs in an environment of mutual support.

12

Your Practice Philosophy and Power as Role Model

- Do you have a practice philosophy that your staff can explain?
- Does your philosophy make a patient orientation and service commitment priority one?
- Do you exemplify behavior that, if your staff emulated YOU, would impress your patients?
- Do you tell your staff periodically the values and goals you hold dear for your practice?

The more *yes* answers, the better.

The leaders of your practice (physicians and any managers you might have) need to communicate a serious commitment to top-notch patient satisfaction. The manager(s) of your practice, including all the physicians involved, need to make a serious commitment to achieving high standards of staff behavior toward patients. Double standards breed resentment and resistance among employees. Your commitment needs to spell out that *everyone* in the practice, not just the lower-paid staff, are expected to conform to the highest standards of behavior, so that the practice is successful and generates a deserved superior reputation in the community.

You can lay the groundwork for this by establishing an explicit and clear practice philosophy that you communicate, reiterate, and exemplify to your staff. Then, you can make it real by practicing this philosophy in your own behavior.

A PRACTICE PHILOSOPHY

Big corporations make their mission and values public—to the external public and to their staff. They call staff attention to it repeatedly and often. Their reasoning: if employees know where you're heading, they're much more likely to act in ways that help you get there. Without clear knowledge of what you're in business for and what your values are, employees do their own thing.

Just because your practice might be a tad smaller than these companies, it doesn't mean you can't benefit similarly by thinking through and making explicit a philosophy that states in no uncertain terms what you believe in and want to achieve in *your* business.

Here's an example from Kaiser Permanente Medical Center in Santa Clara, California, a medical center with an enormous amount of ambulatory activity and a high priority on service values.

Service Matters

Our Promise to You, Our Health Plan Members
In every encounter, with every person, in every part of our organization, you will experience:
- *Confidence* in the quality of care you receive.
- *Caring*, courteous, and prompt service in your interactions with our physicians and staff members.
- *Convenience* as you use our system.
- *Choice* of your personal physician.
- *Confidentiality* and respect for your medical information and condition.

Thomas R. Seifert   Christopher Chow, M.D.
Medical Center Administrator   Physician-in-Chief

And here's the philosophy statement from one small medical practice:

We exist to provide top-notch, state-of-the art medical care in an atmosphere of caring, compassion, patience and attention to our patients as people. We know this is only possible by providing an atmosphere for our staff that helps them be productive and satisfied in their work.

If you don't have a practice philosophy, consider developing one. It helps to start by interviewing your staff about what they "think" it is. By finding that out, you can more easily clarify what you need to think through and make clear.

Ask yourself, What is your practice philosophy?

- Why are you in medicine?
- What values do you want to motivate your staff's behavior?

Now, put this in words and try it out on your colleagues. Ask:

- How does this make you feel about our practice?
- What do you like and what don't you like?
- What would you add if you were the exclusive owner of this practice?

After you collect this information, draft your practice philosophy and make it public. Post it in your waiting area, announce it at a staff meeting, and give it to each staff member on a reminder card.

CREDIBILITY BY EXAMPLE

A policy that reflects your service commitment is a start, but the leaders in your practice must make it credible by example. If you tell your staff that you want them to act in ways that make patients feel special, but then you yourself don't, you have installed a double standard. And double standards breed resentment and resistance among employees. Your commitment needs to spell out that *everyone* in the practice, not just the lower-paid staff, are expected to conform to the highest standards of behavior, so that the practice is successful and generates a deserved superior reputation in the community.

13

Clear Expectations and Staff Accountability

- Does your practice make it clear what behavior on the part of all staff is needed to satisfy patients?

- Do your employees have job descriptions that spell out customer relations expectations?

- When you hire new people, do you screen for interpersonal communication skills and demeanor in addition to technical skills?

- Do you orient new people to the value your practice places on excellent customer relations and the behavior you expect of them in their particular position?

- Do you have a performance appraisal process that you use regularly and meaningfully as a way to shape employee performance?

- Do those who supervise staff give feedback about "service" behavior regularly?

- Do those who supervise staff coach and counsel employees who are not exemplary in terms of customer relations?

- Do you take interpersonal behavior and courtesy so seriously that you are willing to fire people who don't get high marks in the eyes of patients?

- Have you seen to it that there is no one on your staff who is notoriously annoying to patients or co-workers?

- If we asked your patients, would they say that you manage your staff in a way that makes excellent customer relations an ineluctable job requirement?

The more *yes* answers, the better.

A global statement of policy and commitment to patient satisfaction is an essential beginning. But you also need to establish clear expectations for staff behavior, so each person does not define appropriate behavior in their own ways, but instead, in ways that you define as "excellent." Some people might be wonderful in their behavior toward patients—instinctively. But if you have staff members who are not, then you have to get specific. Then, after setting standards, you have to hold people accountable, putting "teeth" into your expectations so that people fulfill them.

It isn't enough to emphasize the need for a good attitude, because attitude is elusive. You've undoubtedly seen a frontline staff member in a service business who moves maddeningly slowly, sighs when you ask for something, and rolls his or her eyes in annoyance. Behavior like that tends to enrage the customer. However, when a person who behaves like that is confronted by a supervisor with the words, "I want to talk with you about your attitude problem," the worker typically gets defensive and disagrees vehemently that an attitude problem exists, especially if he or she did fulfill the customer's request. Attitude is elusive. The effective supervisor has to describe the problematic behavior and its consequences *and* describe the behavior desired instead of the behavior exhibited.

This means you have to decide what behaviors will satisfy your patients. Then, you have to define those behaviors as key elements in each person's job.

You can build behavioral expectations into people's jobs using standard personnel management tools, including codes of conduct and job descriptions. Then, you can hold people accountable to these standards using performance appraisal, feedback, and discipline.

CREATING A BEHAVIORAL CODE OF CONDUCT

Customer service training programs often emphasize behaviors that seem trite and insulting to employees, such as smiling and being courteous and kind. To go beyond these euphemisms, you need to delineate explicitly the behaviors expected of staff. In our work with medical practices, we recommend development of "House Rules" that apply to everyone in the practice.

Since most people would rather prevent employee behavior problems than have to confront employees who've demonstrated them, it pays to describe *in advance* what you expect of staff in behavioral terms. You prevent many behavioral problems, and, if you do have a problem with a staff member later, you can refer back to the clear "rules" in operation.

Here's an example of House Rules (developed by The Einstein Consulting Group) used by many medical practices as a baseline set of staff expectations relating to interpersonal communication and courtesy.

House Rules

1. *Welcome warmly.* First impressions last. Make eye contact. Extend a warm welcome. Introduce yourself. Call people by name.
2. *Put people at ease.* Reach out with friendly words and gestures. Extend a few words of concern. Convey confidence. This is what people remember.
3. *Keep people informed.* Tell people what to expect. Invite questions. Check back. Apologize for delays. People will be calmer and grateful.
4. *Anticipate.* You'll often know what people need before they have to ask. Don't wait. Act first.
5. *Respond quickly.* When people are worried and waiting, every minute is an hour.
6. *Privacy and confidentiality.* Watch what you say and where you say it. Protect a person's rights.
7. *Dignity.* That person could be your child, your relative, your friend. Give choices. Cover up. Knock as you enter. See the *person*.
8. *Take initiative.* Just because it's not your job doesn't mean you can't help or find someone who can.
9. *Treat patients as adults.* Your words and tone should not insult.
10. *Keep it quiet.* Noise disturbs when people are anxious. Remember where you are. Show consideration. Remind each other. Keep it professional.
11. *Listen.* When people complain, don't be defensive. Hear them out. Show understanding. Give alternatives. Do all you can.
12. *Help each other*, and you help a patient.
13. *Take care on the phone.* Our reputation's on the line. Sound pleasant. Listen with understanding. Help.
14. *Professional Image.* You're part of a long, proud healthcare tradition. Look the part.
(The Einstein Consulting Group, York and Tabor Roads, Philadelphia, PA 19141; ©1986 and reprinted with permission.)

You can develop House Rules like these in a meeting with your staff, or present these to your staff in the context of a discussion of your service-oriented practice philosophy and the value you place on patient satisfaction.

Job-specific expectations

In addition to generic House Rules that apply to everyone (including you), you also need to get specific with staff about the service aspects of their particular job. The generic House Rules don't go far enough.

For instance, consider the person who handles the phone. There are obviously specific behaviors that matter to patients when they call. That staff member who handles the phone should have a clear definition of the behaviors that constitute excellent phone behavior. For instance:

- Answer within three rings.
- Have a smile in your voice when you say "hello."
- Identify yourself with, "Good morning, Barker Orthopedics, Mary Perkins speaking, may I help you?"
- When you leave a caller to find out something, put phone on "hold."
- Thank people for waiting after they've been on hold.
- Take complete messages.
- And so on.

The nurse has a different set of expectations, because the nurse's job is different. The same applies for every other position in your practice.

The fact is, the more specific you can get about what constitutes excellent behavior, the more likely you are to see it *without* having to intervene. And if you have a problem and must intervene, because you have a clear description of expected behavior that the employee was aware of, the employee is very quick to run out of excuses when confronted.

"Teeth" and Accountability.   Once you have issued explicit behavioral expectations, the people with supervisory responsibility in your practice need to hold employees accountable by appraising employee performance at least annually in a formal way and, on an ongoing basis, providing the monitoring, coaching, feedback, and counseling required to ensure conformity to expectations.

PERFORMANCE APPRAISAL

Do you have a formal performance appraisal process? The best performance appraisal process involves a rich, careful, two-way discussion of the employee's performance in relationship to each item on that employee's job description.

Some practices have a quantitative performance appraisal process in which the supervisor rates the employee on key job dimensions on a scale from 1 to 10 (10 reflecting excellence). If you use a quantitative approach, you need still to provide discussion and comments. The "grading" of adult behavior isn't sufficient to reinforce positive behavior and eliminate negative behavior. You need to get specific about the behaviors you liked and didn't, and discuss these with the employee.

In the Semi-Annual Performance Appraisal shown in Table 13–1, you'll find an example of a combination quantitative and qualitative performance appraisal form that focuses on key job dimensions of one physician's receptionist. Twice a year, both the receptionist and the physician complete this form about the receptionist's performance and then they sit down and discuss their views in depth.

Table 13–1. Semi-Annual Performance Appraisal.

Date of Review _____

Name _____ Position _____

KEY JOB DIMENSIONS	POOR EXCELLENT
1) Manages telephone calls, so that callers reach the appropriate person and receive needed answers. *Comments:*	1 2 3 4 5 6 7 8
2) Manages the appointment system, so that people are seen in a timely fashion, the physician has appropriate time with the patient, and those with priority needs are seen most quickly. *Comments:*	1 2 3 4 5 6 7 8
3) Extends courtesy, warmth, and concern to all patients, their family and friends; conforms to the House Rules. *Comments:*	1 2 3 4 5 6 7 8
4) Is responsive and helpful with co-workers; helps others meet patient needs. *Comments:*	1 2 3 4 5 6 7 8

The goal: to recognize positive aspects of performance and set goals for whatever improvements are needed.

Ideally, the appraisal form for each position differs, because the responsibilities differ. The key point is to make sure you include customer relations responsibilities, not just technical skills, required on the job.

FEEDBACK, COACHING, COUNSELING, AND DISCIPLINE

To put "teeth" into service standards, management also needs to give the employee consistent feedback on his or her behavior, reinforce the positive behavior, and, when necessary, implement a counseling and discipline process that might in some cases result in eventual termination. If the supervisor does not monitor staff behavior, you run the risk of problems and inconsistencies in staff behavior toward patients and co-workers, and you run the risk of watching your standards and patient satisfaction levels sink.

Effective feedback

Feedback, both positive and negative, is the most powerful shaper of staff behavior. Constructive feedback has these characteristics:

- Effective feedback is concrete and behavioral. It describes performance; it doesn't interpret it. For instance, here's an example of concrete, behavioral feedback: "When the patient approached the front desk, you did not look up and greet them. They had to say 'excuse me' in order to get your attention." This is in contrast to feedback that is interpretive that fails to detail the actual behavior that was unacceptable. Example: "When that patient approached you, you were rude." People define *rude* differently, and being accused of being rude makes people defensive. It works better to say, in effect, "Here's the behavior I saw that works against patient satisfaction. Instead, I want to see behavior like this . . . ."
- Effective feedback is timely. You shouldn't pile up dissatisfactions with staff behavior; instead you should offer feedback every time the behavior is problematic. You nip problems in the bud, instead of waiting until they escalate, and you have a litany of complaints to express when you've reached your boiling point.
- Effective feedback has to be constructive; it needs to relate to characteristics or behaviors that the staff member can change.

Tried-and-true feedback model

When you see employee behavior that is undesirable, you have to confront that behavior or it might become normal and routine. The following format is excellent for providing feedback about employee behavior that affects patient satisfaction.

Step 1. Describe the problematic behavior. Example: "When Mrs. Maxwell approached you, you said 'hello' in a bland, lifeless voice. You did not call her by name even though you know her name, and you did not introduce yourself."

Step 2. Articulate the consequences of the problematic behavior—for the patient, for the physician, for the practice. Example: "This behavior is a problem, because it makes the patient feel unwelcome and unknown. It reflects on me (the physician) because, from the patient's point of view, I am permitting you to behave in a disinterested fashion. And it affects the future of this practice by creating a dissatisfied customer who will certainly not rave to her friends about us."

Step 3. Express a pinch of empathy. Healthcare workers by and large are caring, idealistic people. Very few treat people poorly intentionally. Sometimes there are pressures that make it difficult for the employee to be as good as they know how. By expressing a pinch of empathy, you acknowledge that other circumstances might be making courteous behavior toward each and every patient a real challenge. Example: "Now I realize that this has been an extremely hectic day for you and that you're under pressure."

Step 4. State the behavior you expect in the future in no uncertain terms. Example: "Still, from now on, I expect you to greet each patient warmly—with a smile and by name." (The Einstein Consulting Group, York and Tabor Roads, Philadelphia, PA 19141; ©1985 and reprinted with permission.)

Here's how the four parts sound when integrated.

> When Mrs. Maxwell approached you, you said 'hello' in a bland, lifeless voice. You did not call her by name even though you know her name, and you did not introduce yourself.
>
> This behavior is a problem, because it makes the patient feel unwelcome and unknown. It also reflects on me (the physician) because, from the patient's point of view, I am permitting you to behave in a disinterested fashion. And it affects the future of this practice by creating a dissatisfied customer who will certainly not rave to her friends about us.
>
> Now I realize that this has been an extremely hectic day for you and that you're under pressure. Still, from now on, I expect you to greet each patient warmly, with a smile and by name.

Complete and comprehensive, this statement leaves no stone unturned. It states the problem concretely, along with its consequences. It shows that you are not an unfeeling person, and it goes on to say clearly what you want to see happen in the future.

Counseling, discipline, and termination

You're probably familiar with the progressive discipline process. When you see a behavior problem, you give the staff member feedback. *Usually*, they change their behavior as a result. If they don't, you need to escalate the attention and consequences you pay to the behavior. First, you counsel them and discuss the problem and how it might be solved. You document what took place in your discussion with them and when it took place. You give them time to show improved behavior. If they don't, you counsel them again, this time stepping up your disciplinary action to a "warning." Again, you troubleshoot what's in the way of improvement and how you might help by providing support, training, or whatever. Then, you give them time to show improvement. If they don't, you terminate their employment, but you have done it fairly and only after offering substantive, recurrent feedback, coaching, support, and opportunities to improve. If you are not used to a progressive discipline process, hopefully it's because you've never had a problem employee. If that's not the reason, you might greatly benefit from a training workshop on how to handle problem employees fairly and constructively. Such workshops are offered by numerous management development companies, management consultants, and universities.

The point is that you have to be prepared to go the limit with accountability—all the way to termination if you're genuinely serious about achieving unequivocally high standards of employee behavior.

14

Hiring and New Employee Orientation

Another pillar that supports a service orientation on the part of your staff should start on day one of a staff member's affiliation with you: hiring and new employee orientation.

When you interview job applicants for *any* position in your practice, you need to emphasize your concern about patient satisfaction and make explicit the fact that you're looking for people who have the technical skills needed, but not only the technical skills. You must emphasize that you also are seeking a person who has a service orientation, patience, calmness, and a dedication to meeting patient needs in a courteous, compassionate manner.

After stating this, then you need to screen applicants for their interpersonal style and communication skills. Some practices do this by posing small case situations and asking the applicant to react then and there. For instance:

> *Interviewer to Applicant:* Let's say there are five people sitting in the waiting room. The physician is running late because some patients took longer than anticipated. The person who has been waiting longest loses his patience, and complains to you in such a loud, angry

tone that everyone can hear. Let me be that patient for a minute, and I'd like you to try to handle the situation. Here I go: "I've had it with this place. I had an appointment and I came on time, missing work to come here. And here I sit. This doctor values his time a lot more than he values mine. I should send him a bill!"

How would you react?

Given that applicants are equal in technical skills, the reactions you see to simulated scenarios like this will make it quite clear which applicant has the best interpersonal or communication skills.

When hiring a receptionist, or anyone who will spend considerable time on the phone, it's also a good idea to conduct your initial interview with them over the phone. An interview conducted in this manner will give you a good idea of how well this person "thinks on the phone"—how adept he or she is at answering questions without the benefit of eye contact.

Also, since the telephone distorts and magnifies the voice in much the same way as a tape recorder, you can also listen for a clear voice, good diction, and friendly tone during your phone interview.

This brings us to the question of new employee orientation. The first question is, do you have one? Many practices don't. New employee orientation doesn't have to be fancy, but you do need to think through how you want to inculcate new people into the philosophy, procedures, and style that you want everyone to reflect in your practice. If you orient people up front, you have to do vastly less correcting and troubleshooting. This applies to customer relations skills as well as it applies to technical procedures.

The following sequence of events will help your new people pay attention to patient satisfaction and service concerns.

HOW TO ORIENT A NEW EMPLOYEE

1. Tell new people about how you value patient satisfaction, why you care about it, the impact on your pride and the success of your practice.

2. Lay out the behaviors or House Rules that you want everyone in your practice to follow. Discuss them. Invite questions.

3. Now, discuss the job-specific expectations that reflect courtesy, empathy and other service factors.

4. Ask the new person if they see any obstacles interfering with their ability to meet these expectations (skill gaps, office layout, etc.). Trouble-shoot and figure out ways to remove these obstacles.

5. If your practice is large enough, introduce your new person to an exemplary person you've identified to be their mentor/role model/coach—a person

you want the new person to observe and consult when dealing with everyday and difficult situations— for advice, and fine-tuning of skills.

The point is that you can heighten behavioral effectiveness by new employees by taking the time to orient them to *high* standards of behavior and the resources for achieving them. The result: you have fewer problems to correct, because you've prevented the kinds of attitude and behavior problems that drive patients *and* employers crazy.

15

Training and Development in Key Interpersonal Skills

- Are you clear on which interpersonal skills on the part of staff matter most to patients?
- Do you provide information and enrichment to your staff about the key skills they need to impress patients?
- Do you pay tuition for staff interested in upgrading their interpersonal communication skills?
- Do you actively recommend training opportunities to staff who are less than superb in their interpersonal skills?
- If you have a large practice, do you ever provide in-house training to upgrade the customer relations skills of all your staff?
- If you hold in-house training, do you show the high value you place on it by seeing that all levels of staff participate?
- Do you budget for staff training every year, so that people see it as a serious option?
- Do you devote staff meeting time to build patient relations skills?

The more *yes* answers, the better.

Many staff feel, "I already know how to be nice." And they may be right. But for many people, excellent interpersonal skills are not that easy. In healthcare, where the patient is often concerned, anxious, pained, or otherwise vulnerable, sophisticated skills are called for, (e.g., handling complaints without defensiveness, calming an upset patient, dealing with angry people, easing a long wait, listening actively, and communicating disturbing information).

No matter how clearly you set expectations, some people need information, training, and practice with feedback because they just frankly don't have it in their skill repertoires to be excellent without help from you. Training can help staff members identify and seize opportunities to satisfy patient needs and concerns.

IDENTIFY KEY INTERPERSONAL SKILLS

Patients point out the importance of staff behavior in their satisfaction with a medical care provider. Fortunately, excellent staff behavior is a win-win proposition because, while it impresses patients, it also engenders in staff a sense of pride in their work. People who, day after day, meet the public with grace and warmth on the outside will appreciate the dignified self they have on the inside.

Every human being is capable of demonstrating excellent service-oriented behavior as a matter of routine if it's expected of them. They do in McDonald's and at airline ticket counters and good restaurants.

Yet, in healthcare, where people are more often than not nervous and vulnerable and *really* want to be welcomed warmly, few front-desk people exhibit these behaviors on a consistent basis. Frustration with front desk staff isn't appropriate, because if they don't engage in these behaviors, it's because they haven't been told by the leaders of the practice that these behaviors are required.

If you have problems in this area, you need to develop explicit standards that, in essence, *require* staff to apply these behaviors consistently. That's the first and foremost step.

When patients are asked to identify staff behaviors that matter to them, they most often cite these as having the highest impact.

Specifically:

- Welcoming behavior and the use of small talk
- Staff use of names
- Professional dress
- Personal attention, empathy and listening
- Dealing calmly and skillfully with angry people

* Handling tough situations with aplomb
* Keeping the peace with co-workers

The following section addresses each of these key areas very briefly, providing you with guidelines and resources for use with your staff.

START WITH A SELF-AUDIT

Before focusing on training, engage your staff in a self-audit that taps their perceptions of their own patient relations skills (see Table 15–1).

WELCOMING BEHAVIOR AND THE USE OF SMALL TALK

Patients want staff to be approachable and welcoming. There are a simple few behaviors that cause patients to perceive staff this way. Specifically,

* Look up from what you're doing as the patient approaches (or even before).
* Make eye contact.
* Smile.
* Say hello.

On small talk

Small talk or friendly, easy patter is a critical skill because it makes people feel welcome and noticed, not invisible or alone; it significantly eases patient anxiety; and it makes the time go faster. It warms up what might feel to many patients like a scary environment.

In short, small talk breaks the ice, but, for most staff members, it may not be easy.

What are no-fail small-talk openers for patients?

* Comments about the weather, e.g., "Nice day out there" or "What a storm this is!"
* "Busy place, isn't it?" "I hope you haven't had to wait too long!"
* The opener that wins the prize for getting a conversation going with a patient: "How are we treating you here?"
* "Have you been to our practice before?"
* "Hi, I'm June Ross. I'm the lab technician here."
* "Welcome. I hope you're finding our service satisfactory."
* "I'm sure you must be anxious to be seen."
* "How are you feeling today?"

Table 15–1. Self-Audit on Patient Relations Skills.

	Never	Occasionally	Most Of The Time	Always
1) Patients find it easy to talk to me.				
2) I act warm and welcoming to patients.				
3) I'm eager to help patients and their companions.				
4) I consciously avoid engaging in behavior that irks people.				
5) When someone has a problem, I solve it or find someone who can.				
6) I make it a point never to interrupt a patient.				
7) I care about whether patients think well of me.				
8) I care about whether patients think well of this practice.				
9) I am challenged by people who are angry or upset, and I do all I can to calm and help them.				

- "Do you live near here?"
- Pick up on cues for conversation starters: "I like your bracelet. Do the charms stand for something special?"
- Try some personal comments, "I like your coat" or, "That's a very distinguished suit."
- Just start with "Hello" or "Good morning."

In talking with family and friends of patients, these openers work well:

- "Have you been here before with your family?"

Table 15–1. *(Continued)*

	Never	Occasionally	Most Of The Time	Always
10) I consider patient problems my problems.				
11) I am keenly aware that a dissatisfied patient can hurt our practice.				
12) I take initiative to satisfy patients and hopefully increase their loyalty to our practice.				
13) I have ways to handle my own frustrations and bad days, so that they don't affect our patients.				
14) I work hard to be a cooperative and supportive member of our staff team.				
15) I derive satisfaction from being a calm, skilled, caring professional in my dealings with patients.				

- "It must be very difficult waiting."
- "Have you been to the lobby restaurant?" Or, "Have you noticed the new magazines over on the far table?"
- Personal identification can be helpful: "Someone close to me was sick. It was very difficult for me."
- "Hi! Is there anything I can do for you while you're waiting?"
- "Are you from our city?"

STAFF USE OF NAMES

Publius Cornelius Scipio is said to have known the names and faces of all citizens of ancient Rome. Themistocles knew the names of 30,000 Greek citizens. George Washington called every soldier in his army by name. Napoleon did, too. Andrew Carnegie, Charles de Gaulle, and Franklin D. Roosevelt are also acclaimed for their memory and use of names.

These people were leaders. By using people's names, you too can win followers, motivate others to work with you, influence people (think of politicians!), enjoy people more ("A show of interest usually turns into the real thing"), save time (having made good personal contacts, you'll be able to rely on people more), weaken resistance, soften opposition, and dilute or prevent antagonism. Above all, calling patients by name personalizes care.

The challenge is to develop a protocol that dictates how you and your staff should address people—and how you can meticulously avoid addressing people in ways perceived to be inappropriate (see Figure 15–1). The fact is, that even though you never mean to offend, some staff members unwittingly presume a too familiar form of address. By following a few simple guidelines, you can avoid such situations.

The professional norm is to address adults by their last names, prefaced by Mr. or Ms.—until corrected or invited to do otherwise. Many people consider a stranger using their first name as too forward. Don't use a first name until invited to do so, and then take the invitation as a compliment.

About "honey" and "sweetheart" and other taking of liberties

This point is very controversial, but shouldn't be. It's as simple as this. Professionals who call patients "honey," "sweetheart" or some other diminutive always mean well. Let's accept the fact. And let's accept the fact that some people like being called "honey" or "sweetheart." They feel that the professional is being endearing. But what about the people who are offended by it? And these people are increasing in number. Why risk offending some of the people, when you can offend no one if you choose a low-risk alternative.

Consider this analogy. Pretend you have a sick patient. Two drugs exist to cure the disease, Drug A and Drug B. Drug A always cures the disease and has no side effects. Drug B always cures the disease, but *sometimes* has negative side effects. Which would you prescribe? Undoubtedly Drug A, because why take the risk of negative side effects? The same applies to names. If you call people by their last names until invited to do otherwise, and then you call them what they prefer (and people don't say, "Oh, don't bother calling me 'Ms. Jones.' Please call me 'sweetheart' "), you avoid negative effects.

Avoidance of diminutives also should apply to nicknames. For instance, when addressing teenagers, avoid nicknames liked "Katey" for Katherine, or

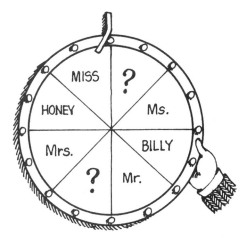

Figure 15–1. Addressing patients by name.

"Billy" for William, unless asked to use these particular names. When in doubt, ask the person what he or she would like to be called.

> The Principle of Lowest Risk: Always address someone in the most respectful form. Some names might offend; others won't. Always choose the lowest-risk alternative.

What's in a name? It seems like such a little thing. But addressing someone in a way perceived to be offensive can be upsetting however slightly. And especially in a doctor's office where most people don't want to be in the first place, people will often stew over little upsets and become, without saying a word, angry and resentful. By applying the Principle of Lowest Risk, you can play the name game and win.

In a nutshell:

- *Do* refer to people respectfully and in a professional manner.
- *Do* call patients, their friends, and family by their last names until invited to do otherwise.
- *Don't* slip into calling patients "honey," "doll," "sweetheart," "dear," and so on. Be especially aware in your care of older people.
- *Do* call people what they want to be called. To find out, start with "Mr." for men and "Ms." for women. For women, start with "Is that Ms. Jones?" If she prefers something else, she's apt to tell you, and then you can respect her preference.

- *Don't* make assumptions about people's marital status.

Those points are what current standards of etiquette recommend.

But what if you can't remember?

Most of us realize how powerful and personal it is to call people by name, but we say, "I'm terrible at it .... I have a bad memory.... I just *can't* remember names!"

Not so! The ability to remember names can be enhanced by office systems and by sharpening your memory muscles. It's a matter of helping and training your memory.

A system of name prompts

Instead of relying entirely on memory, establish first a system for prompting staff on the names they'll be sure to need during each day. Many practices have a policy of circulating daily a list of the patients expected that day. Then, staff who will surely interact with these patients can read and reread their names before their arrival. You might also consider the secret procedure of many high-class hotel chains. The first staff member to greet a patient repeats back that patient's name in their conversation with them. Then, when that receptionist or other frontline person passes the patient to another staff member, he or she refers to the patient by name. For instance, "Nice to see you again, Mrs. Jones. Please have a seat, and Mary Parker, our nurse, will be with you in about five minutes." Then when Mary Parker is ready, the receptionist says, "Mary, Mrs. Jones is ready for you now." Then, Mary Parker can say, "Hi, Mrs. Jones. Thanks for waiting."

Why rely on memory when you can have a routine that helps every staff member call every patient by name?

Toning up your muscle for remembering names

Many courses exist on how to remember names. In summary, here's what they teach:

Rule 1. Start saying and thinking to yourself, "I have a great memory for names." Stop telling yourself, "I never remember names." Whatever you think about yourself will come true.

Rule 2. Be sure to *hear* the name. The major reason why we don't remember a name is because we don't really listen for and *hear* the name in the first place.

It's not a matter of forgetting. It's a matter of "not getting." If you don't hear the name, admit it and ask the person to repeat it. They won't mind. Say, "Would you pronounce your name again please?" or "How do you spell your name?" or "Am I pronouncing your name right?" Usually, people find it flattering when you ask about and repeat their name.

Rule 3.   Use the name immediately, and again during your initial conversation. Right after you meet someone, repeat the name right away. "It's nice to meet you, Mr. Barry." Experiments show that people who repeat a name immediately after hearing it improve their ability to recall the name later by as much as 34 percent. Then, during your conversation, use the name two or three times more and make a remark about it. "Is that an old family name?" Spell it to yourself or out loud. Through repetition, you make the new name familiar.

Rule 4.   Use the name when you part. Always say, "Goodbye, Mrs. Jacob," not just "Goodbye," or "So long, Helen," not just "So long." People receive it as a compliment. And if you still have problems even after you follow the advice above, try these mental association exercises:

- Associate the name with something. Connect a characteristic of the person with the name. Or think of a familiar association that reminds you of the name. For instance, for Virginia, think of basking in the sun in beautiful Virginia Beach. For Mitch, think of Mitch Miller conducting sing-alongs. For Graham, think of Graham crackers. For Hudson and Jordan, think of rivers.
- Create a silly or ridiculous picture in your mind that connects with the name and person. For Mr. Chandler, picture a chandelier hanging from Mr. Chandler's nose. (You'll see this in your mind's eye. Mr. Chandler won't know!) Most people remember what they *see* more than what they hear, so if you can associate the name with a visual image, you're more likely to remember it.
- Break the sound of the name down into similar sounds that mean something to you. For Blumenthal, think "bloomin' tall"; for Chesnavik, think "Chasin' a witch"; for Greenbaum, think "green bomb."
- At the end of the day, write down all the names you learned that day and they're more likely to stick.

These tricks work for people who really apply them, and many people need to, since remembering names requires attention and concentration. After all, Honey Hazelnut, or is it Henry Hazlitt, said, "Our thoughts are so fleeting, no device for trapping them should ever be overlooked."

PROFESSIONAL STANDARDS OF DRESS

Now, a few words about a very unpopular subject—dress. Over the past several years, it has been fashionable to dismiss the notion of dress codes as a relic of an uptight past. Informality has replaced formality. Individual freedom has replaced authority-imposed uniformality. All that is probably for the better. Healthcare deliverers needn't look rigid and intimidating. But unfortunately, many patients report a shocking lack of professionalism in the appearance of their healthcare staff.

For one thing, casualness of dress creates confusion among many patients as to who's who. They often can't distinguish a doctor from a patient from a technician, because everybody's dressed alike.

Some patients grow anxious about hygiene when they watch staff members in sandled, unsocked feet. And most significant, extremely informal dress on the part of healthcare professionals can cause a crisis of confidence.

It's very difficult for already apprehensive patients (both young and old) to put their trust in healthcare personnel who attend them dressed in jeans, t-shirts, and torn sneakers, or still worse, in sweats after a five-mile run!

Some of us resent restrictions of dress and simply want to wear what's most comfortable. But to foster patient satisfaction, we should want to wear what generates the most confidence in us among the people we serve.

ON PERSONAL ATTENTION, EMPATHY AND LISTENING

Some people, when they walk into a room, seem to say, "Here I am!" They want the attention to focus on them. Others, when they walk into a room, seem to be saying, "There you are" and make you the center of attention. That's the way you should feel when a patient enters your office. Instead of focusing on how important you are to them, make it understood that they are the most important thing in your life as long as you're with them.

To achieve that effect, you need to listen to patients and understand them, taking their feelings seriously. What may seem like a small matter to you may be of monumental proportion to your patient or their loved one. You may recognize the problem as simple, but as long as they think it's important, it is important.

In dealing with people and their needs, showing understanding is often more important than solving their problems.

Remember how you felt when...?

There have been times in your own life when you've felt confused, hurt, frustrated, angry, anxious, afraid. These experiences, whether you realize it or not, represent rich resources for understanding how patients feel when they call or visit your practice. When you let patients know that you understand these feelings, you ease their burden and show you care.

Genuine interest must be cultivated and communicated. Speak the patient's language. Using words and expressions specific to a healthcare environment or to your specialty when dealing with the public only causes confusion. You have to translate, find the words the patient will understand. Your purpose is to communicate, not to show off your knowledge.

People have unseen powers for reading how others feel toward them. Insincerity and rejection can be sensed behind a false smile that tries to convey warmth but only conveys indifference.   On the other hand, people respond positively to signs of respect—simple courtesies, being called by name, being listened to and patiently heard through.

People can accept "no" for an answer more readily if they've been affirmed as a person. But when rejected—even without words—they want to respond in kind.

Sure, you see lots of patients in any working day. But each patient sees you only once. So make each patient feel important.   Learn their names quickly, and use them. If you have other work to do, put it aside promptly. If you're really pressed, explain this difficulty to patients and let them know you will finish this one task as quickly as possible and return immediately.

Listening is a skill

Good listeners aren't born; they're made. And you can learn to be a good listener with a little practice and attention to the following tips.

1. Listen with purpose. Ask yourself what it is you want to find out and what it is you expect or want to hear. What might the patient say that will affect your preconceived ideas or plans?

2. Listen for meaning. There are several levels on which patients communicate. There are the words themselves, the implications behind the words and nuances, and tone of voice. And there are nonverbal cues, like posture, facial expression, and gestures. It's important to listen with your eyes as well as your ears, to listen for what is not said, but felt, as well as for what is said.

3. Whenever possible, eliminate distractions. You need to give undivided attention to the patient, and you want the patient to have the opportunity to express feelings without distractions.

4. Don't jump in. Try not to reply too quickly. Instead, briefly restate what you heard to make sure you understood it. Then formulate your reply and give it. This takes a little extra time, but with practice it will become quicker.

5. Be an active listener. Involve yourself in the listening process. Be aware of your own listening barriers and guard against them. Take time to be aware of your thoughts and reactions.

Dealing calmly and effectively with angry people

Long waits? A miscommunication about their appointment? A delayed doctor? An irritable three-year old pulling on mom for attention? Anxiety about what the doctor will say? Transportation difficulties on the way to the doctor?

Some patients enter your practice in a hostile or belligerent mood, bringing their own tensions and hidden anxieties with them or reacting to circumstances caused by your practice that they feel you should have avoided.

Some staff members are warm and professional in their dealing with patients, until that angry patient approaches them. The pressures of a busy day, and the energy they know they've expended for patient after patient, make it difficult to stay cool and nondefensive in the face of a complaining or angry patient.

Whenever an organization is in the business of dealing with people, difficult situations such as these will occur.

Patient anger and hostility in a difficult situation is often made worse by the following:

- *Becoming defensive*—Comments such as, "I only work here," "It's not my fault," or "It's our policy" tend to turn most patients off. These and other defensive statements usually make the situation worse.

- *Poor listening*—Failure to listen intently to a patient's complaint will almost always increase patient hostility.

- *The runaround*—Passing the buck or referring to higher authority with statements such as, "You'll have to see my supervisor," "There's nothing I can do about it," or "I'm too busy right now to look into the problem" are other sure ways to further alienate patients.

- *Arguing*—Aggressively pressing your or the practice's point of view in these situations usually does little to de-escalate the emotion involved in the situation or encourage problem-solving.

- *Nonverbal behavior*—Nonverbal gestures that tend to make matters worse include fidgeting, appearing rushed, looking at your watch, looking away from the patient, becoming preoccupied by reading, writing, conducting other paper transactions, or turning your back.

These circumstances make people more upset and angry.

When patients lose their cool, what can you do to keep yours and build your practice's relationship with patients? How can you lower the emotional pitch of the situation and defuse hostility that is inappropriately aimed at you?

Just remember that every complaint and, in fact, every angry person, is an opportunity to improve your relationship and your practice's relationship with a patient. To handle anger well, the staff person first needs to respect that the source of the patient's anger is not them personally—that patients have valid, deeply felt reasons for being angry. Second, it doesn't help to get defensive or angry at the anger expressed at you. Instead, it helps to follow a rational step-by-step process for handling anger constructively for both you, the patient, the people in the waiting area who are eavesdropping and for the staff member himself or herself.

Here's a tried-and-true process that you can teach to staff and practice applying in roleplay situations.

Seven Steps. These steps will help you deal with a patient, or any person, who is angry.

1. Try to get the person to a private place and make him or her comfortable. Get on the same level by shaking hands and introducing yourself.

2. Listen with concern, and don't argue or interrupt. Let people tell their story. The best medicine for upset patients is letting them get their frustrations off their chests—without getting you upset! Draw them out with noncommittal remarks like "Uh-humm" or "I see how strongly you feel about that." This not only has a calming effect, it also will help to reveal points of agreement important in leading to a solution. Allow the person to verbalize and ventilate. Use positive body language by staying relaxed and maintaining eye contact. Act as if you have all the time in the world to listen. Sitting passively while the patient talks is not enough to establish rapport. You also have to listen with your mind, looking for paths that lead to understanding and problem solving. And that means leading the speaker with apt and timely questions, sometimes turning the speaker's questions back to him or her so that he or she will tell the story fully.

3. Investigate: gather information and ask questions that will clarify the situation. Try to understand the other person's viewpoint and perception of the situation.

4. Apologize if appropriate. Apologize for problems created by the organization. Convey sympathy for the person's situation and feelings of frustration. The words "I'm sorry" usually have a calming effect. However, do not overuse the words and make them sound insincere.

5. Suggest realistic alternatives, and be as flexible as possible. Consider how you and the organization can meet the person's needs.

6. Direct the person to the right resources, if necessary. If you cannot solve the problem yourself, direct the person to someone who can. Do not give the

person a number to call or a person to see without trying to smooth the way as much as possible.

7. Provide a target time, and follow up. Give the person a specific target date or time in which the problem will be handled. If the problem cannot be dealt with on the spot, the person needs to have a realistic understanding of when he or she can expect the problem to be resolved. Most important, make sure you do what you say you are going to do for the person. Make notes to yourself and put them on your calendar. At all costs, do not disappoint the person further by promising something and failing to deliver.

Other tips:

- Get on the same physical level as the angry person. Stand if the person is standing. Or, if it seems more natural, invite the other person to sit down, then you sit down, too.

- Let your facial expression, body position, gestures, and tone of voice show your concern for the upset person. Adopt a sympathetic tone of voice. Nod in agreement in appropriate places. It lets the person know that you are on their side.

- Give the person your undivided, active attention. Show your sincere interest. Make eye contact. Sit forward in your chair. All bodily movements should be directed toward the other person.

- Even if you believe the complaint is basically in error, acknowledge whatever is right about it. For example, "Yes, that is our policy," or "You are correct in saying. . . ."

- If a mistake has truly been made, admit it. Don't excuse the error or minimize it. "Mistakes do happen" may sound good to you but *not* to an irate patient! Instead try, "You're right, that shouldn't have happened. Let me see what I can do to help."

- *Never* admit the complaint is widespread or even that it has happened before; for example, "Uh-oh, Dr. Bumbler is at it again," or "Our billing system never seems to run smoothly."

- When an interaction with a patient is allowed to drag on, it loses effectiveness. Once the problem had been resolved, you can courteously and tactfully end the contact. This should be done firmly but pleasantly. Often, simply extending your hand and saying, "Thank you for speaking up. I'm going to follow through as I promised," is all that is needed.

- Be honest with yourself. It may be okay to bluff in poker, but it doesn't work in patient relations. If you don't have the information needed, don't "fake it."

Go find out the information or, at least, refer the patient to somebody who does have the information.

And remember: often when patients complain, they are venting their frustrations about being where they don't want to be in the first place—in a doctor's office. They may simply need to talk to someone. Listen!

THE ASSERTIVE ALTERNATIVE

"If 'the customer is always right,' does that mean that the employee is always wrong?"

Assertiveness training teaches people to handle uncomfortable and potentially explosive situations in a calm, constructive, and authoritative way—a way that satisfies the patient and simultaneously allows the employee to maintain self-respect.

Consider the angry patient complaining loudly because he thinks your office has overcharged him. Here are the typical passive, aggressive, and assertive responses to this patient's situation:

The Passive Response.   Allow the patient to yell and scream while you apologize profusely and take the blame upon yourself. Or, sit there saying nothing but seething inside.

The Aggressive Response.   Yell back at the patient, become defensive and argue that it's not your fault, and is either the patient's stupidity or some co-worker's problem.

The Assertive Response.   Listen carefully to the patient's complaint. Get a good understanding of the problem and respond in a supportive, empathetic way. Use statements such as, "I can see this is frustrating for you. . . ." or, "I'm really sorry that we've inconvenienced you. . . ." Once you begin to address the complaint, if the patient continues to be abusive, let him or her know that you want to help and will do all you can to resolve the problem when he or she calms down.

There's nothing wrong with saying "I'm sorry" on behalf of your practice. That's not always passive; it's often appropriate. You can apologize and still maintain your dignity. It's all in the way you handle the problem.

HANDLING TOUGH SITUATIONS WITH APLOMB

Even if you have basic communication skills, you'll still be confronted by characteristically difficult situations—dealing with long waits, confidentiality problems, and more. Anticipating them and being equipped to deal with them coolly can nip a bad day in the bud for both you and your patients.

Situation. A waiting room is filled with patients; the doctor is delayed.

Don't wait for patients to ask about the delay. First, screen the patients and see if another caregiver can provide for them. Tell patients in the waiting room that their doctor is delayed. If appropriate, tell them briefly the reason for the delay and when the doctor is expected. Be sure to apologize for any inconvenience. And stop by to give frequent progress reports. Give patients the option to continue waiting, to reschedule or to be seen by someone else, and thank them for their cooperation. Also, offer patients use of a telephone, if needed.

Situation. A patient is dissatisfied with the care rendered and let's you know it.

In a setting of privacy, and as tactfully as possible, try to find out exactly what happened. Remain calm, show concern, and try to offer solutions. Do all you can. If that's not enough, refer the patient to the office manager or key physician. Show sensitivity and concern without taking sides.

Situation. A patient is dissatisfied with your service and is threatening to go elsewhere.

Remain calm. Find out what the problem is and be helpful and sympathetic. Getting the patient to calm down may be the most important thing you can do initially. Take careful notes. Determine whether you can help resolve the problem. If not, refer the patient to someone in your practice who might be able to deal more effectively with the problem. Express genuine regret that they have been disappointed and ask for the chance to resolve the problem.

Situation. Sometimes a patient will say he or she has an appointment when, in fact, none is on record. Should you schedule another appointment, or should you see the patient anyway?

Tactfully, tell the patient that no appointment is recorded for him or her at this time, but that if they'll take a seat, you'll check into the matter. Give the patient the benefit of the doubt and resolve the problem as quickly as possible, either by having the caregiver fit the patient into the existing schedule or by scheduling the patient for another time. If you suggest that the fault was with the person, you will create very negative feelings in that person and those overhearing the interaction.

Situation. Asking patients to disrobe for examination can be a sensitive issue. What's the best way to deal with a patient's embarrassment?

Above all, be professional and go all out to respect the patient's privacy. Reassure the patient and explain to him or her exactly why disrobing is necessary, which clothing to remove and what the intended procedure will be. Give the patient the proper cover-up garments and explain how to use them. Then tactfully close the curtain or leave the exam room. Tell the patient how to signal when they're ready and reassure them that you won't reenter until they signal. Then, even after they signal that they're ready (e.g., by opening the door or using a "ready latch"), knock when you return.

Situation. Privacy is so important in medical practice. How do you ensure that a personal discussion is not overheard by others?

If the patient is already in the examining room, be sure the door is closed. If the patient is not in the examining room, bring him or her back in there or in some other private area to talk or to give instruction for specimen collection or preparation for a procedure. If there is no suitably private area, lower your voice so that the conversation is less likely to be overheard.

If it's a telephone conversation, be sure the phone is in a private area, and try to phrase questions so they require only yes and no answers. Try not to repeat the patient's name so that it can be overheard by others. And, if someone walks into the area where you are talking with the patient, stop talking and politely ask the other person to wait until you are finished with this conversation. Never conduct private conversations in open areas, such as busy hallways or elevators.

KEEPING PEACE WITH CO-WORKERS

Smooth co-worker relationships are critical to the smooth operation of your practice. The way staff members interact can color the entire personality of your office. A harmoniously cooperative staff is an efficient staff. And co-workers who treat each other with dignity and respect are more likely to extend these courtesies to patients. So, it's in everyone's best interests if staff members interact cooperatively and courteously.

We all know people whose behavior on the job drives us crazy! And, most likely, our behavior drives our co-workers crazy, too. The wear and tear created by less-than-wonderful relationships with each other makes each of our jobs much more stressful. In a medical practice, problematic relationships also tend to be apparent to the patient.

Consider setting guidelines for co-worker relationships. By getting clear on the co-worker behaviors that reflect support among staff and convey a positive image to patients, you improve your practice's effectiveness *and* your staff's job satisfaction.

Here's an example of one practice's guidelines:

Code for Quality of Work Life
1. *Cooperation is contagious. When you give it, you get it.*
2. *Every job is unique . . . take care of yours. Let others take care of theirs. We're not here to judge.*
3. *Keep complaints constructive. Speak to the source of the problem.*

4. *Negativism not only drains you; it depletes others. Hit the high notes!*

5. *Build supportive relationships. We all need them.*

6. *Be generous with appreciation. It pays great dividends.*

7. *Look and act the part of the professional. You are this practice.*

8. *Be aware of interrupting. It distracts and causes tension.*

9. *Keep conversations with co-workers brief. Lengthy discussions irritate.*

10. *Be a role model. Make this practice better because you're in it.* (The Einstein Consulting Group, York and Tabor Roads, Philadelphia, PA 19141. ©1984 and reprinted with permission.)

CONFRONTING PROBLEMS IS THE ONLY CURE

If you have problems with a difficult co-worker, it's certain you're not alone. But there are steps you can take to make matters better.

Typically, we spend about 40 hours a week at work, and sometimes that means spending a lot more time than we'd choose to with someone we don't get along with. If the person at the next desk turns out to be the kind of person that jangles your nerves, it's really up to you to learn to deal with this person in such a way that your differences don't interfere with your work and, at the same time, don't keep you on the edge of your seat with irritation, anger and resentment.

- First, pay attention to what makes you happy. Instead of concentrating on this irritating person—for argument's sake, we'll call her Gretchen—and all the ways in which she irritates you, take a good look at what you do like about your job: the satisfaction you get from doing your work well, the friends you have made there, the little things you do during the day that bring pleasure. And let Gretchen, for the most part, go her own way.

- Enlist her help. Gretchen may be a born complainer. And one of the things that annoys you most is how she's always complaining about how the office is run and, in particular, about how you do your work. Listen to her. Or better still, ask her advice. She may have some legitimate suggestions, and when you thank her for them, she'll probably be flattered and may be easier to work with.

- Flattery can get you somewhere. Everyone appreciates a compliment, and Gretchen is probably no different in that respect. Tell her what a great job she's done on something—but make sure she deserves it so you'll come across as sincere.

Sometimes a Gretchen's behaviors go beyond causing just mild irritation. If your co-workers' actions and attitudes disturb you to the point where you can't do your work right, or if she does something concrete to interfere with a job you're doing, it's time to take more drastic measures. Invite her to lunch. In the process, get everything out in the open. Tell her exactly the kinds of problems you're having with her. This kind of communication, perhaps in a setting away from the office, can be just what's needed to establish lines of communication that can go far toward making a good working relationship.

If all else fails, take it to the top. Let's say you've tried everything you could think of to ease the tension between Gretchen and you, and still her behavior is interfering with your ability to do your work. It may be time for "the court of last resort"—the boss. It's an obvious route to take, but too often people don't go about doing it in the right way.

First, don't rant and rave, and leave personalities out of it. Second, do your homework. Develop a case of actual documented incidents in which Gretchen's behavior has interfered with your ability to perform your duties optimally. Perhaps there was a day when Gretchen misfiled charts, resulting in your spending the entire afternoon looking for what you needed. Or, maybe she's lax about reporting phone calls to you, causing major delays in getting you and patients needed information.

Small incidents can add up quickly, and your boss will appreciate that your resulting inability to perform your duties properly is interfering with the productivity of the entire office.

State at the outset that you're having a problem and, in confidence, ask your boss's help in solving it. Tell your boss what you've already done to try to remedy the situation and that you're willing to do anything in your power to keep things running smoothly. Hopefully, your boss will acknowledge that you are a valued employee and will recognize the importance of high morale and teamwork among the staff. And, hopefully, he or she will intervene to rectify the situation.

In the best of all possible worlds, co-workers would work together happily and productively. Unfortunately, in reality that's not always the case. So if you're having a problem with a co-worker, do what you can by yourself to right the situation. But if all else fails, take the matter to your boss.

It boils down to this

The basic measure of your practice, naturally, is the quality of your service, extended by you and your staff. Staff shortcomings can spoil the image of even the most efficient healthcare provider. Try to assess how your staff is doing on interpersonal dimensions by asking yourself:

- How do patients feel after seeing your staff?
- Has the patient's personal dignity and uniqueness been confirmed by staff actions and attitudes? Or does he or she feel like a number in a faceless crowd?
- Does the patient want to return to your practice? Or are the patient and their family left feeling that they want to punish you and your practice by turning to a competitor and telling others of the frustrations they endured at your hands?
- Do the patient and family go away praising your practice? Or do they instead want to berate you and your service because they felt mistreated?

HOW TO STRENGTHEN STAFF SKILLS THROUGH TRAINING OPPORTUNITIES

There you have information about essential skills of the service professional. But most people are not "naturals" who need training. And, increasingly, medical practices are figuring out ways to provide that training so that they can achieve their patient satisfaction objective.

There are many ways to provide training, through books and other print resources, by paying people's expenses to enable them to attend programs in the community or out of town, by providing time off with pay for people who take initiative to improve their job-related skills, by creating a clear mentoring or coaching system for one-on-one training by a particularly skilled staff member, or by bringing to your practice special training programs that fit your practice's specific needs.

Books and Other Print Resources. The bookstores and libraries are replete with self-help and how-to books that focus on improving interpersonal skills—on handling complaints, on building positive relationships, on tactful assertiveness, and more. Also, there exist hundreds of curriculum materials on customer relations skills, including films, programmed instruction materials, training designs and tapes. The best way to learn about these is to call the training department of businesses in your community; for instance, banks, airlines, and hotels are good examples of businesses rich in training materials. You can probably borrow useful materials or at least find out which ones they recommend.

Subsidize Your Staff's Attendance at Commercially Available Programs. The training industry is a $6 billion industry. A huge part of that industry consists of a rich array of training programs available in central locations nationwide. People can sign up to go for a day or two of enrichment and skill-building on any subject you want. A particularly popular program is on "Customer Relations Skills." Some programs focus on healthcare clients, others, on people from all service sector businesses. In either case, your staff will mix with individuals who possess sophisticated customer relations skills that certainly are relevant to interactions with patients in a medical practice. Watch your junk-mail, community newspapers, and professional association bulletins for opportunities. Also, call the hospitals you're affiliated with and ask if they will make their ongoing training programs available to your staff. Since hospitals want your loyalty, they'll probably say 'yes' and happily.

Bring Training In-House. Through your local hospital or independent training consultants or universities, you can find excellent training program providers who can tailor programs specifically to your staff's needs. Increasingly, medical practices are sponsoring training events at least semiannually to build teamwork among their staffs and to upgrade the professional skills they all need to ensure a loyal patient following. The Einstein Consulting Group in Philadelphia offers excellent programs of this kind for healthcare audiences, or you can call your local hospital for appropriate resource people. Many hospitals offer within their guest relations programs or service strategies special training opportunities for physicians' office staff, usually at no charge.

Here's a model for a service excellence workshop for office staff provided by Allan Geller, a consultant experienced in providing practice enhancement programs for medical practices:

Practice Enhancement Workshop for Medical Practice Goals
- Increase awareness of the need for service excellence as an unbeatable competitive strategy.
- Define standards for employee behavior in interactions with customers.
- Sample techniques for positive interactions.
- Provide a forum for taking stock of service strengths and weaknesses, and discussing what people can do to strengthen their practice's service reputation.
- Strengthen teamwork and cooperation.

The Plan
   I. Introductions, Objectives, and Agenda
   II. Warmup Exercise. Partners talk about themselves and their work. This gives participants a chance to focus on the workshop's objectives and to interact with people they might not know.
   III. "Think of a Place." Ask people to think of a place where service is terrific and to identify the behaviors demonstrated by its staff. In the large group, invite sharing about the key components of excellent service and what it takes to achieve these.

IV. "Why Focus on Patient Satisfaction?" Present a lecturette and a group discussion on the need for service excellence as a major strategy to achieve patient satisfaction. This can include a review of the multifaceted aspects of service in successful organizations—the need for quality of work life, positive image and reputation, malpractice prevention, patient retention, quality care, and financial success. This discussion draws attention to healthcare as a service industry and the practical reasons why a service commitment is so important for the office practice.

V. "How Are You Doing?" In small groups, take stock of how well people are already doing in providing excellent service. This is an opportunity to give and get a pat-on-the-back for the work people are now doing and to learn new ideas for enhancing service delivery.

VI. Service Goals. A lecturette on the Patient Satisfaction Matrix examines who your customers are, compares your current level of service to a usable model, and determines future needs for strengthening your reputation for outstanding care. These goals will help build a practice enhancement strategy that allows the office practice to be proactive in meeting patient needs.

VII. "The Behaviors That Matter." Using anecdotes and demonstrations, the leader presents a set of key behaviors (e.g., House Rules) that affect patient satisfaction. During this awareness-raising experience, the leader stresses the importance of consistent practice of these key behaviors.

VIII. Skills Modules. If there's time, you can focus in on a basic skill needed in excellent patient interactions, using group and individual exercises that explain and reinforce coping with multiple demands, working with the angry patient or co-worker, making people comfortable, or handling complaints. This important component gives assistance to office personnel in making their job more manageable.

IX. "What Do We Need More Of?" Conduct a group brainstorm of future training needs.

X. Thank You's and Evaluation of the Session.

(*Guest Relations in Practice*; (3), 1988, pp. 1–4. The Einstein Consulting Group, York and Tabor Roads, Philadelphia, PA 19141; (215) 456–7065; ©1988.)

You might have staff who can conduct a session like this, or you might consider the many experienced consultants available.

One-on-One Training.   If your practice is large, you probably have within it some people who are superior in customer relations skills. Make those people your in-house training squad. Give them explicit responsibility for coaching and mentoring other staff to achieve high standards of performance. Consider paying them extra and making this responsibility a very serious, important, recognized dimension of their job.

Staff Meetings that Improve Staff Behavior.   The highest potential and least tapped source of skill-building and awareness-raising is staff meetings. Short-sighted practices don't have them, but far-sighted practices do. The fact is that you can dramatically improve staff behavior toward patients and one another and build more effective helping relationships among staff by designing purposeful, meaningful staff meetings. Here are three examples of staff meeting formats that can strengthen staff behavior:

- *From Good to Excellent:* Ask staff to make a group list of patient interaction situations they handle everyday. Divide into groups of two. Have each group choose one situation and develop two short skits that show the best and worst ways to handle that situation. Not only do the "worst" skits raise awareness of staff behaviors that drive patients crazy, these skits are also inevitably hilarious and enable people to let off steam. Then, the "great example" skits can be used to identify the fine points in human interaction that distinguish inoffensive behavior from greatness. After each pair of skits, you ask people to think of ways the staff behavior could be even more impressive. Push for other alternatives and missed opportunities. The goal: to engage the group in helping one another expand their repertoires of interpersonal skills that satisfy patients.
- *The Problem Clinic:* In this meeting, you invite people to brainstorm sticky situations. Then, working with one at a time, invite group *enactments* of various ways to handle each situation. Discuss each until staff feel they have optimal alternatives for handling the situation.
- *Peer Training:* Develop a list of key interpersonal skills; invite interested staff to develop a short training plan for reviewing this skill with his or her colleagues. If you have people who will do this but lack resources, refer them to a hospital training department for relevant books, sample training plans and curricular materials.

The point is that some staff won't achieve excellent behavior toward patients without some investment in them on your part. If they don't know *how* to be wonderful, if they don't know the many tiny behaviors that impress patients, they won't engage in them. Consequently, your practice suffers. If you set up a system for helping staff explore missed opportunities and build their skill repertoires, they win, your patients win, and your practice wins.

16
Reward and Recognition

When given a choice of all affordable methods of reward and recognition (including merit pay, pats on the back, merchandise awards, prizes, certificates, and more), the vast majority of all employees chose "a pat on the back from my supervisor" as the single, most powerful, meaningful way they believe they can be recognized on the job. The sad fact is that most employees also say this method is the least common, even though it's the only method that costs absolutely nothing.

This tells us something. Employees at every level in healthcare want to be noticed and recognized when they reach out to patients and perform well. A comfortable environment and a reasonably long lunch hour are comfort factors that employees appreciate. But feelings of satisfaction come from doing a job well and getting recognized for it by physicians, the office manager, and others with a stake in making the practice successful.

If you want to enhance your practice by optimizing staff behavior toward your patients, harness the power of recognition of staff behavior as a far-reaching method for strengthening staff performance.

START SIMPLE

Simple positive feedback is the most powerful method. This should be included, of course, in any performance appraisal with employees, where you need to focus on their positive accomplishments and specific contributions to your practice. Also, on a daily basis, you should be generous with positive feedback.

Here's an excellent format for giving staff positive feedback about their behavior toward patients. You'll notice its similarity with the negative feedback model presented earlier.

Step 1: *Describe the positive behavior.* Example: "I noticed that you left your desk to sit down with Mrs. Pendleton to talk with her and ease her obvious anxiety."

Step 2: *Articulate the consequences.* Example: "I'm sure she felt much better to know you cared, and you eased the time she had to wait by treating her specially and kindly. This is the kind of behavior that makes our practice stand out as having very caring people, and I'm sure word gets around."

Step 3: *Express a touch of empathy.* Example: "I realize you were very busy this afternoon, and taking that extra time with her put extra pressure on you."

Step 4: *Express appreciation.* Example: "I want you to know I really appreciate what you did. Thank you."
(The Einstein Consulting Group, York and Tabor Roads, Philadelphia, PA 19141: ©1984 and reprinted with permission.)

You can increase the power of this even more by putting it in writing as, for instance, this Appreciation Telegram:

Dear Martha,

I noticed that you left your desk to sit down with Mrs. Pendleton to talk with her and ease her obvious anxiety. I'm sure she felt much better to know you cared, and you eased the time she had to wait by treating her specially and kindly.

This is the kind of behavior that makes our practice stand out as having very caring people, and I'm sure word gets around.

I realize you were very busy this afternoon and taking that extra time with Mrs. Pendleton put extra pressure on you.

I want you to know I really appreciate what you did. Thank you.

Sincerely,
Brad

OTHER RECOGNITION DEVICES

Medical practices of various sizes use a rich variety of methods for rewarding and recognizing employees.

Merit Pay.   Employees appreciate receiving a pay differential tied to their performance. Generally, people find it to be quite unfair to receive the same raise as a colleague who works less or extends oneself less to meet patient and colleague needs.

Incentive Bonuses.   This is an increasingly popular option. At year end, you give staff members bonuses based on your perception of their contributions to making your practice successful. Typically, a practice will develop a bonus pool as a percentage of their annual profit and dispense it according to criteria like these:

- Was this person reliable and trustworthy?
- Did this person efficiently and competently demonstrate the technical skills needed for the job?
- Did this person go all out to satisfy our patients?
- Did this person demonstrate exemplary teamwork and support of physicians and other colleagues as he or she went about his or her job?

Some practices give minimal bonuses as gestures of appreciation. Research shows that if the bonuses are minuscule in the eyes of staff, they are worse than none. If you are going to give bonuses, make sure the amount is not insulting.

Annual Recognition Events.   Many practices hold annual dinners or celebrations at which they don't just have a group dinner, but they develop awards to exchange with one another based on appreciations they feel for one another's work. This can be a tremendous morale booster, which you can enhance even more by giving out as a party favor $25 or $50 merchandise certificates to a local department store.

A System of Appreciation Notes.   People sometimes save notes of appreciation for years because they find them meaningful. You can mushroom the number of appreciations that are expressed among your staff by making available, perhaps in your waiting room and office, a stack of printed Appreciation Telegrams that anyone (patient and staff alike) can fill in and bring up to the front desk for delivery to the intended party.

Public Thanks. In your staff meetings, as a warm-up or wind-down activity, invite people to go around the room, focusing on one person at a time, and expressing compliments and appreciation statements to them about behaviors or actions they had witnessed over the last few weeks. You can make this a powerful, moving ritual for what can otherwise be business-only meetings.

In short, there are so many ways to recognize staff if you decide to do it. But in the hustle and bustle of a busy practice, it's easy to take the wonderful people for granted, instead of refueling them with kind words and recognition that say you noticed all they're doing to make your practice successful and your patients happy.

17

Employee Involvement and the Employee as Customer

The success of your practice depends on your staff. And how your staff performs has a lot to do with how you relate to them. People who enjoy working together work well together. But they can't do this without help and support from you.

That's where the "Five A's and a B" come in—small points to remember, but big steps in helping your employees feel good about working for you, about working for your practice, and, most important, about giving their all for your patients.

- *Affection.* Your employees want to know that you care about them, that you see them as individuals, not just as members of a workforce.

- *Attention.* Pay attention to what your employees are saying. Listen to them and be responsive.

- *Appreciation.* Notice when they've done something especially well, and give them recognition for it.

- *Acceptance.* Help your employees know that they belong, that they fit in with your practice and with the other employees.

- *Accomplishment.* Employees need their workload constructed in such a way that they can go home feeling they've accomplished something during the workday. Too heavy a workload leaves them feeling overburdened and resentful; too light a workload will leave them feeling bored and unfulfilled.

Those are the "A's," and this is the "B":

- *Believe in your employees.* People who feel their bosses believe in them make things happen. (Source Unknown)

In an atmosphere of caring and respect for them, your employees become perhaps your most powerful practice enhancers—if you invite their involvement. Opportunities for employee involvement in practice enhancement abound. First of all, you need to proclaim and then reiterate periodically the key role staff play in patient satisfaction. You can do this through recognition of exemplary staff, expressions of appreciation, reminders at staff meetings, posters, awareness-raising memos, and more. The point is to repeat yourself in myriad ways, so that excellent customer relations on the part of your staff become a pervasive theme in your practice. Here are two examples of printed methods for making this point:

Consider the wisdom of this old typewriter:

Xvxn tho my typxwritxr is an old modxl, it works wxll xxcxpt for onx of thx kxys. I wishxd many timxs that it workxd pxrfxctly. It is trux that thxrx arx timxs whxn fortythrxx kxys function wxll xnough, but just onx makxsall thx diffxrxncx.

Somxtimxs it sxxms to mx that our practicx is somxwhat likx my typxwritxr—not all thx pxoplx arx working to satisfy our patixnts.

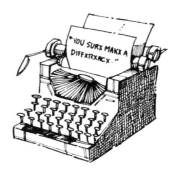

Figure 17–1. Each one of us is key.

You may say to yoursxlf," Wxll, I'm only onx pxrson. I won't makx or brxak this practicx." But you do makx a diffxrxncx, bxcausx our practicx, to bx xffxctivx, nxxds thx activx participation of xvxry mxmbxr. So, thx nxxt timx you think that you arx only onx pxrson and that your xfforts arx not nxxdxd, rxmxmbxr my old typxwritxr and say to yoursxlf, "I am a kxy pxrson in this practicx, and I am nxxdxd vxry much. Any timx I don't work right, it surx makxs a diffxrxncx"

And here's another that you might consider hanging on a wall near your office staff:

You Are This Medical Practice.
You are what people see when they arrive here.
Yours are the eyes they look into when they're frightened or worried.

Yours are the voices people hear when they try to forget their problems. You are what they hear when they come for appointments that could affect their destinies.

Yours are the comments people hear when you think they can't.

Yours is the intelligence and caring that people hope they'll find here. If you're noisy, so is our practice. If you're rude, so is our practice. And if you're wonderful, so is our practice.

No patients or their companions can ever know the real you, the you that you know is there, unless you let them see it. All they can know is what they see and hear and experience.

And so we have a stake in your attitude and in the collective attitudes of everyone who works in this practice. We are judged by your performance. We are the care *you* give, the attention *you* pay, the courtesies *you* extend.

Thank you for all you're doing.
(Albert Einstein Medical Center, York and Tabor Roads, Philadelphia, PA: ©1982 and adapted with permission.

Raising awareness and emphasizing the essential value of every person on your staff in making your practice successful by meeting patient needs—that's the first step. With that as a critical backdrop, you can then engage your staff in establishing behavior expectations for staff performance. By engaging staff in identifying pivotal behavior, you prevent the resistance often generated by a more authoritarian approach to the setting of expectations. You can show your respect for staff as experts and adults who are well equipped to identify key staff behaviors. If you engage staff, you are also much more likely to generate commitment to the behaviors identified as key. The result: less need for policing by you and a higher level of consistent excellent performance. Employees will recognize their own influence and will be less likely to balk at new "rules imposed from on high."

Another powerful and far-reaching way to involve employees in enhancing your practice is to engage their creative imagination in identifying possible ways to enhance your practice. Management needs not only to respect employee views but to invite them to offer complaints and ideas about your practice's service problems and opportunities. This way, employees feel invested in your practice enhancement strategy and respected by you as key players in the process. When they see you act on their ideas, they feel influential and important, and a sense of ownership in your strategy to optimize patient satisfaction.

Effective vehicles for employee feedback and participation are needed. The underlying message: "Every one of us is important to the future of this practice. We need you and we care what you think." Suggestion boxes, weekly rap sessions on "How Can We Make Things Better?" and periodic team-building retreats for the entire staff are examples of effective ways to involve employees in identifying and solving your practice's service problems.

EMPLOYEE AS CUSTOMER

Involving employees in your practice enhancement strategy builds investment and ownership. But there are other ways you can harness employee motivation and energy, if you adopt a mind-set that allows you to see your employees as customers whose needs must be met in order to create employee satisfaction and effectiveness.

Research on workers in all fields show that the number one motivation of employees is "doing a good job." Many employees in medical practices develop resentment against the key physicians because they feel that office practices and procedures are inefficient and frustrating, creating barriers to doing that good job.

To tap employee potential, you might benefit from looking at your office's practices (your hours, your scheduling methods, your resources, your suppliers, etc.) and making sure that these are not disabling to your employees. Hassled employees don't have the stamina or goodwill to extend themselves to patients as you need them to. The remedy: remove the hassles and barriers and create a work environment that is enabling, comfortable and empowering.

To move in this direction, talk with your employees. Invite them to identify systems problems and procedural hassles that need attention in order to improve patient satisfaction *and* their own ability to be patient, courteous, and responsive to patients. If the management of your practice is unwilling to examine these factors, escalating pressure on staff to behave better will not work in the long run and your staff will resent you. They will accuse you to your face, or more likely behind your back, of trying to put a paint job on a machine that needs body work.

THE POWER OF A TEAM

Staff members tend also to be most effective and most loyal to your practice if they feel part of a team. Regular staff meetings, annual team-building retreats, a staff recognition dinner paid for out of your budget, a daily "huddle" to review the day's priorities with everyone together—all of these are excellent ways to build teamwork and the kind of esprit de corps that makes your practice a warm and friction-free environment for patients and staff alike.

IV

The Essence of Patient Satisfaction: The Physician-Patient Relationship

The following chapters are our attempt to review in some depth the specific behaviors that create positive patient-doctor relationships and offer you ways you can develop these behaviors. For many readers, this section reviews behaviors that you already do well. For some, it will hopefully trigger a realization of why some of your current behaviors work or don't work. And, for others, it may suggest opportunities to substitute new behaviors for ones that you acknowledge have produced disappointing results.

To identify the key behaviors on the physician's part that foster patient satisfaction, we interviewed 16 physicians identified by patients and peers to be highly effective in their interpersonal skills. In Chapter 18, "The Interpersonal Skills of Successful Physicians," Elizabeth Dunn, Ph.D., presents highlights from these interviews.

After providing these highlights from physicians themselves, we will proceed to examine in depth a repertoire of effective ways to build each critical aspect of the physician-patient relationship. Specifically, we will examine:

- Establishing rapport initially and forever
- Communication is a two-way street
- Dignity and how to preserve it
- Sensitive handling of feelings
- How to handle sticky situations

In each section, we present the (1) rationale for developing the skills addressed, (2) specific examples and cases that illustrate effective behavior, and (3) options—ways you can apply the skills to your reality.

We realize that there is no simple cookbook approach to creating positive relationships with patients. Each physician has his or her own style and each patient encounter presents new needs and conditions. Instead, we believe that you can benefit from a *repertoire* of options that will enable you to build effective relationships with various patients in a vast range of circumstances.

18

Interpersonal Skills of Successful Physicians

The definition of *good physician interpersonal skills* varies widely from person to person. So, we decided to pursue a practical approach to defining excellence in physician-patient relationships. Through word-of-mouth recommendations, we identified a select group of physicians recommended by more than four people as effective and successful, people who have solid reputations in their communities for having both highly successful practices *and* excellent interpersonal skills. Gail Scott, Elizabeth Dunn, and Wendy Leebov each interviewed several physicians from the resulting list.

Our premise is that these physicians must be doing something right. And, if we can crystallize what it is that they are doing right, we will have a somewhat generalizable or at least interesting understanding of what constitutes excellent interpersonal skills. Admittedly, the research design (namely, interviews with a

This chapter was written by Elizabeth Dunn, Ph.D., Vice President of Marketing and Planning, West Jersey Health System; Camden, New Jersey. As an experienced market researcher, Dr. Dunn designed the physician interview protocol, conducted two of the interviews, analyzed the results, and wrote this chapter.

select number of select physicians) is weak, but it yields rich qualitative results. As physicians interested in practice enhancement and enlargement, you can check your own skills and attitudes against those of these successful physicians and decide on the validity.

We identified 16 physicians successful on human and business dimensions. Those interviewed reflect a variety of specialties. Once we identified our physicians, we interviewed them, asking them questions ranging from their views on the changing role of physicians to how they deal with difficult patients.

Our gratitude goes to the physicians who shared their views with us. The behaviors and opportunities we present in detail in chapters 18 through 23 derive largely from their knowledge and insights. The physicians include: Allen Arbeter, M.D., General Pediatrics and Infectious Diseases; Jose Castel, M.D., Family Practice; Lillian Cohn, M.D., Internal Medicine; Howard Elefant, M.D., Internal Medicine; Harris Gerber, M.D., Internal Medicine and Geriatrics; Marvin Gershenfeld, M.D., Medicine, Allergy, Immunology; Richard Greenberg, M.D., Rectal Surgery, Surgical Trauma, General Surgery; Sandra Magos, M.D., OB/GYN; Dahlia Sataloff, M.D., General Surgery; Mark Singer, M.D., ENT; Courtney Snyder, D.O., General Medicine; Marjorie S. Stanek, M.D., Cardiology; Margo Turner, M.D., Internal Medicine; Shahriar Yazdanfar, M.D., Cardiology; Robert Weinstock, M.D., Family Practice; and Gary Levine, M.D., Gastroenterology.

In this chapter, we begin by quoting 12 of these physicians whose views we feel create the context for the more thorough treatment of key physician skills in the next chapters. Before we share highlights from our group of successful physicians, consider your own answers to these questions:

1. What does today's patient want or expect from their physician?

2. What particular things do you do to "break the ice" with patients or make them feel comfortable?

3. What particular things do you do to protect a patient's dignity?

4. What is your philosophy on the use of names? What do you like to be called, and what do you call patients?

5. To what extent do your patients seem to want more of your time than you can give them? How do you handle time issues?

6. What particular skills do you use to deal with a pushy or demanding patient?

7. Other than clinical skills, what would you say are your best skills?

8. If you were going to teach medical students about interpersonal skills, which ones would you focus on? What do you really wish they would all learn?

9. Some people say good physicians are born and not made. What do you think about this? Can physicians improve on their interpersonal skills?

10. How important are interpersonal skills to the success of your practice?

FROM THE MOUTHS OF SUCCESSFUL PHYSICIANS

Related to each of the above questions, here are highlights from the physicians we interviewed. When we reviewed these interview results with other physicians, they pointed out that unsuccessful physicians might say some of the same things. The difference is that the successful physicians probably practice what they preach! You decide.

Question #1: What do today's patients want or expect from their physicians?

Dr. Singer: Today's patient expects magic. They expect that you will be able to cure everything.

Dr. Gerber: Patients today want more than just medical care. They are willing to pay for understanding, empathy. They want to be treated honestly, and want a doctor who takes time.

Dr. Sataloff: Today's patient is less willing to go to a technically excellent physician if that physician has a bedside manner that's abysmal. Instead, the patient will go to someone who is good and who also deals with patients well interpersonally.

Dr. Gershenfeld: Many patients are more demanding now for medical care of various sorts. They want tests to prove why they are sick, they're impatient, and they're certainly more medically sophisticated.

Dr. Arbeter: The majority of the patients that come in have very high expectations . . . . it's not unusual for a patient to have a shopping kind of approach and, although they have that right, it has eroded rapport in patient–physician relationships . . . . The patients that come in here from the suburbs demand a lot of care and attention and are medically sophisticated. They are aware of the disease processes far more than several years ago, they're better read, and you cannot do a song and dance around them. You have to be straight up with the information that you give them.

Dr. Castel: I think patients want to be taken seriously no matter what it is that they have. They want the doctor to care about them as a person and not just see them as a heart attack, or whatever. Somewhere along the line, they hope that you are competent to take care of them—I don't think that's as high on the list as wanting to be understood, listened to, and have their complaint taken seriously. And they want some reassurance.

Themes loom large. From their physicians, patients want:

- Superior interpersonal skills, including empathy, understanding, willingness to listen, and personal attention
- A willingness to share substantial medical information
- A very high level of technical excellence

It is important to note that almost all of the physicians recognized the importance of these factors. Technical excellence in and of itself is definitely not sufficient to attract and hold the sophisticated patient of today. This observation is reinforced by consumer studies that indicate that patients select physicians primarily on the basis of interpersonal skills—skills they have the ability to evaluate.

Question #2: What particular things do you do to "break the ice" with patients or make them feel more comfortable?

Dr. Sataloff: I tend to touch patients more than other physicians do. I shake their hand or put my arm around them.

Dr. Gershenfeld: I schedule enough time to be able to listen to them. I try to give them enough of my time and enough of my energy to create a positive atmosphere for the relationship. Some physicians have a knack of seeming always to be busy, always wanting to get on with the next situation. By their attitude, they don't like questions to be asked, and the patient has to push themselves in if they want to get a question asked.

Dr. Arbeter: I often start out by complimenting something about the way the child is dressed, like their barrettes or their snow boots. And, when the child is on the examining table, I will go and sit next to the child on the table and take my history sitting on the table with the child . . . . I look at people, I touch them, I let them tell me how they feel, I give them a chance to talk.

Dr. Castel: Most people like to feel some kind of connection with the doctor besides the medical visit. They like to be related to as a person, not just somebody with a cold or a heart condition. It changes the whole nature of the relationship when you can interact on different levels, and part of that is knowing something about that person that is separate and apart from the specific reason that they are there. So, I write things down. When I dictate I might say something like "Concerned about sore throat because he is leaving for Florida tomorrow," and that's in my last note. So when I see them again, I say, "How was your trip to Florida?" If you know something separate and apart about the person, it makes them feel better and, actually, it makes me feel better, too. If I can connect with a person in more than just the fact that they are here to see me for their illness, it is a greater satisfaction for me as a physician. I like to think that anybody who comes in has something interesting to offer. I may see ten people with sore throats in a row, and you might think that must be boring, but it's not ten sore throats, it's ten people, each one bringing something a little bit different.

Dr. Greenberg: I think it's important for me to portray a sense of confidence in myself because I think that good results are dependent upon the patient's psyche as well as technical outcomes. I talk to my patients and try to relax them and let them know that I'm going to be able to get along with them, that I'm not going to raise their anxiety level any higher than it is. I talk to them in a relaxed voice with a fair amount of eye contact. I listen to what they say to me and repeat it so that they really understand that I'm listening to them, and I really care about what they say.

Dr. Snyder: I walk out to the patient and introduce myself without having the patient have to walk back. It's very important to listen carefully to what the patient is telling you. Physicians of the older age, like some of the ones I saw during my residency, don't talk *with* patients, they talk *to* patients.

Dr. Cohn: I'm more open with my own experiences than many doctors. I have pictures of my kids on the wall, and that lets people know that I'm not just a doctor—I'm also a mother, and I live in a house like they do. Sharing personal experiences with patients makes them feel more comfortable, and they can relate to me better.

Dr. Gerber: I try to create a subdued, warm environment. I use Impressionist prints and pleasant music. I have also trained my office staff to behave in ways that contribute to this relaxing environment.

Dr. Castel: I think it's important that both the physician and the office staff greet the patient by name. People like to be recognized. If you go to a store and they say, "Hi, how are you, Mrs. Jones," you will keep going to that store, because people like to be known. It's the same principle with any kind of service to the public. If you get to be known in the place, you feel comfortable going back there. In fact, you want to go back.

Themes loom large:

- Patients aren't happy with you unless you treat them as a whole person, not a disease.
- You can make patients comfortable or break the ice or reduce fear by using some very specific, very simple behaviors that matter to the patient.

Question #3: What particular things do you do to protect a patient's dignity?

Dr. Stanek: There's a whole variety of things you can do to help protect a patient's dignity: addressing them by their last names, not asking them uncomfortable questions in front of others, maintaining eye contact when talking with them. I also have a philosophy that I use, even with difficult patients—I never fight with a patient, because the patient is always right.

Dr. Sataloff: It helps a patient's dignity if he or she participates in his or her healthcare. My role is to explain why things should be done in a certain way based on my expertise, and then the patient and I decide what to do. That preserves a lot of dignity because people feel terrible if someone just tells them what to do. It's bad enough being ill, but to take away their control is worse.

Dr. Arbeter: Number one is not to treat them as if they are inferior. When I start a new group of residents in the clinic, I give them a spiel about physicians and about caring for the kind of people that we care for. You absolutely have to respect everybody. You have to give them space to be what they are and not change them into what you are. The more unsophisticated, the more in need they are, and the more you do this. So if it's a 14-year-old with a baby, you don't treat that person as if she is a diminutive character. You talk with her, you look at her, you get her ideas. The first thing you do is make a person feel that they're a person, valued and not judged. I will unequivocally tell you that there are an awful lot of patients that I'm terrified of what they are doing, how they're doing it, why they're doing it, and some of the social aspects of what they are doing to themselves, but I can't approach it from judging these people. I may come out of there with a knot in my stomach, but I can't let them know that I disapprove.

The second part about their dignity is to ask them questions in a language that they understand, to use phraseology that they understand, in a tempo that they can tolerate. Don't just rattle off—bang, bang, bang—"What's the answer?" You have to be able to give them time.

From there, you get into issues of how you are examining them in a way that they won't feel or be exposed. It could be a six-year-old child, who has no biological reason to be embarrassed. They're sitting there in nothing more than their underpants. But, the truth of the matter is that they know for themselves that they're embarrassed, and that's no way to take care of a patient.

Dr. Elefant: If I recommend a procedure, and someone doesn't want to have it done, I say, "You should have it done for this reason, but if you don't want it now, go home and think about it."

Dr. Cohn: I talk with them while I'm examining them so they don't feel like they're being invaded by a physician. If you explain what you're looking for as you go along, it makes the patient feel more comfortable.

Key themes loom large:

- Dignity requires sensitivity to what people might feel is uncomfortable, and preventive measures to avoid these situations.
- You can minimize their discomfort and embarrassment if you care to, and if you take actions—some of which take time.

Question #4: What is your philosophy on the use of names? What do you like to be called, and what do you call patients?

Dr. Turner: I did my training at this hospital, and everybody called me by my first name. When I went into practice, most people continued to call me by my first name. I regret that now. For the majority of patients, the professional relationship where I am the doctor and you are Mrs. Smith is something that we should maintain, because it conveys a certain meaning to our relationship in the office that is different than what happens outside. For all patients that I'm meeting now, I introduce myself as Dr. Turner and call them by their last name. Patients take my information much more seriously when Dr. Turner gives it than when Margo says something. It's true.

Part of the relationship that I have is free and easy and very approachable—there are no boundaries to it. But I want this to happen within a framework where it is clear that you are here because I am the physician and you came for something that I have to do or to say to you. A professional use of names seems to keep the relationship clear and within limits.

Dr. Elefant: Most of the time I address my patient as Mr. or Mrs. unless I've known them for a while. I don't care if my patients call me Howard, Howie, or Dr. Elefant. Most of them call me Dr. Elefant, because that's the way they address their doctors. I go in and introduce myself as Howard Elefant—then they choose. Younger people are the ones that will call me Howard.

Dr. Snyder: Some patients want to be called by their first names. I try, until I get to know a patient, to speak on a more professional basis, but some patients call me by my first name. Some take that privilege more so than I would give it out.

Themes loom large:

- There are no hard and fast preferences.
- The key is, keep it professional and parallel. If you want to be called Dr. X, then call your patients Mr., Ms., Mrs. Y.

Question #5: To what extent do your patients seem to want more of your time than you can give them? How do you handle these time issues?

Dr. Greenberg: I never look at my watch. My internal clock can tell me how I'm doing time-wise. If I find something terrible like cancer in a patient, the clock just stops, and I spend as much time as that person needs, and I hope that things will be all right in the waiting room at that time. The office is small enough that people can see me come and go out of my office into the examining room, and I'll say something like "I'm here, and I'll be with you really soon."

Dr. Cohn: I take as long as is necessary to make patients comfortable that we have resolved the majority of their problems. If necessary, I apologize to people in the waiting room. If patients take advantage of my time, I educate them as to what they should consider a "problem."

Dr. Singer: I work in a very high-volume office where there is pressure all the time. I see 45 to 60 patients a day, and I find that patients appreciate quickness. If a patient wants and needs more time, I move them to the lounge and return to them to discuss prognosis and treatment. I don't leave patients stranded.

Dr. Gershenfeld: I think it's just a question of trying not to have patients wait. I'll use the example of the family practice where there is never an appointment on time, and it's not unusual for an hour to an hour and a half wait. I just think that this is an abuse. I think that there are certainly situations, if somebody walks in who is obviously sick, that you take them out of turn. Most patients understand this. But, for the doctor to be continually late coming to office hours or continually schedule everybody at one o'clock and not finish until five or six is an abuse. I think this is just a question of your secretary trying to call patients and say "Please come in later."

Dr. Turner: Patients do demand a lot of time! They do, and it's because the practice of internal medicine and family medicine is filled with people who are depressed and come to talk. The presentation of those problems is often a medical problem or complaint, but underneath, it's often someone who needs to talk. I don't dismiss them when I can't find a disease. I try to help them understand what my perception of things is. So, if it means a follow-up visit in six weeks just to talk, that's okay. I don't need to examine you or give you medication to feel you are coming for my service.

If a patient is taking up a lot of time, and there are patients waiting, I often say, "This has been very good discussing this with you today, and I can tell that we have more to talk about. Let's arrange another time so that we can pick up on this."

Dr. Arbeter: Time is a real issue. What has happened in medicine is that there are a lot more regulatory agencies that demand that people work for quality assurance areas, and insurance collections and the problems of running a practice are more and more like running a business. People's time is really very competitive. The pressures on our practices lead to pressures at home which then have a negative effect on how satisfied you are in your practice, and vice versa. And it becomes a vicious cycle.

Dr. Castel: Even if I'm pressured by time, I try hard to make it look like I'm not in a hurry. Do you know when I look at my watch? When I go behind the person and listen to their lungs. I'm extremely conscious about not looking at the watch. I want to appear as if I have all the time in the world. I try to make up time on the simpler things and, when someone needs extra time, I give it to them.

Key themes loom large:

- Different patients inevitably demand or require different amounts of time. Your scheduling should allow that flexibility.
- These exemplary physicians stress the importance of keeping your time concerns under wraps when you're with a patient.
- It's essential to accept the patient's desire for time and attention as understandable and deserved. Otherwise, you resent their demands on your time and they see this.
- Since time is not infinite, you can benefit from *educating* your patients *in advance* about how you view time, the length of an appointment, and the options they have.
- No matter how much you do in advance to prevent time problems, there will always be people who, without your knowing this in advance, truly need lots of time and others who have to wait.

Question #6: What particular skills do you use to deal with a pushy or demanding patient?

Dr. Sataloff: I try not to lose my temper. I try to explain things, because I think being pushy means they are anxious about something, particularly those who are used to being in control of their own lives.

Dr. Cohn: I would define a pushy or demanding patient as one who asks for my advice and then consistently ignores it and does what he/she wants to do. In this situation, I tell the patient that I can't take care of them if they persist in this behavior. The threat of withdrawal is useful.

Dr. Castel: The first thing I do is to not let them get to me. I try to teach our staff on the phone, that when somebody calls and they are angry, they're not angry with you. They're having a problem, and if you get caught up in their problem, you will not be able to help them. If you are attacked by somebody, the normal, social reaction of people is to rear up and attack back. But, as professional people, we need to learn how to say to ourselves, "I'm not going to react to this person. I'm just going to stay cool and react as nicely as I can." It's very hard for people to continue to be difficult and demanding when you are nice to them.

Dr. Turner: I can be a little bit stand-offish when it's appropriate to be so, and I do that when there's someone who needs that. Those patients need structure. They're not being pushy to be pushy. They just need to know their limits.

Key themes loom large:

- Successful physicians recognize that most patients who act out do so because they feel inordinate stress, fright or discomfort related to their health or their visit to the doctor.

- The successful physician stays calm, steady and accepting. He or she does not get defensive or angry.

Question #7: Other than clinical skills, what would you say are your best skills?

Dr. Sataloff: I think that I'm more empathetic than a lot of people. I feel for people. I really do. I feel terrible for them when they get sick. I try to do the best I can to cope with whatever emotional issues they have, whatever it happens to be. And, I spend a lot of time with patients.

Dr. Cohn: The ability to make people feel comfortable about opening up to me.

Dr. Gershenfeld: Listening to people.

Dr. Elefant: I'll let a person talk—even if they are blubbering, they just have to get it out.

Dr. Castel: I like people. I like to interact with people. I like to think that everybody I meet has something to offer, which hopefully makes me nonprejudicial. I also like it when people have a positive reaction toward me.

Dr. Turner: I'm sure there are many doctors more skilled than myself academically, but I have a list of patients that I can't even accommodate because something happens here that doesn't happen someplace else, and it doesn't happen because I have tons of credentials next to my name. I think it's listening to them, letting them feel that they can express things, trying not to be judgmental.

Key themes loom large:

- Technical skills aren't the challenge. Interpersonal skills are.
- These successful physicians gain great satisfaction from their interpersonal skills, which they claim differentiate them from less successful physicians.
- Excellent interpersonal skills satisfy the patient and gratify the physician.

Question #8: If you were going to teach medical students about interpersonal skills, which ones would you focus on? What do you really wish they would all learn?

Dr. Gershenfeld: Students need to understand that patients are not able, for the most part, to evaluate the medical skills of their physicians. Their judgments are based on the other skills of the doctor—how nice the doctor was, how pleasant, and so forth. But if doctors are abrupt, if they don't answer questions, if they don't make themselves available, if they leave their offices at X hour and leave no one else on call. These kinds of things affect the physician's practice.

Dr. Sataloff: I would say that it's important to listen to what patients tell you—verbally, by body language, and nonverbal cues. You can get a sense of how they will respond to anesthesia, or to a diagnosis, or to a procedure if you're really open to what they're communicating.

Dr. Turner: We can all learn a thousand facts and regurgitate them back, but I don't feel that's necessarily what makes people better. Being supportive and being available and being someone that the patient can talk to can help the most grim situation seem different.

Dr. Cohn: I tell students to listen to patients. They can be the most brilliant physicians, but if they can't listen to patients and make them comfortable, they'll be worthless.

Dr. Snyder: The one striking difference between the training process and what I see now as a physician is the difference between technology and bedside patient management. We work with residents now, and their desire seems to be to know as much technology as possible—the specifics of case management—regarding high-tech apparatus. That's really very important. But what happens is that that's not what one sees in general in private practice. The patients don't see the technology—they just want to get better. There's a big disparity between technology and day-to-day patient management.

One key theme looms large:

- The key skills are listening and seeing the patient as a whole person with a life apart from their ailments.

Question #9: Some people say that good physicians are born and not made. What do you think about this? Can physicians improve on their interpersonal skills?

Dr. Turner: Some things can be taught. Eye contact is important. Not having a thousand interruptions, not having a telephone in the examining room. Having a policy that when you're in a room examining a patient, you're not to be interrupted unless there is a life-threatening situation going on. These kinds of things can be taught.

Dr. Cohn: I think about 25 percent of the necessary interpersonal skills can be taught, but the rest is innate. I think we need to change the way we select people who are going to become doctors. Medical schools need to spend less time seeing who graduated with honors and more time seeing who is a good person.

Key themes loom large:

- Many skills can be taught. Whether they're learned or not depends on the attitude of the physician and whether or not that physician strives to excel on the human dimension.
- Medical schools accept students too much on the basis of their academic skills and not enough on the basis of their ethics and interpersonal skills. If this weren't so, we would have more physicians who don't need to be educated on the interpersonal dimension.

IN CONCLUSION

We selected the physicians to interview by asking people to recommend physicians who were successful on business *and* patient satisfaction dimensions. These physicians all emphasized the power of interpersonal skills, communication, and personal attention to create patient satisfaction. Drs. Snyder and Castel boil it all down to this:

Dr. Snyder: If I had to pick something that has to be right to make the practice grow, I would say that it is discussion—with patients or with family members. If you don't discuss things, you aren't going to make the right diagnosis, you're not going to take good care of the patient, and the patient will walk out the door. And, you're not going to get the family members' support, because you haven't set up a good relationship from the beginning with that patient.

Dr. Castel: The days of being the only physician in town are gone. No matter how much knowledge you have, if the patient doesn't have a good interpersonal experience, they're not going to come back to you no matter how good you are.

Dr. Snyder: Marketing means that you talk, and if you don't talk, that's it.

19

How To Establish and Maintain Rapport

When you greet a new patient, you have an all too brief opportunity to start off on the right foot by making a positive first impression. Then, once you get to know the patient, you need to nurture the relationship to achieve long-term rapport. This chapter examines three aspects of creating a positive impression and perpetuating it through attention and acknowledgement of the patient throughout your relationship. Specifically, we will examine:

- How you handle introductions
- Taking a history
- Establishing rapport

We will consider each area, describing your behavioral options and their consequences for patient satisfaction.

HOW YOU HANDLE INTRODUCTIONS

In most doctor–patient interactions, the first "live" encounter is the one where the doctor says who he or she is to the patient. It is important to note that this brief 20- to 40-second interchange triggers a great many feelings on the part of the patient, and these feelings affect the chain of events that follows.

Consider the possibilities:

Dr. Grunt: A middle-aged patient walks unescorted into a physician's office. The doctor, seated behind a desk, says, "Have a seat, Tom. I'm Dr. Grunt."

Dr. Jones: Young Dr. Jones enters the waiting room, walks up to a patient saying, "Tom Smith *(shakes hand)*. Nice to meet you. I'm Dick Jones."

Doctor Haley: Dr. Haley gets up from behind a desk to meet and greet Sara Smith, an elderly patient, saying, "Good morning, Mrs. Smith. I'm Dr. Haley. Won't you take a seat?"

Methods for introducing yourself abound. Yet, in each scenario there are positive and negative implications for the relationship. The difficulty with Dr. Grunt is the unequal status given the patient. "How come he gets to call me by my first name when I must call him 'Doctor'?" is a sentiment often expressed by patients—to their friends. The scene is worsened when the physician is younger than the patient. Consider also the opportunity to make contact that Dr. Grunt missed by remaining behind the desk, by putting physical distance between him and the patient.

The physician in this case didn't see it that way at all. He was using the patient's first name as a way of becoming familiar, and remained at his desk to review the charts and histories before each patient's visit. In short, to his way of thinking, he was doing a fine job.

In the second case, young Dr. Jones feels that it is important to escort each patient personally into the room. Also, since Dr. Jones and the patient are about the same age, he wants to give the patient the choice of calling him "Dick" or "Dr. Jones." If the patient uses "Doctor," he will not use the patient's first name. Although Dr. Jones' intentions are admirable, some patients are uncomfortable with that level of choice or control. Perhaps in this case the doctor could ask Tom if he would mind being called "Tom" adding, "You may call me Dick or Dr. Jones. I'm comfortable with both." This leaves little room for discomfort on the part of the patient.

In the third case, Dr. Haley feels it important to call her elderly patient by her last name. This doctor wants to make Mrs. Smith feel welcome and, at the same time, convey professionalism and respect.

Based on his research, reported in the *Bulletin of New York Academy of Medicine* (57 (1), 1981), Dr. Hans Mauksch says, "Increasingly, people want their doctors to call them by first names only if they can do the same with their doctors."

Do's and don'ts of names

- *Do* refer to people respectfully and in a professional manner.
- *Do* call patients and visitors by their *last names* until invited to do otherwise.
- *Don't* slip into calling patients "honey," "sweetheart," "dear," or "doll." Be especially aware in your care of older people.
- *Do* call people what they want to be called. To find out, start with "Mr." for men and "Ms." for women. That's what current standards of etiquette recommend. For women, start with "Is that Ms. Jones?" If she prefers something else, she's apt to tell you and then you can respect her preference.
- *Don't* make assumptions about people's marital status. "When you call me Miss or Mrs., you invade my private life. For it's not the public's business if I am or was a wife."

The point: introductions and the behaviors that accompany them have significant ramifications.

Ask yourself:

- Do you personally escort patients into your office?
- Do you have your receptionist or nurse show the patient in and deliver the introductions?
- What names do you use and how do you refer to yourself?

You have options. You need to decide what message you intend to convey to your patients, how you want to be perceived, and how you want your patients to feel.

Nonverbal attentiveness

Of course, what you call a patient and whether you choose to escort your patients from the waiting room are only part of the opening scenario. Your nonverbal behavior also says a great deal.

Table 19–1 shows seven indices related to your nonverbal behavior. This index is adapted from "Enthusiasm Awareness Index" by Patricia Sanders, *Training and Development Journal*, June 1985.

Patients prefer doctors who:

1. Maintain eye contact;
2. Smile often;
3. Appear relaxed, not rushed or nervous;
4. Lean in toward patients during conversations; and
5. Assume a relaxed posture while interviewing.

Statistics show that individuals being interviewed for a prospective job are sized up positively or negatively in the first 30 seconds by the way they enter the room, shake a hand, and take a seat. So are you, and you don't get a second chance to make a first impression.

TAKING A HISTORY

It is the art of medicine that you bring to play when you begin the patient interview. This interplay between physician and patient forms the fabric of what hopefully will become a productive relationship in which the physician can come to understand the patient's needs, and to evaluate and treat them.

The explosion of medical technology, with its emphasis on testing and procedures, has unfortunately overshadowed the importance of the art of the interview and yet, in the patient's mind, this is an experience that shapes their relationship with you.

Let's start with three key questions:

• Why take a history?
• Should this be primarily a medical history?
• Should you be the one to take the history?

Let's examine these questions by looking first at the most rudimentary methods of obtaining patient histories. Most physicians use some method of obtaining basic medical information from a first-time patient. For many, this method consists of two pieces of poorly duplicated paper on a clipboard, given to the patient by a receptionist who says, "Please take a seat over there, fill this out, and bring

Table 19–1. Level of Attentiveness.

	LOW	MEDIUM	HIGH
	1 2 3	4 5	6 7
1. Eye Contact	Avoids eye contact; unfocused gaze or blank stare; or dull look.		Maintains excellent and constant eye contact while avoiding staring; shining, wide-open eyes.
2. Facial Expression	Expressionless, deadpan, or frowning; little frowning; closed lips.		Demonstrative; exhibits many variations and frequent changes in expression; agreeable looking.
3. Gestures	Arms kept at sides or folded; rigid; infrequent use of arms		Demonstrative movements; calm, open movement or hands.
4. Body Movements	Stationary; standing or sitting; seldom moves from one spot.		Moves freely, naturally but slowly; uses frequent instructional motion.
5. Vocal Delivery	Monotone; minimum inflection; poor articulation; little variation; looks at client while talking.		Pleasant variations in pitch, tone, cadence, and volume; good articulation.
6. Overall Energy Level	Lethargic; inactive; sluggish; appears tired or sleepy.		Maintains an even and moderate level of energy; occasional bursts of energy.

Scoring: In general,
- a score of 35–42 indicates a very high level of attentiveness.
- a score of 20–34 indicates moderate levels of attentiveness.
- a score of 6–19 indicates a low level of attentiveness.

Source: ©1985, *Training and Development Journal*, American Society for Training and Development. Reprinted with permission. All rights reserved.

the form to me when you're finished." The patient sits in the waiting area checking an endless series of *N.A.'s* since the "history" has little relevance to the patient. Somewhere it asks, "Have you been hospitalized?" and "Are you taking any medication at this time?" Great! Something the patient can respond to. At best this approach gets to the bare bones—the medical basics—that the physician needs to know, but it certainly gives very few clues as to the patient's complete medical profile. It reveals nothing about what these diseases meant to the patient, how serious they were, what the methods of treatment were, and so on. Nor does it begin to help the physician understand the patient on a personal basis and set the stage for building trust. Furthermore, the process of having the patient complete the information alone misses the opportunity to establish early contact or communicate personal interest in the patient either by the physician or the support staff.

Your options

Some doctors do get personally involved in history-taking for the reasons cited above. *They* want to ask the pertinent medical questions and hear and observe the patient's own descriptions and reactions. This gives them the opportunity to ask clarifying questions about diseases or experiences and understand more of what being a patient means to this individual. Many physicians specifically set aside 45 minutes or even more for each new patient because they feel it takes an investment of time to establish a strong foundation with this patient. The history-taking process becomes the vehicle for getting to know the patient as part of the initial interview.

Expanding the history

Some physicians go one step further in history-taking and include questions about family history, careers, hobbies, recreational choices, and more. Their goal: to learn as much about the person as possible and to record this information so they can draw from it key information about the patient's lifestyle and its relationship to health, and also use it to break the ice and establish rapport early and quickly.

M. McGoldrick and E. Carter, in *Genograms in Family Assessment* (New York: W. W. Norton and Co., Inc. 1985), discuss a model for getting patient information. This diagram or "genogram" allows doctors to elicit and record family history, as well as a medical profile for relevant members on the patient's family tree. The genetic problems of heart disease, cancer, and more are accurately recorded for the physician's use, as well as symbols for nonmedical descriptions of people and relationships.

The genogram is extremely helpful. It:

1. Organizes the family history;
2. Identifies the support system;
3. Displays symptom constellations and pallors;
4. Focuses anticipatory guidance;
5. Facilitates diagnosis of difficult medical problems;
6. Provides a tool for dealing with psychosocial problems;
7. Helps the physician to understand the patient;
8. Improves the physician's clues to engaging the patient.

The physician interested in establishing rapport and setting the stage for an ongoing, mutually satisfying and trusting relationship should consider these questions and make a conscious, deliberate decision that will optimize patient satisfaction:

- How much medical information do I want and need from the patient?
- How much nonmedical information do I want and need from the patient?
- What would be the best method of obtaining this information based on my feelings about myself and my practice?

Clearly, your answers will differ from practice to practice and from specialty to specialty. The point is to know that you have practice options and each option has costs and benefits for you and your patients.

ESTABLISHING RAPPORT AND PUTTING PATIENTS AT EASE

Building rapport begins with introductions and history-taking. But rapport over the long haul must be nurtured. It is achieved as a result of many small understandings and micro-interactions or "moments of truth." Each time a patient enters your office, you have a moment and a chance to display caring, friendliness, and recognition of the patient as an individual. At that moment, you need to "break the ice," put a person at ease, and convey, "I see and respect you as a person!"

Patients enjoy being recognized as an individual with a life beyond their illness or physical well-being. They respond positively when you remember something personal—that they just got married, that they took a vacation, that they changed jobs. Just the mention of one of these relevant topics brightens many people's days. And, when used as an ice breaker, this recognition has other positive effects. First, it says to the patient, "My doctor actually cares enough about me to remember this; I'm not just a number." This builds trust.

Also, if you and the patient spend a few moments discussing something important to him or her, it sends a deeper message—you aren't concerned only with the patient's physical problems.

Finally, these moments can serve to relax the patient and ready the patient for what may be a more anxiety-provoking discussion: the real reason they came to see you. Clearly, the more relaxed and comfortable the patient, the easier it will be for you to get the information you need for an accurate diagnosis.

As you know full well, not all patients are in control of their emotions and ready to discuss their illness the moment they enter your office, in spite of their relationship with you or your good nature.

Not all physicians agree

Some members of the medical community consider these brief encounters or moments of small talk to be unnecessary. They think, "Let's get down to the business of medicine and cut the chit-chat."

Some physicians admit to being shy—uncomfortable in social situations and far more comfortable talking about medicine about which they have more knowledge and control. Other physicians admit that they don't like initiating conversations that are too open-ended. Others say they are afraid of picking the wrong topic and upsetting the patient more. The challenge, then, is to find appropriate topics and have a versatile repertoire of openers that make shyness, the need for creativity, and risk less of an impediment.

Finding appropriate topics

Safe Subjects. There are a host of safe topics that can be used as ice breakers with patients with whom you have had very little experience or understanding. Weather, sports, geography, are all considered neutral. Local events—the neighborhood arts fair or parade, the opening of a store or mall, a town hero—are also easy topics to discuss. Certainly, the more information a physician has about a patient over time, the easier it becomes to initiate safe discussions around hobbies, family and common interests.

In many cases, it is ideal to pursue a topic, medical or nonmedical, that emerged during a previous visit. This may be about family members—"How's your husband doing with his diet" and "How's your ankle been"—may be openers and safe, if you are aware of the history and remember or note it.

Controversial Subjects. Discussions about current events or politics, unless you are aware of the patient's views, are certainly riskier, since you probably don't want to get into an intense discussion or debate with a patient. Even asking patients to share their views on subjects like movies, plays, and TV shows can make some people uncomfortable. They may be nervous about sharing their opinions because they fear your disapproval.

Comments on Appearance. Comments about appearance can be very risky, depending on how well you know the patient. If you know that your patient has been working hard to lose weight and is succeeding, it might be appropriate to remark, "Your diet seems to be working. You look wonderful." A less carefully worded, "Wow, have you lost weight" might imply, "And you really needed to." Even comments that convey your evaluation of obvious changes, e.g., "I love your hairdo" can be touchy. Whereas,"You changed your hair style. How does it feel?" tells the patient that you noticed something different, but lets the patient give more information. There is always the possibility that the patient hates the new 'do and feels unattractive.

Some physicians feel that greater liberties can be taken with either very young or older patients—patients who are perceived to be less or nonsexual. A physician who would not say, "You're really the type to wear short skirts" to a 40-year-old woman may feel that it would be appropriate to make this comment to a 12-year old.

If you listen to patients, you'll find that nothing could be further from the truth. Comments like these are out of line, regardless of the patient's age, and they tend to generate resentment.

Self-disclosure: When does it work?

Sometimes, revealing information about yourself, especially if you think the patient would relate to it, may be useful in initiating conversation. If you know the patient is from Boston, stating that you just got back from New England can be a nice opener. Remembering a hobby in common and using that as a springboard—"Planning on skiing out West this winter? I just got back from Vail"—works well. Needless to say, the extreme in self-disclosure is inappropriate—when doctors share their marital status, problems, and more. The danger in talking about yourself is greatest when you are really using the patient to talk about your own accomplishments, acquisitions, and problems. Further, discussing your expensive car with a patient who drives a used wreck certainly drives an unnecessary wedge in the relationship. Sound extreme? Patients can cite endless examples of offensive bits of self-disclosure on the part of doctors.

Comments about this visit

If a patient has been waiting an unusually long time, it is insensitive to make no reference to the wait and launch into "How's your tennis game?" A simple, "I'm sorry you had to wait" or "I hope this wait didn't create a big problem for you" shows that you are at least sensitive to the patient's feelings and respectful of their time. Offering excuses like, "Sorry about the wait. I had a patient with a real emotional problem," invites the patient to compare his or her problem with the problem of the previous patient. In many cases, the patient will feel less important and hurt.

Switching the focus

Ultimately, you must focus the conversation on the medical problem or objective of the visit. In most cases, this means you need to make a conscious transition. It's easy if the conversation has centered on medical issues; you can ask, "Is that why you're here today?" But, sometimes, transitions are more difficult, especially if you feel pressed for time. In that case, you might say, "Sounds like you had a great vacation, but I know you came here with something else on your mind" or "So, I'm curious to know, what brings you here today" Sometimes, you can make a transition by a few words of empathy, followed by a comment that's task-oriented, based on information in the patient's chart: "Sounds like you've been through a great deal lately. I notice that you're here because you haven't been sleeping. Do you see a connection here?"

Other ways to switch the focus, if the patient needs prompting:

- "I'm sorry I don't have more time to hear...."
- "Seems like a lot's going on for you. What do you want to focus on today?"
- "What brings you here today?"

Finally, if you feel unable to focus the conversation, you might consider leaving the room for a moment to do or get something. This will create a new chance to start afresh on the medical issue.

Pitfalls in switching from person to problem

What you hope to avoid is having the patient feel rejected or cut off by your redirection.

> A woman complains about being so upset about her husband's death that she is unable to sleep. The physician asks her if she had her blood pressure checked. The physician switched the focus, leaving the patient hanging, and probably missed some valuable information that needed to be pursued.

If you're sensitive to the patient's needs, and appreciate the effect of emotions on health, you need to find a more appropriate method.

Ask yourself: How do you feel about ways you introduce patients, get patient information, break the ice and put people at ease?

- Do I have a system for introducing patients that fits with my style and philosophy?
- Am I aware of the importance of my nonverbal behavior in putting people at ease?
- Do I have a system for taking a history that gives me the information I need about my patients?
- Am I comfortable initiating nonmedical conversations about the weather, etc.?
- Do I have a repertoire of safe subjects which I use to break the ice?
- Do I have a system of obtaining nonmedical information about my patients?
- Do I often bring up nonthreatening but personal pieces of information about my patients during the interviews?
- Do I know how to steer the conversation to the medical issue without offending my patients or leaving them stranded?

The little things you say and do speak volumes to patients. It's important to decide how you want people to feel when they meet you, and then carefully plan and monitor your practice so that the outcomes match your philosophy and personality. Everyone is different, and doctors will have different ways of putting patients at ease. The key question is: "Is it working for you and your patients?"

20

Communication Is a Two-Way Street

Much of the relationship that develops between a patient and physician is dependent on positive communication. In fact, three of the top five qualities that patients value about their physicians have to do with the physician's ability to communicate. Certainly a great deal of this communication takes place during the medical interview where the physician needs to get as much information as possible so that an appropriate diagnosis can be made and a course of treatment outlined. Each party, the patient and the physician, has a very important role to play if this interaction is to be successful. The physician's job is to create an environment where the patient feels safe enough to tell the physician extremely personal and/or painful things that he or she is feeling physically and emotionally so that this physician can treat the problem appropriately. The patient's job is to describe, as best as he or she can, symptoms and feelings related to these symptoms.

Sounds simple? Not really. The reality is that the basic communication model is so complex that even under ideal circumstances, there is an enormous margin for error and complication. Consider this example from Edward Krupat ("A Delicate Imbalance," *Psychology Today*, November 1986, p. 22):

> A middle-aged man has recently noticed a mole on his left shoulder. Uncertain whether it is just a minor skin problem or a sign of something serious, he makes an appointment with his physician. Arriving at the office, the man decides to begin by talking about his arthritis. His physician quickly picks up on this complaint and checks the patient out. He reassures the man that the medication he has prescribed will relieve some of his discomfort and begins to usher him out the door. A bit overwhelmed, the man looks for an opening to mention his real concern, but finds that the physician's efficient manner leaves him no room. His attempts to expand the conversation seem to fall on deaf ears. The patient leaves the office flustered and upset.

There are many things wrong in this example: the patient's inability to describe his real concern, the physician's inability to tell the whole story, the physician's seeming insensitivity to the patient's attempts to discuss the mole, and more. According to patients, the man's story typifies what can and does go wrong during many medical interviews that depend on the patient's ability to communicate with the physician and the physician's ability to interpret what the patient has said.

Unfortunately, because of the imprecise nature of this exchange and others like it, many physicians would prefer to rely as much as possible on technology, concluding that personal observations won't yield much. This is not a great solution, especially when you consider that getting accurate information is only part of the picture. There still is the issue of building a relationship, getting to know the person and handling the treatment, or therapy, all of which are dependent on communication skills. What makes more sense is to learn some of the key skills needed in communication and to refine especially those which you know cause difficulty. These skills are learnable. The pay-offs for you are fewer misunderstandings, fewer complications, and a great sense of personal achievement.

This chapter examines two sides of the communication coin:

- Communication from the patient to you, and
- Communication from you to the patient.

COMMUNICATION: FROM THE PATIENT TO YOU

Starting with all you need to learn from the patient, we'll examine skills: (1) listening, (2) asking questions, and (3) avoiding shutting the patient off.

Skill #1: Listening

It has been proven that the average person's listening effectiveness is only 25 percent. That means that we only really listen to and absorb 25 percent of what we hear. One reason for this is that the average person can process information at a rate of 75 miles per hour while most people only speak at a rate of 25 miles per hour. There is, then, room for us to be doing things other than "listening" when someone is talking to us. This "other activity" can be rehearsing what we're going to say, judging, wandering, problem-solving, or subliminally snoozing.

Becoming aware of traps

A first step to developing greater listening skills is to become aware of what you do during conversations with patients. Most people have a tendency to fall into one or more of the traps shown in Table 20–1.

If you fall into these traps, and *most* people do, catch yourself. You can consciously monitor your listening behavior and strengthen it.

Why bother?

Listening skills are crucial. Think of the benefits for the patient when you listen well. The patient:

1. Feels accepted as a person.
2. Is able to express himself or herself.
3. Feels less anxious or tense.
4. Feels good about you.
5. Becomes clearer about what is on his or her mind.

You reap just as many benefits. The doctor:

1. Develops a positive relationship with the patient.
2. Gains additional insights and understandings which enhance future communication.
3. Obtains a complete, accurate message and can act on it correctly, if action is needed.
4. Saves time in the long run by listening in the short run.
5. Gets to know problems, attitudes, feelings, interests, ambitions, hobbies, and many other things that can help you treat the patient.

Table 20–1. Listening Traps.

CHECK YOUR TRAP		
YES	NO	
		1. Does your mind tend to "wander" and think about something else when you are supposedly listening to a patient?
		2. Do you tune the patient out in order to prepare your response?
		3. Are you often so wrapped up in your own feelings that it's impossible to get outside of yourself to really listen to your patient?
		4. Do you tend to jump ahead of the patient and reach conclusions before you've heard them out?
		5. Do you often figure you know what the patient is going to say, before you have listened?
		6. Are you anxious to contribute your ideas to the conversation, or relate your experiences or observations when the patient is trying to talk?
		7. Do you have a tendency to finish sentences or supply other words for the patient?
		8. Do you get caught up in insignificant facts and details and miss the emotional tone of the conversation?
		9. Do you listen with half your attention tuned toward giving advice, solving the problem, or figuring out what to say to make the patient feel better?

Elements of good listening

You know when you've been listened to well by another; and you can probably point to people who are great listeners. But listening is not a simple skill. It involves a set of subskills, each of which can be learned. Consider first the nonverbal behaviors often associated with good listening.

Nonverbal Behaviors.

1. Looking and acting interested
2. Facing the speaker with an open posture, at a fairly close distance
3. Leaning forward
4. Making good, warm eye contact
5. Nodding your head to show understanding
6. Making a facial expression that matches the speaker's message
7. Using a tone of voice that shows understanding
8. Clearing your own head of distractions

Now, consider these important verbal behaviors—what you, the listener, say.

Verbal Behaviors.

1. *Asking questions*, when needed, to help understand the patient better. This encourages the patient and shows you're listening. (Example: "Is that what you came in for today?")
2. *Commenting* briefly on something the patient said.
3. *"Door openers"*—phrases that show interest and help the patient to open up. (Example: "Go ahead" or "Tell me what's on your mind")
4. *Paraphrasing*—reflecting back to the patient in your own words what you understood the patient to have said. This is a *very important* verbal behavior. (Example: "You say that a lot is going on for you and you have several concerns . . .") When you paraphrase, you let the patient know you've understood the message. Or, if you haven't, it gives you and the patient the chance to achieve clarity.
5. *Empathizing*—listening with the heart and reflecting back to the speaker what you think he or she is *feeling* behind their verbal message. (Example: "You sound pretty excited . . .") Empathizing involves putting yourself in the role of the other in order to feel what the other seems to be feeling. Sometimes, in reflecting it back, you hit the speaker's feeling right on the nose! Other times, you might not get the feeling quite right, but then the speaker has the chance to say how he or she really feels. And, you've increased the understanding and trust between you and the speaker.

Recall the patient with the mole, this time interacting with a physician who is truly listening.

> *Patient: (anxious)* Boy, am I glad I could see you today, Doctor!

Doctor: You sound pretty concerned. What can I do for you?

Patient: I've got a lot on my mind. I've been under pressure at work. I'm concerned about a few things—healthwise—and, of course, my arthritis hasn't been making it very easy for me.

Doctor: You say that a lot is going on for you and you have several concerns, including your arthritis. Is that what you came in for today?

Patient: Well, not really. I mean, there are several things. I'd like to check the medication for my arthritis, but that's not the only reason. I'm not sure. . . ."

Doctor: I can certainly check your medication, but it sounds as though you're concerned about some other problem, too.

Patient: Well, kind of. Really, one problem. I mean, I don't know if it's important or not. I just want to know if it's something for me to worry about.

Doctor: So, you'd like some clarification. Fine. Tell me what's on your mind.

Patient: "Well, I have this mole, and I know that they can be serious if they change size or color.

This doctor was able to help the patient focus on the real problem. The doctor:

1. Asked questions to help the patient become clearer.
2. Repeated the patient's phrases for clarification.
3. Shared understanding of the patient's feelings and emotions.

Roadblocks to listening

There are several pitfalls that can interfere with effective listening to patients. To avoid these:

1. Don't interrupt the patient.
2. Don't offer advice or solutions until you have listened, and unless it's asked for.
3. Don't get off the track by telling *your* story, when the patient needs to tell his or hers.
4. Don't morally judge the patient.
5. Don't deny what the patient is feeling. (Example: "Oh, don't be upset. Calm down, there's nothing to worry about," or "You shouldn't feel that way.")

6. Don't doodle, tap, or shuffle papers. Give your full attention.

When you listen well, you encourage patients to share more easily the things they want to talk about. The opposite is also true. If you don't listen, you impede the flow of information *you* need to do *your* job.

Also, by listening to patients, you create a climate in which your patient will be *more willing to listen to you.*

Skill #2: Asking questions

Another important skill needed to elicit information from patients involves asking questions. As Edward Krupat reports in "A Delicate Imbalance," *Psychology Today*, November 1986, p. 24: "In one of the most comprehensive studies of its kind, Patrick Byrne and Barrie Long, physicians in the Department of General Practice in Manchester, England, collected and analyzed 2,500 medical interviews conducted by British, Dutch, and Irish physicians. They identified four distinct styles of interaction, ranging from physician-centered to patient-centered. The physician-centered style fits the high control, "I'm in charge" approach. The physician asks direct questions requiring yes or no answers that follow a predetermined concept of what information is important. The cadence of the interview is clipped, involving a good deal of one-syllable responses from the patient.

This conversational style derives from a disease-oriented view of healthcare, according to epidemiologist Moira Stewart and her colleagues at the University of Western Ontario. The goal is to establish a relationship between the patient's complaint and some form of organic pathology, and the best way to do that is to let the expert determine what is relevant and what isn't.

At the opposite extreme is the patient-centered style in which patients are questioned in an open-ended manner so that they can determine what is important to relate. The physician avoids jargon, asks for clarification and permits (even encourages) joint decision-making. In essence, the physician tries to understand the meaning of the illness from the patient's point of view. Not surprisingly, patients are more likely to adhere to medication or behavior-modification programs when approached in this way. The skill: Open-Ended Questioning.

A not insignificant difference

Consider the case of the open-ended question versus the closed-ended question. How much freedom or restriction does the question offer?

- Did you sleep well last night?—Yes/No (Closed)
- How did you sleep last night?—Fine/OK/Not so well (Better, you've offered alternatives.)

- Tell me about your night. "Well, I was somewhat restless because of the arthritis pain, but after the night nurse gave me my medication, I slept soundly and I'm less tired today." (Open)

The open question affords the patient an opportunity to select the answer from a vast array of possible answers. You have, therefore, communicated that the patient has freedom, control, and responsibility for participating. This allows the patient to reveal a frame of reference and select the elements of greatest concern.

Here's another example of open versus closed questions:

- Do you think there are some advantages in having this operation? (Closed)
- What do you see as the advantages or disadvantages of having this operation? (Open)

When to use open vs. closed questions

Frequently, the situation calls for an initial open-ended question to yield the greatest amount of information, followed by more specific questions to fill in the details.

For instance, sophisticated people with a clear grasp of their role respond well to open-ended questions. Other respondents may need more structure and respond better to closed-ended questions. Obviously, the admissions clerk with 15 minutes to complete a long form would not ask open-ended questions, so discretion must be used according to job type and situation.

Watch yourself closely to see if you are forming leading rather than neutral questions. Leading questions will communicate some expectation about the nature of the answer; for example, "Have you had any pain?" The neutral question would generalize, "Tell me about any physical changes you've experienced lately." The leading question, "Well, you're making terrific progress, don't you think?" vs. "What progress, if any, do you think you are making?"

Additional tips

- Questions that ask "why" are tough to answer. Most people don't know why and get frustrated trying to explain. Ask "what" or "how" instead.
- Try not to ask "double-barreled" questions; for example, "Do you have insurance and do you have your card with you?" The answer could be "Yes, yes," "Yes, no," "No, no." Multiple questions like that confuse both the asker and the responder.

- Beware of asking "leading" rather than neutral questions. Leading questions communicate an expectation about the nature of the answer. The leading question, "You're making terrific progress, don't you think?" vs. "What progress, if any, do you think you are making?"
- Allow plenty of time for response. You asked the question, so listen to the answer. Don't cut people off.
- If the patient's answer wanders, redirect their ideas and provide focus by kindly asking, "Could we talk about ... now?"
- If the answer is not clear, ask for additional information or clarification. "When you said ... did you mean ...?"
- Elicit feelings. "You seem to be very upset about your medication."
- Provide alternatives. Ask, "Have you considered ...?" Above all, invite the patient to ask you questions.

You may get some unexpected and highly rewarding open-ended results.

Pitfalls in questioning

As reported by Anthony Astrachan in "Five Ways to Blow a Patient Interview" (*Medical Economics*, June 20, 1988, p. 116), research shows that in the most crucial moments of an interview—at the beginning and at the point when the patient describes the problem—most doctors interrupt or dominate the conversation. The result: the patient stops sharing information. This does more than impede the physician's ability to diagnose accurately. It also alienates the patient, diminishing the probability that the patient will cooperate with the treatment—and increasing the likelihood of malpractice suits later.

In explaining why they interrupt, physicians point to:

- The need to focus
- The need to redirect
- The need to get specific
- The need to give answers
- The need to remove anxiety

And many point to what may be a most pressing need: the need to save time. Unfortunately, little time in the long run is saved and much may be lost by interrupting the patient.

Twenty ways to shut people up

Consider these twenty surefire techniques for shutting up patients—inappropriately (adapted from "Communication Workshop" by Muriel Schiffman, *Explorations*, 13, 1967.)

1. *Reassuring rather than showing understanding*
   Example: "Oh, I didn't think you would take it so hard."
   Hidden Message: You're pretty stupid to feel that way.

2. *Justifying one's self*
   Example: "Now look, I didn't mean it that way."
   Hidden Message: You've no right to feel that way about me.

3. *Being Condescending*
   Example: "Tell me about it, dear, so I can help you."
   Hidden Message: I'm so strong and you're so weak.

4. *Blackmailing*
   Example: "Do you *have* to make people so nervous?"
   Hidden Message: You're so downright insensitive.

5. *Responding too soon*
   Example: "Oh, OK, I know how you feel; you don't have to spell it out."
   Hidden Message: I don't want to hear you. Please stop feeling.

6. *Interpreting*
   Example: "What you mean to say is . . . ."
   Hidden Message: I'm so clever and you're such a clod.

7. *Punishing*
   Example: "Oh, yeah! Well, let me tell you how *I* see it."
   Hidden Message: I'll get you, you dirty rat.

8. *Pretending to be stupid*
   Example: "That's your problem."
   Hidden Message: I'm not interested. Why don't you shut up.

9. *Passing the buck*
   Example: "That's your problem."
   Hidden Message: Don't count on me for help. I don't want to get involved.

10. *Responding to content rather than to feeling*
    Example: "That's certainly not a very good reason for feeling that way."
    Hidden Message: If it isn't rational, it doesn't count.

11. *Playing Lawyer*
    Example: "When did I say that? What were my exact words?"
    Hidden Message: Your impression isn't important. It's the facts that count.

12. *Joking as a response to feelings*
    Example: "You remind me of a wilted vine."
    Hidden Message: You're not worth taking seriously.

13. *Scolding*
    Example: "That's very rude."
    Hidden Message: You're a vulgar child.

14. *Showing inattention*
    Example: "My mind wandered. What were you saying."
    Hidden Message: You're really not very important to me.

15. *Deadpan*
    Example: No response.
    Hidden Message: Either say something important or keep quiet.

16. *Priming the pump*
    Example: "Don't you think that ....?"
    Hidden Message: I want to use you as a foil to make my point.

17. *Interrupting with your own point*
    Example: "That reminds me of what happened once to me."
    Hidden Message: Let me in the conversation on my terms.

18. *Scolding an aggressor*
    Example: "Just a minute, George. You can't talk to Sam like that."
    Hidden Message: You're evil, George. You're weak, Sam. I'm strong.

19. *Helping too soon*
    Example: "Now hold it. I think I can clear this up"
    Hidden Message: I'm coming. Give up and let me save you.

20. *Changing a subject before it is fully explored*
    Example: "This isn't going to get us anywhere. Now what I think is ...."
    Hidden Message: You're not doing anything worthwhile, and I know better than you what is worthwhile.

When physicians engage in these behaviors, patients tend to falter in their disclosure.

PUTTING IT ALL TOGETHER

Here is an example of how good, active listening, coupled with appropriate questioning, helped a troubled patient unravel a complicated story.

> Margaret Lorkin is an intelligent, articulate woman in her late forties. She came to Dr. Potter with a concern about a small, festering sore on her elbow. In response to Dr. Potter's questions, Ms. Lorkin said that she had this lump for more than five years, ever since she

had been struck by a golf-ball. She added that the sore had been festering for about two weeks. Ms. Lorkin said she knew she should have seen a doctor sooner, since she suspected there was a bone splintered or some other bone problem. By astutely observing her nonverbal signals, Dr. Potter surmised that Ms. Lorkin was distraught far beyond the distress expected with a sore like this and asked if anything else was bothering her. She answered, "Anything else? Not that I know of. No, not really, nothing at all." After a short silence, she added, "Well, I have been quite tired lately." She then spoke about feeling exhausted, anxious, and not eating well for more than a month. She attributed this to changing her job, even though that change had occurred almost a year earlier. Gradually, through calm, accepting questioning and supportive listening, Dr. Potter learned that Ms. Lorkin had, only a month earlier, lost a brother to cancer after very sudden onset and several months of painful and rapid decline. While Ms. Lorkin had visited her brother twice a month during his long illness, even though she lived more than 300 miles away, still she suffered profound distress because she had not reached him to be with him when he died.

This relatively brief interview, sensitive, nonjudgmental questioning, and empathetic listening by the physician made possible the diagnosis of cancer-phobia, a problem for which the patient did not know how to seek help. Instead, the patient visited her physician to be treated for the sore, a problem legitimate in the patient's eyes.

Communicating with patients is indeed an art and one that requires substantial skill and attention. It may take time and patience to practice and develop these skills, but the payoff in the long run is appreciative patients who feel listened to, valued, supported, understood, and involved.

Ask yourself:

- Do I understand the importance of being a good listener?
- Am I aware of what it takes for me to be a good listener?
- Do I demonstrate positive nonverbal behaviors while listening to patients?
- When listening to patients, do I ask appropriate questions and avoid questions which will detour or side-track?
- When listening to patients, do I know how to paraphrase what patients say and respond with empathy?
- Do I know the difference between open and closed-ended questions and use both effectively when needed?

- Do I know what behaviors "shut people up," and do I monitor my own behavior and responses?

FROM YOU TO THE PATIENT: HOW TO COMMUNICATE INFORMATION

The other side of the communication coin involves communication from you to the patient. To feel confident and clear about what you can tell patients about their concern, and to comply with your recommendations, the patient must understand you. This means you need to convey information well and make sure the patient has absorbed it or received the message you thought you conveyed (see Figure 20–1).

This chapter examines the four components involved in this process: (1) explaining, (2) checking for understanding, (3) body language, and (4) following up on the patient.

Explaining a diagnosis and treatments

The key to explaining to the patient the diagnosis and your recommended course of treatment is to think on a complex level, yet speak simply. There is just as much room for misunderstanding and confusion when you explain a diagnosis to a patient as when the patient explains his or her symptoms to you.

Although certain techniques can make the transformation of information easier for both the patient and you, a great deal rests with your basic philosophy. How much information do you want to give? How much information does the patient need, want, and deserve to know? And what methods do you feel comfortable using to convey this information?

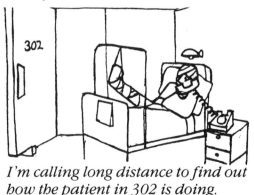

I'm calling long distance to find out how the patient in 302 is doing.

Figure 20–1. Communicating information to patients.

The four step model for explaining

Consider this four step model for explaining a diagnosis:

Step 1: Review and summarize what's been done and the outcome of these procedures. This step gives the patient a sense of history and places your findings in context. Example: "Mrs. Jones, as you know we did your tests. . . ." Label each action and its result. That certainly gives more information than "Mrs. Jones, you have . . ."

Step 2: Label the condition and explain what it means. Example: "Mary Walker, you have a small fibroid mass in the uterine wall. This is a type of tissue, like scar tissue, but it tends to increase in size over time. The tissue is nonmalignant, and we will be observing it when you come in for your regular examinations."

In most cases you need to explain fully what the condition is. It is extremely important at this point to use language and examples that make sense to the patient. This is difficult for many physicians, because they feel that the explanation will be too complex, and that it will only confuse the patient or cause unnecessary anxiety.

But because of the urgency that the patient understand his or her situation, you need to experiment with ways to convey information fully. Here are options:

- Ask the patient if he or she would like more information.
- Show a model of the relevant body parts and illustrate the problem.
- Draw pictures for the patient.
- Keep a file of short, easy to understand readings that will further the patient's knowledge.
- Ask the patient directly what he or she has heard about the condition, or if he or she has ever known anyone with the problem. Start from their—patients— understanding. This allows you to visualize the patient's knowledge base and lets you untangle any myths or misconceptions. Invariably, these medical myths affect the patient's ability to either comprehend your explanation of the disease or follow your treatment plan. Keep in mind that patients will not feel comfortable sharing this information with you if they are made to feel stupid in any way. You need to assume a position of neutrality and interest no matter how misguided the information.
- Help patients seek better information.

Dr. Sheldon Greenfield, in a study at UCLA Medical Center (reported in Anthony Astrachan, "Five Ways to Blow a Patient Interview," *Medical Economics*, June 20, 1988, p. 125), found that patients could be educated to ask questions about their ailments, thereby taking more of the responsibility for getting needed information. In his study of 87 peptic ulcer patients, the group that received training had fewer episodes of ulcer pain and fewer limitations to their work. In short, they had a greater understanding of their disease and what it meant to their lives.

Explaining an illness is complicated, and this phase often takes more time than the physician can spend at one visit. It's important, however, not to leave the patient stranded. Arranging for another appointment time—a time to talk—can help in two ways. It can give the patient time to digest what you've already said and to collect questions; it also gives you time to figure out what this patient may need in order to understand better and act on their condition.

Step 3: Explain the course of treatment. After the patient understands his or her condition, outline the treatment plan, clarifying what you will do and what the patient needs to do. Often, this is a good time to include family members, especially if the treatment involves any lifestyle or relationship changes. If the course of treatment is complicated, having another person present might help achieve understanding. Many physicians use written instructions at this point, since, clearly, there is a great deal of room for error and misunderstanding.

Does "take this pill every four hours" mean take it six times a day including during the night? Or does four times a day mean every six hours? Many doctors are unclear about this procedure, and patients feel uncomfortable asking questions. Instructions for further tests and studies can be equally confusing. Patients should be told when and where to complete the tests and instructions, when and how to call for results, and what to do to follow through.

Understanding involves a partnership

The point is that only if you and your patients have established a true partnership and only if your patients feel secure in their understandings will they follow through as you intend.

The studies on compliance are really quite astounding. The numbers of patients who ignore instructions, fail to take their medications, and confuse the physician's guidelines are staggering. Obviously, this leads to a great deal of frustration for both patient and physicians.

A study done by Hulka and associates examined the level of compliance and concordance between patients and their physicians who prescribe medication. What they found was that "neither characteristics of patients nor the severity of disease were influential in determining the extent of medication errors. For patients with congestive heart failure, good communication of instructions and information from physician to patient was associated with low levels of all types of errors" (*American Journal of Public Health*, 66, 1976, pp. 847–853).

Many doctors don't trust the patient's ability or willingness to do what it takes to get better. Physicians' biases can influence how they outline the course of treatment and how much time and energy they devote to discussion and explanation. Often these biases are unfair and are used as an excuse for the physician not to be more careful.

The problem of medical jargon

A patient is in the hospital and he's scared. He's in a strange environment, surrounded by people he doesn't know and all kinds of ominous machinery. All he wants to know is more about his condition, when a doctor walks in and asks, "So you say that your symptoms include post tussive thoracic myalgia compounded by acute costochondritis with radicular dysaethesia?"

"My God, no!" he replies. "All I said is that my chest hurts from coughing and my ribs are sore."

"That's what I just said," the doctor answers.

That is what the doctor had just said. Patients are not medical experts. They don't know the jargon, nor should they be expected to. Specialized terminology confuses, intimidates, and frustrates. It also may create a barrier that is difficult to bridge. It's the physician's responsibility to *facilitate* communication, not obscure it. If you listen to a patient's chest and tell the patient that you want him to get an ultrasound for heart to confirm a suspected microvalve prolapse, the patient may jump to conclusions and suspect major heart problems when you are testing for a heart murmur or floppy valve.

Ergo, it is herewith promulgated that obfuscating verbalism be expurgated from all articulations.

Which is to say, *talk straight*.

Step 4. Check back for understanding. Your goals in explanations are simple. Give the facts in a way that will:

1. Educate the patient about the condition.
2. Explain what steps can be taken, so that compliance is likely.

Because there are so many roadblocks to communication, it is necessary to go to extra lengths to ensure that patients really understand you.

How to check for understanding

To make sure you've been understood, two techniques are particularly helpful: (1) using direct questions and (2) asking patients to repeat.

Using Direct Questions. To ascertain patient understanding, ask patients to respond to a simple closed-ended question. "Did you understand or follow what I've said so far?" or "Are you with me?" This method is only effective if you know you can trust their response. It does give them a chance to express confusion or ask questions.

An open-ended question like "What did you understand about this description/explanation?" tells you much more. It invites the patient to frame the information in his or her own way, and you can listen for confusion, inaccuracies, or omissions.

Asking Patients To Repeat. A more targeted approach is to ask patients to repeat for you what you have told them. In this way, you are taking an even greater step to test for clarity. You might say, "I've tried to explain what I think is important for you to know about your condition. Would you mind telling me what you've understood me to say, so I can make sure I've been clear?"

Disclaimers Make It Easier. Some physicians feel awkward asking patients to repeat what they've heard. They feel this might insult the patient's intelligence or put them on the spot. You can avoid these possibilities in three ways:

1. *Blame it on the content:* "This regimen is really confusing and I want to make sure that you understand all of the instructions."
2. *Place the patient in good company:* "Many people are confused by this explanation."
3. *Blame it on your explanation:* "I've just given you a great deal of information, and I want to make sure that I was clear."

But I Told Them Already. The bottom line is that patients need to understand fully:

- The tests they've been given and the results
- The complete diagnosis
- The treatment plan
- What is required of them

If they don't fully grasp this key information, problems arise, either in the form of noncompliance, further attempts by patients to achieve clarity (e.g., through phone calls), and an increase in anxiety and frustration.

You need to *plan* ways to deliver information to patients not once, but several times, and in several different ways, oral and written. Then, you need to make sure the information you conveyed was absorbed by the people who need to act on it.

Encourage questions

The more questions patients ask and get answered, the more involved they feel, and the more you know about their understanding. But this is easier said than done.

A physician shared a frustration: "I'm always hearing, 'Let patients ask questions,' and I think I do. I always say, 'Do you have any questions?' But often they don't, or they don't share them with me. Then, I hear later that so and so said I didn't answer any questions. It's a no-win situation. If they don't ask, I can't answer. What am I expected to be—a mind reader?"

Absolutely not, but you are expected to understand why patients may not be asking questions and what you can do about it.

1. *They are on overload.* Sometimes, patients have so many questions, they may not know what to ask first. This is very common after a complex diagnosis has just been explained. The patient has been bombarded with information and needs time to sort it out. A good thing to say is, "I've just given you a great deal of information, and you may want to think first to get your questions together."

2. *They are in shock.* Sometimes, patients need permission to collect themselves. They also may need you to help define the appropriate way they can ask questions. "You've just been given some hard news" or "This has been quite a shock, and you probably have many questions, but now may not be the best time."

3. *They are afraid of getting confused or not asking the right questions.* Often it helps to suggest that they write the questions on paper first.

4. *They are afraid they won't hear the answers.* Again, writing can help. You can give them something in writing to clarify the explanation.

5. *They are afraid of looking foolish.* You need to let them know that it takes courage to ask. Foolish people assume or guess.

6. *They aren't sure you want them to ask questions.* One good reason patients may not ask questions directly is *bad history*. They haven't had success getting straight, easy to understand answers, so they are turned off.

Information is power

In short, your effectiveness rests in large part on your ability to convey needed information and, in so doing, to spark purposeful, responsible action and compliance on the part of your patients. By taking pains to give careful explanations using whatever medium the patient can understand, you save time and anguish—yours and the patient's.

And, since even the best explanations sometimes may not be grasped or absorbed by the patient, you can benefit from building into your communication process a feedback loop from the patient to you—a feedback loop that tells you not what you said, but what's been heard.

Body language

"Actions speak louder than words." In the area of physician-patient communication, "how you say what you say" is even more powerful than "what you say." In this chapter, we examine nonverbal behaviors and gestures, often subtle and subliminal, that have a demonstrated impact on patient comfort, confidence, and satisfaction.

Imagine this: you are visiting a patient in the hospital—you rush in, pick up the chart, glance quickly at the patient in the bed, and say, "I'm glad to see you this morning." You may be, but the patient won't believe you because your body language says something else.

If, on the other hand, you enter the a patient's room, pull up a chair or sit on the bed, look the patient in the eye, place your hand on their arm, and say, "I heard you had a rough night. Why don't you tell me about it," the patient believes that you want to hear his or her story, that you care about them.

Your gestures are powerful and can work for you or against you. It pays to examine the messages you send nonverbally and make certain you are "saying" what you really mean. Table 20–2 should help you identify the way in which patients interpret particular nonverbal signals.

Nonverbal behaviors fall into two categories: those that offend or repel others and those that encourage or attract others. Each of these behaviors can be helpful and appropriate in certain situations.

Behaviors That Offend. Certainly, there are times when you want to choose body language that says "stay away." Perhaps you feel the patient is getting too close and dependent or too hostile and aggressive. At times like these, you might want to gain control of the situation by turning away, standing up or even leaving the room.

Behaviors That Attract. Eye contact, smiling, and head nodding when patients are talking are all ways to say "you're important." Also not to be underestimated is the importance of touching and hand-holding.

Table 20–2. Patient Interpretation of Nonverbal Signals.

TYPES	POSSIBLE INTERPRETATIONS
Eye Behaviors	
eye contact	
a. steady, warm	a. I'm listening (or I like you)
b. staring	b. You're weird (or I hate you)
c. none or fleeting	c. I'm bored (or I'm anxious or I'm resistant)
peering over glasses	I'm skeptical
one eyebrow raised	I disapprove (or I don't believe you)
Gestures	
drumming, tapping pencil	Hurry up, I'm impatient (or you bother me)
clenched fist	I'm angry (or I'm tense)
relaxed	I'm open to you (or I feel relaxed)
a. firm hand on other's hand, arm or shoulder	a. I care about you (or I feel you're important)
b. none	b. I want to keep my distance
pointing finger	I'm blaming you (or now, you get this)
Postures	
direction	
a. facing other	a. I like you (or, I'm straight with you)
b. turned away from other	b. I want to avoid you
slouched	I'm relaxed (or I don't take this conversation seriously)
erect	I'm on edge or I take this coversation seriously
forward lean	I'm interested
backward lean	So what . . .
open arms or legs—	I like you (or, I'm relaxed)
closed arms or legs—	I don't like you (or, I'm feeling defensive)

Table 20–2. Patient Interpretation of Nonverbal Signals *(cont.).*

TYPES	POSSIBLE INTERPRETATIONS
Physical Distancing	
closeness	I feel warm and friendly (or, I'm trying to intimidate you)
far away	I feel distant (or I feel superior)
above the other	I am superior
below the other	I am beneath you
at same level	We are equals
Head Behaviors	
nodding	I agree (or, I understand)
head shaking	I disagree (or, I'm confused)
cocking head to one side	I doubt it (or, I'm amused, or I'm listening)
Facial Expressions	
smile	I like you (or, I want your approval)
frown	I'm confused (or, I don't like this, or I don't like you)
clenched teeth	I'm tense (or, I'm feeling threatened)
open mouth	I'm relaxed (or, I'm suprised or in wonder)
curled lip	I'm disgusted (or, I'm mocking you)
Vocal qualities (pitch, volume, rate, quality of voice)	
high pitch	I'm nervous (or, I'm angry, I don't really believe in myself)
low pitch	I feel firm and confident
fast rate, no stops	I'm excited (or, I'm afraid someone will try to interrupt me)
softness	I feel affection (or, I'm afraid of offending anyone)
monotone	I am bored
cracked voice	I'm nervous

Following up with patients

"My six-month old baby woke up one night with a fever of 103°. I tried everything to get her fever down and calm her. Nothing worked. Out of desperation, I called my pediatrician at 4:00 AM at home. Was I surprised when she answered the phone! She gave me instructions, and told me to call again in several hours. At 7:30 AM, the phone rang. 'Mrs. Smith, how are you and the baby?' "

Another patient describes a message her physician left on an answering machine. "Hi, Ms. Landen. This is Dr. Jones. I'm calling to see if the tetracycline worked for your strep throat. I guess it did, since you're well enough to be up and about. Glad to hear it."

Some physicians might consider these actions on the part of physicians as either time-consuming or insignificant. However, the personal touch or "check back" may be just the thing to help the patient feel important, to check on compliance and results, and to remind the patient of the need for a return visit.

Many patients are told, "Take this medication and make an appointment to see me in two weeks." The patient might take the medication, but how many don't make the appointment?

Certainly not all of your patients need a personal call, but many doctors initiate several quick check-up calls to patients each day.

According to physicians who swear by them, these calls differ from return calls initiated by patients. These check-back calls are your spontaneous way to say, "I care" and "I'm taking responsibility for helping you become or remain healthy."

The Bottom Line. Effective communication from you to the patient—it requires commitment, skill, and initiative.

Ask yourself:

- Do you explain what you're doing to the patient to ease their anxiety?
- Do you review and summarize what's been done and the outcomes?
- Do you explain the condition and what it means?
- Do you explain the course of treatment and what the patient can expect to experience?
- Do you avoid obscure, intimidating terminology and ask the patient direct questions to ensure understanding of what you've said?
- Do you ask the patient to repeat back to you what they need to do?

- Do you encourage patients to ask questions?
- Do you consciously use nonverbal behaviors and gestures?
- Do you use multiple methods to explain things, so you are sure to be successful?
- Do you feel so committed to giving your patients thorough information in a form they understand that you devote time and energy to it, without resenting their need to know?
- Do you take initiative?

Effective communication—from you to the patient—requires, first of all, commitment. If you're concerned about patient satisfaction and patient involvement in their own care, then thorough, careful communication is a must. And this takes skill, time, and creative initiative.

21

Dignity and How To Preserve It

A 64-year-old male suffered a severe stroke, paralyzing the left side of his body. His family, including his wife and 30-year-old daughter, worried, "Will Dad get better? How will we afford his care? Is Dad getting the best medical attention? Is this paralysis temporary?" and more. The family was accustomed to the hospital routine, many rotating physicians, endless questions, countless pushing and probing, and very few answers from those who were handling the patient's case. The family waited interminably for a kind word or a glimmer of hope. One afternoon, two weeks after the attack, their daughter experienced what she described as the ultimate violation to her father's dignity.

> Dr. Smith, the chief attending on the case, entered the room during visiting hours, followed by nine physicians in white coats. We were seated by the bed. Dr. Smith grimaced in our direction and said to his entourage, "Come on in; step around!" He didn't introduce the others. He never spoke to us. He said to the others, "This patient had a stroke two weeks ago. He's conscious of his surroundings, but isn't able to open his eyes at this point." Dr. Smith never addressed

my father. He then proceeded to pick up my Dad's arm, raised it as high as he could, and suddenly let go of it, allowing Dad's arm to fall with a *thud* on the bed. He made a point of exclaiming to the other *physicians*, "Can you believe that? Did you see that?" The group "oohed" and "aahed." Then, they turned and left—without ever acknowledging us. We sat at the foot of Dad's bed and cried, horrified at what we had just witnessed. Then, we had to explain to Dad, who was indeed conscious, what had happened, since he could hear the words that were said, but had no idea who said them and why.

A young woman went for a prenatal ultrasound. Her physician entered the room where she was lying, undressed, and cheerfully introduced her to Bud Smith (a young gentleman wearing a white coat), who would be watching the exam. Later, in her physician's office, she asked, "When did you bring on your new assistant?" meaning Dr. Smith. Her physician laughed, "Oh, he's not a doctor. His company makes the ultrasound equipment!" The patient was humiliated and prayed that she would never see Bud Smith again.

An elderly patient visits her doctor. Because the patient cannot drive, she is brought in by her daughter. The doctor asks the daughter to be present during the examination. The physician ignores the patient, instead directing all questions to the daughter, giving her all explanations, and handing her the medication instructions.

In these examples, physicians neglected to recognize the patient as an individual with feelings and needs (see Figures 21–1 and 21–2). In the first example, the patient felt like a specimen, a useful tool for the purpose of educating future doctors. In the second example, the young pregnant mother had to suffer the embarrassment of being exposed in front of a nonphysician. And, in the final case, the elderly patient was viewed by her physician as being incapable of logic and reason.

These are negative stories and there are many more. But there are certainly many positive stories, too.

A stroke patient had a gag reflex problem and was afraid to try to swallow any liquids. He was visited one evening by his doctor. "If you could have *anything* to drink now, what liquid would you wish for?" his physician asked. "A Rolling Rock," muttered the patient dreamily. "Hang on," was the doctor's reply. The doctor returned 15 minutes later with two cold beers, sat down next to the patient, and said, "Glad you thought of this. I needed a break today." The doctor also put instructions on the chart for the patient to be given a beer the following evening.

An obstetrical patient was extremely impressed with her experience delivering her first baby. Her doctor was present for most of the 18 hours, even though

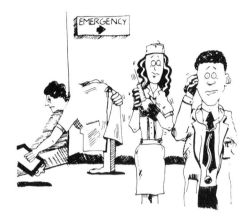

Figure 21–1. Preserving patient dignity.

he hadn't seen his family for more than 24 hours. He actually had his wife and kids come to the hospital for dinner, saying to the patient, "Please don't be frightened. I'm not leaving you. I'm only a beeper and one floor away."

Examples abound of patients being treated as individuals with dignity and respect. But it's the negative instances that stick in people's craws. And they can be avoided.

This section examines steps successful physicians take to preserve the dignity of their patients. We address issues of privacy and confidentiality, when and how to involve patients in their care, ways to give choices, and how to prevent patients from feeling like just a number.

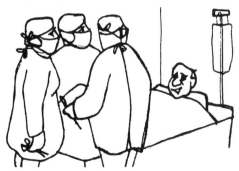

I don't mean to pry, but would you mind telling me how I'm doing?

Figure 21–2. Providing the patient with information.

RESPECT FOR PHYSICAL PRIVACY

Patients complain bitterly about what they believe to be unnecessary violations of privacy and the feeling they get from some doctors that patients "shouldn't be sensitive." The fact is, patients *are* sensitive about being exposed and vulnerable, and physicians can let their patients know they understand and respect this feeling. Four strategies, each extremely simple, help patients avoid exposure and the embarrassment that might result:

- Knocking on doors
- Covering up
- Separating the exam and the consult
- Limiting the people viewing the patient

Knocking on doors

Whether in your office or in the hospital during rounds, it is respectful to knock on doors and to announce that you are entering a room. Patients would rather lie on the table in the exam room, covered only by a paper sheet, than to be observed in the process of getting undressed. A simple "May I come in?" works fine.

Covering up

Regarding undressing, ask patients to undress or uncover as little of themselves as possible. "You only need to undress from the waist up" is far more respectful of privacy than asking patients to take off unnecessary articles of clothing that are really not in the way.

If a patient must disrobe completely, use the gown or sheet to cover parts of the body not being examined. Your message: "I understand that it's uncomfortable for you, and I want to do all I can to put you at ease."

Separating the exam and the consult

When you suggest, "Get dressed and come into my office," you allow your patients time to collect themselves before conversing with you. Dressed, patients feel more equal, more composed, and better able to concentrate on the discussion. When they are not fixated on being undressed, they can give and receive information, ask questions, and complete their visit more effectively.

Limiting the number of people viewing the patient

Generally, patients don't like being on exhibition. If a patient must be seen by others such as students or residents, it's important to pay attention to these points:

1. Ask the patient's permission.
2. Introduce all other staff.
3. Describe the procedure or exam before beginning.

Also, most physicians agree that it's advisable to have a female nurse present when a male physician is conducting an internal examination on a female patient. Patients have said that the female nurse makes them feel more comfortable, and it also protects the male physician.

INVOLVING THE PATIENT

Beyond steps you take to protect a patient's physical privacy, you can go further to protect their dignity and convey respect by involving them in their case. It is important to involve patients in their care because: (1) they have the right, (2) you need their attention and cooperation, and (3) you show respect.

Some of the burden physicians feel in working with patients is brought on by the physicians' notion that they are entirely responsible for what transpires between them and their patients. The language used to describe these medical encounters betrays this attitude. We "do a physical." We "take a history." The patients "get a treatment."

What is obscured by this language is the fact that you actually rely on the patient to help you in the medical encounter. You and the patient together develop a history. An examination is a process in which the patient's participation is vital. Treatments do not occur in a vacuum; not only must the patient show up, but often they are part of the treatment and are required to follow complex instructions.

When you think of patient involvement as a positive exchange that helps you, you can engage the patient in more positive ways. And most patients want this approach. So often, negative encounters with their physicians stem from the lack of awareness of their involvement, their feelings, and their ability to add something to the exchange.

Implicit in involving the patient is the idea of giving the patient a choice. Certainly when you recognize the patient's active role, you see the importance of asking permission before barging ahead with procedures, questions, and the exam. Consider the case of a patient who had suffered a stroke and appeared unable to eat. Since her ability to verbalize was limited, treatment plans were developed in a vacuum. After she moved to a nursing home, the question was raised as to whether she was competent to make decisions for herself. She had already pulled out one feeding tube. What was overlooked was that this patient could write. Although her communication was limited, with some creative efforts on the part of the staff, she was able to indicate her willingness to try limited liquid feedings that were progressively increased. Communication opened up other productive avenues of communication with this patient. When last seen, she was adequately nourished and working on regaining some motor strength.

Consider another patient. This patient constantly questioned his doctor about the adequacy of his potassium level and the suitability of various potassium supplements he was taking. This patient was a pharmacist confined to the hospital for a number of weeks due to heart failure. The initial response of staff was annoyance with him because they felt he was meddling in his own care. This patient's preoccupation with his potassium was his way of fighting off his fears of being so passive. Once the physician recognized this point, he could more freely discuss various pharmaceutical choices with the patient and progress to the patient's other concerns and fears. Predictably, the patient then centered on his fear of not recovering, his concerns for his family, and his ability to support them financially.

It is not only the physician who hampers patient involvement. Sometimes patients themselves regress into a passive mode that misleads their physician to think that they don't need to be included in their care.

Consider the woman who came to her general practitioner with cardiac symptoms. She insisted that her husband be present throughout the interview, examination, and follow-up discussion. During the discussion, she directed all responsibility for understanding the questions of treatment to her husband. Once her physician recognized this style of interaction, he was able to disengage from it and to open discussion with her of her possible role in her healthcare. What evolved was a revelation of her fears that her condition was terminal and that death was imminent. In essence, she was already giving up on herself. The dialogue that followed was critical to her stabilization and cooperation in her own care.

The discussion that follows centers on specific ways to encourage active involvement and responsibility on the part of your patients.

GIVING CHOICES

Whenever possible, give your patients an opportunity to make choices. Most physicians agree that it's better to present objectively the pros and cons of a course of treatment and guide the patient, rather than directing the patient—even though some patients are not comfortable with choices and may push you to make their decisions.

A young gynecologist comments:

> It's difficult sometimes to open up the choice of treatment to patients
> when you know in your heart that one method would produce infi-
> nitely better results. A post-menopausal patient came to me with
> complaints of hot flashes that were severe enough to keep her up at
> night. I inquired about other symptoms—dryness, etc. She concurred
> that they were also a problem. I explained to her that there were
> several things that women her age needed to be aware of, including
> osteoporosis. I outlined several treatment plans for her condition and
> went into detail describing the estrogen/progesterone regimen that
> she could pursue to control the flashes, the exercise plan, and cal-
> cium pills she could take. After much discussion, this patient decided
> that she could not follow a complicated schedule of taking medica-
> tions. She opted for the calcium pills and said she would rely on
> lubrication to ease the discomfort during sex. I will admit that I was
> a little disappointed with the patient's choice, but I felt good about
> our relationship and the level of trust and honesty.

It is difficult, but important, for physicians to be flexible and creative. When
you are insistent on one treatment plan and reject other options, the patient may
reject help altogether. A patient's ability to accept change or follow a strict
course of therapy is a key factor in his or her compliance. Sometimes, it's better
to modify your own expectations in order to get patients to begin and perhaps
demystify a course of action.

DNR

One of the most trying choices facing doctors and patients is the question of
DNR (do not resuscitate). Moral implications aside, many doctors feel uncomfortable leading their patients in any one direction. One family member reports:

> My mom was approaching 90. She had suffered five heart attacks in
> one year and experienced frequent and acute episodes of angina.
> Aside from the heart problem, she was a vital woman in control of
> all of her faculties. During her sixth stay in the hospital, her doctor
> approached us with the DNR issue. He came to visit my mother in
> the hospital and explained that there were many things medical sci-
> ence could do to prolong the life of a patient and all of these proce-
> dures have implications. He then described the resuscitation tech-
> niques, the use of respirators, and other life support systems. He
> wanted her to know what could take place so that she could make the

most informed decisions about her treatment. He then met with me and explained what he had told my mother. The next day, Mom and I had a very open discussion about her life and her death. She had led a full, rich life in every way and was not afraid to die. What she feared most was lying in a hospital bed, unconscious, hooked to tubes and machines—at the mercy of modern science. She was relieved to learn that she had the choice—the final control—and could say, "No, that's not for me."

Choices—whether small or large, insignificant or ultimate—encourage patient responsibility and convey your respect for the patient's own intelligence and goals.

Confidentiality

Patients feel strongly about confidentiality. They don't want to go to an office where personal information is made public. They feel that this violates privacy and shows disregard for the extremely private and precious nature of health and lifestyle information.

Three keys to confidentiality are particularly important to patients:

1. Keeping Records Confidential. Patients need to know that their medical records are seen only by the physician and appropriate staff. In situations where patients are likely to be concerned about this, you should take initiative to state that the patient need not worry about confidentiality and to clarify your policy that will ensure theirs.

2. Discussing Cases in the Office. Many patients don't like the idea that their physician would discuss their condition with the office staff. Because of this, care must be taken in public areas to keep all mention of patients strictly professional. If Mr. Harmon hears you discussing Mrs. Jones' mastectomy with the receptionist, he can't help but wonder what you will say when he leaves.

3. Discussing Patient Cases with Another Patient. This may seem extremely obvious, but patients state that doctors sometimes drop casual comments like, "I saw so and so the other day." This information may seem harmless, but patients begin to wonder about the physician's discretion.

OBJECTIFYING PATIENTS

We are on attending rounds with the usual group: attending, senior resident, junior residents, and medical students. There are eight of us. Today we will learn how to examine the knee properly.

The door is open. The room is ordinary institutional yellow; a stained curtain between beds. We enter in proper order behind our attending physician.

The knee is attached to a woman, perhaps 35 years old, dressed in her robe and nightgown. The attending physician asks the usual questions as he places his hand on the knee: "This knee bothers you?"

All eyes are on the knee; no one meets her eyes as she answers. The maneuvers begin—abduction, adduction, flexion, extension, rotation. She continues to tell her story, furtively pushing her clothing between her legs. Her endeavors are hopeless, for the full range of knee motion must be demonstrated. The door is open. Her embarrassment and helplessness are evident.

More maneuvers and a discussion of knee pathology ensue. She asks a question. No one notices.

More maneuvers. The door is open.

Now the uninvolved knee is examined: abduction, adduction, flexion, extension, rotation.

She gives up.

The door is open.

Now a discussion of surgical technique. Now review the knee examination. We file out through the open door.

She pulls the sheet up around her waist. She is irrelevant. ("The Knee" by Constance J. Meyd, *Journal of the American Medical Association*, 248(4) July 23/30, 1982, p. 403. ©1982, American Medical Association and reprinted with permission.)

Objectifying patients or making the individual feel like "just another case" is a reliable way to ensure patient *dis*satisfaction. To avoid objectifying patients, albeit unintentionally, consider these tips:

1. Use the Patient's Name.   Always use a patient's name to identify his or her case. No one wants to be thought of as the hysterectomy in Room 303 or the gall bladder down the hall. In an office, it's even inadvisable to say to your nurse, "How many colposcopies do we have left?"

2. Avoid Labeling the Patient.   Illness sometimes triggers unpleasant behavior on the part of patients. Often due to fear and anxiety, these behaviors are certainly annoying. But patients resent being thought of as "difficult" or "crabby" or even "sensitive." They want to be thought of with an open mind. One hospitalized patient remarked that her doctor warned everyone that she was picky and demanding. The physician's intention was to alert staff so that they would be more attuned to her needs. But this labeling backfired because staff treated the patient with an edge of defensiveness and patronizing behavior. Consequently, the patient confronted her physician.

3. Avoid Stereotypes. It's important to find out what each person is like and what special techniques will work with that individual. Cultural and economic differences cause many people to come up with some simple solutions to more complex and individual problems.

4. Address the patient. Avoid discussing a patient with other people as though that patient weren't present. Whenever possible, direct questions and explanations to the patient rather than to other family members. This is a particularly sensitive issue for the elderly and for younger patients. Some physicians, treating a 75-year-old man, will direct all comments to his 50-year-old daughter, despite the fact that this man is the patient *and* is perfectly capable of grasping the facts of his condition. Some physicians speak to other family members because:

- They doubt the patient's ability to answer questions or receive information.
- They feel that the patient would be more cooperative or comfortable communicating with the family member.
- They need the third party because they, the physician, feel more comfortable. But the fact is, many patients don't see it that way. They would feel more respected and involved if the physician directed questions to them. After all, it's their body and their problem.

DIGNITY IS BASIC

Ask yourself:

- Do I place a high priority on preserving the dignity of all of our patients?
- Am I sensitive to patients' need for privacy?
- Do I regularly knock on patients' doors?
- Do I try to cover patients as much as possible during examinations?
- Do I limit the number of people who view patients undressed?
- Do I think it's important to involve our patients in their care?
- Do I try to present treatment options to my patients?
- Do I try to be sensitive to how certain treatments affect a patient's lifestyle?
- Do I try to be open to compromises and alternatives?
- Do I place a high priority on confidentiality?

- Do I not discuss a patient's condition in public or with inappropriate people?
- Do I not think of my patients as "another case?"
- Do I make an effort to call people by name?
- Do I avoid stereotyping by race, economic status, and gender?
- Do I address patients directly whenever possible?

When patients don't feel respected, they not only tend to feel angry; they also lose confidence in their medical caregiver who, they fear, is not really focusing on them as an individual, deserving of individualized attention, concentration, and respect.

22

Handling of Feelings

- Mark, a 16-year-old boy, suffered a severe concussion fracturing his skull and cracking the mastoid. His recovery was slow and, throughout, the boy lost a great deal of weight. Mark also experienced depression and an inability to concentrate. After seeing a series of physicians, Mark was finally diagnosed as having Graves disease and was given medication. Mark's mother believed that the head injury caused or contributed to Mark's thyroid condition. The neurologists told her she was crazy, saying, "The two couldn't possibly be connected." Only one physician, the one the family is currently seeing, told her instead, "I've actually never heard of this connection, but I wouldn't rule anything out 100 percent." Mark's mother was somewhat satisfied.

- Margaret Lerner was a woman in her fifties diagnosed as having cancer. She became convinced that poor diet caused her condition, and she rejected traditional treatments in favor of a macrobiotic diet. Her physician didn't understand the patient's need to become part of the treatment—to gain a sense of control—and argued with her about what he thought was a mythical connection between nutrition and breast cancer.

- An orthopod confines 40-year-old Harry Preston to "bed rest" for three weeks, based on a back complaint. He doesn't ask Mr. Preston if this is possible or what this would mean to his life. Mr. Preston, a truck driver and father of four, worries, "Who's going to support my family? If I stay home, I'll lose my route." Mr. Preston finds another doctor.

These examples illustrate ways that patients reject physician explanations of causes, diagnoses, and treatments, not because the doctors were incorrect, but because the physicians didn't explore the patient's concerns or take into account the patient's or family members' feelings about their disease and condition.

These examples are not isolated incidents. Myriad cases in which patients either switch physicians or refuse to comply with their physician's course of treatment are rooted in situations like these. The doctor has neither respected nor explored the patient's or family members' feelings. The patients are left feeling frustrated, misunderstood, and ignored.

The feelings that patients experience are varied, often with several occurring simultaneously. These feelings may have different roots and be expressed differently, but all are important for physicians to understand. In this section, we review:

- Feelings about being a patient
- What illness means to the patient's life
- The patient's feelings about the causes of illness
- Feelings about treatment

We explore how patients express these feelings and the impact of your response on patient satisfaction.

FEELINGS ABOUT BEING A PATIENT

We have all heard stories about the corporate executive who ignored the early warning signals of heart disease, suffered a massive attack one morning, and died instantly. Comments at the funeral centered on this man's need for control and power and how it was beneath him to ask for help. He rarely went to doctors, taking responsibility for his health into his own hands. Friends offered condolences to the widow and shook their heads, thinking "foolish man." A classic story.

The fact is that this corporate executive is more typical than foolish. Being a patient is not easy for any of us. It's difficult to be that vulnerable, that "out of control." And it's very difficult to be labeled "sick" in a society that places so much emphasis on being young and healthy. To some extent, sick people have feelings about what it means to be a patient—whether they demonstrate these feelings or not. For many, being a patient means a loss of self-esteem or self-image.

What the illness means to the patient's life

Patients also have feelings about what the illness or symptom means to their lives. The truck driver was afraid of losing his job, and therefore putting his family in jeopardy. An 80-year-old woman who is told that she cannot drive her car is afraid of losing her mobility and autonomy. She feels dependent on her family for her survival. Now she must ask her relatives to take her to the store, to the doctor, to the movies. How can she visit her friends when she wants to? Who will walk her dog and tend to her garden?

Why am I sick?

Patients also have feelings about what actually caused the condition. The woman with cancer believed that poor diet was the contributing factor. Other patients attribute their illness to a particular activity or event. Still others feel that they are being punished for something they have or haven't done. Sometimes, these feelings are obvious to the patient, and they can articulate them. Other times, the feelings may be well guarded and layered, making them more difficult to explore. In either case, most patients have some personal notion of what caused or contributed to their being ill. And, if you ignore it, you have a hard time "selling" your diagnosis and remedies. You also risk insulting the patient's intelligence.

Feelings about the treatment

Patients also have feelings about the treatment or course of therapy. The woman with breast cancer worries about her attractiveness, her sexuality: "Will my mate still love me?" Some people fear side effects and lifestyle changes that may be required and difficult. Cultural issues might also arise. Puerto Ricans, for example, have "hot" and "cold" classifications for diseases, medications, and cures. They believe that a hot disease must be coupled with a cold treatment. If a physician prescribes a hot treatment, the patient will discount the information, believing that "it can't work."

Why explore these feelings?

Reasons for doing so are compelling. On the one hand, you need to examine these feelings to understand the patient's behavior better. Patient behavior stems from these feelings and will certainly influence compliance and future outcomes. The woman convinced that her diet is key to her cancer needs help to explore *why* she feels this way, and she needs information and discussion if her reasoning is faulty.

Aside from any benefits that might accrue from such a diet, this patient is groping for a way to become a more active participant in her fight with cancer. Her physician didn't fully appreciate the importance of her taking charge of her diet. Instead, he immediately analyzed her behavior in terms of its scientific merit. By not paying attention to the patient's need for active participation, her physician missed the opportunity to build a powerful partnership between patient and doctor. A more subtle element in this communication was the patient's growing belief that she had caused her illness by dietary indiscretions. Here again, her physician could have engaged her in a discussion of these beliefs with the hope of warding off further self-blame. Rather than triggering productive exchange of feelings and beliefs between doctor and patient, we see instead a turning away of patient from physician.

Another example of such a breakdown occurred in exchange between the orthopedic surgeon and his 40-year-old male patient who was advised to follow up his back injury with "complete bed rest" for three weeks. His surgeon directed him with firmness and conviction, but did not afford the patient an opportunity to express his resistance to compliance. The exchange ended with the surgeon expecting compliance, while the patient ruminated about its impossibility. The physician neglected to ask, "What problems will these directions create in your life." As a truck driver and father of four, the patient was worried about financial support for his family and what would happen to his job if he stayed home. A productive exchange should have included these feelings and the action alternatives that would address them. An offer from the surgeon at that point to document the medical need for such an absence might be in order. Instead, this became an occasion for the patient to not comply with the treatment needed and to decide against scheduling further visits.

In each case, the physician could have been in a better position either to suggest alternatives or to help the patient more fully understand the importance of the recommended treatment, if the surgeon had explored the patient's feelings, assumptions, and realities.

ENCOURAGING PATIENTS TO SHARE THEIR FEELINGS

John Thomas complains of lower back pain. He is dissatisfied with the results of tests ordered by his physician and is convinced that he needs a CT scan. The physician spends a great deal of time countering this and trying hopelessly to "convince" the patient otherwise. The physician feels frustrated and the patient feels ignored. At no point does the physician come right out and ask, "Why do you think you need a CT scan?" The physician doesn't check out the patient's knowledge of the CT scan and ways it can and should be used. It is more productive in a case like this if the physician takes the position of "Perhaps you have some understanding" and explores the patient's knowledge base. In doing so, the patient can express his underlying concern which is, "Doc, are you really doing everything possible for me?" The doctor shouldn't say, "Sounds like you don't trust my judgment" in response to "I need a CT scan," but he can get the patient to articulate more about why he thinks the test is necessary and what information the patient would get from this test. This gives the doctor a lead-in to respond, "Yes, I think we do need more information, and here's what I'd like to do."

The point: you need to carefully avoid defensiveness in the face of patients who question your judgment and cautiously work to keep communication lines open.

Direct questions

Asking direct questions of the patient in this type of situation, using door-openers in the form of open-ended questions, is very helpful.

> Tell me why you see it that way.
> Tell me what you know.
> I'm interested in your opinion.
> How do you feel about this test?

The key to this line of questioning is to let the patient know you care about his or her opinions and understandings, and that you want to understand the patient's feelings, wants, and needs.

Listening with empathy

One key to getting patients to open up is to be able to put yourself in their shoes and understand as much as possible what the patient is feeling and experiencing. This does not mean that you need to experience your patient's pain and frustrations. It means you need to take steps to understand *why* and *how* patients can feel the way they do. This type of empathy is distinguished from apathy or sympathy as follows:.

Apathy	*Empathy*	*Sympathy*
I don't care.	Looks like you're feeling down today.	You poor thing.

| That's your problem. | Sounds as if you were really hurt by that. | I feel just dreadful for you. |

The difference between a lack of understanding and feeling, which is apathy, and "feeling for" someone, which is sympathy, is empathy, the middle of the continuum. Empathy involves some distance from the feeling. It is the ability to respond to another's feelings without losing one's own identity and feelings.

Physicians need to be able to understand the patient's feelings and let the patient know that you understand. After the patient who wanted a CT scan expressed why he felt it was necessary, the physician might have given this empathetic response: "I understand that you want to know *why* you're experiencing the pain," or "I know you've been through many tests and it can be very frustrating not to have all the answers." Once you've acknowledged the feelings, and reflected that you've heard the patient, it becomes easier to move on to how you want the patient to proceed.

READING PATIENTS' FEELINGS

In describing their feelings, most people use only four "feeling words"—happy, sad, glad, and mad. Usually, these global feelings mask deeper feelings that, if expressed and acknowledged, make patients feel attended to and understood. Also, by helping the patient to pinpoint their feelings more accurately, you have important clues to their problem and their compliance prospects.

To enhance your vocabulary of feelings so that you can reflect back to patients the knowledge that you've read and understood them, Table 22–1 gives an excellent list of feeling words provided by Madelyn Burley-Allen in *Listening: The Forgotten Skill* (New York: John Wiley and Sons, Inc., 1982, p. 105).

The more you tune in to your patient's particular feelings and the clearer you both are about these feelings, the more your patients will feel understood and the fuller your picture will be of the circumstances that affect their care.

PHYSICIANS HAVE FEELINGS, TOO

So far, we've dwelt largely on how to recognize and appreciate a patient's feelings. But how about the physician's feelings? Albert Schweitzer said, "Medicine is not only a science but also the art of letting our own individuality interact with the individuality of the patient."

Letting your own individuality, with its ensuing feelings, interact, can be risky business to someone whose training has demanded that such feelings be set aside. Even the more informative curriculum on behavioral medicine included in some medical schools these days frequently misses the need for medical students

Table 22–1. Feeling Words.

	Anger	*Elation*	*Depression*	*Fear*
Mild	annoyed	glad	unsure	uneasy
	bothered	pleased	confused	tense
	bugged	amused	bored	concerned
	peeved	contented	resigned	anxious
	irritated	comfortable	disappointed	apprehensive
		surprised	discontented	worried
		relieved	apathetic	
		confident	hurt	
Moderate	disgusted	cheerful	discouraged	alarmed
	harassed	delighted	drained	shook
	resentful	happy	distressed	threatened
	mad	up	down	afraid
	put upon	elated	unhappy	scared
	set up	joyful	burdened	frightened
		hopeful	sad	
		eager		
		anticipating		
Intense	angry	great	miserable	panicky
	contempt	excited	ashamed	overwhelmed
	hostile	enthusiastic	crushed	petrified
	hot	turned on	humiliated	terrified
	burned	moved	hopeless	terror-stricken
	furious	enthralled	despair	
		free	anguish	
		proud		
		fulfilled		
		fascinated		
		titillated		
		engrossing		
		absorbing		

to come to know themselves before they can know their patients. The result: you become very good at assessing the technical side of your patients, while the realm of feelings and emotions remain a vast, dark unknown. No wonder that a rise in patient emotion during an interview often triggers a rise in physician tension and defensiveness. This is hardly the way to begin the process of empathy.

But you do have feelings about patients, diseases, treatments and about your ability to deal with them effectively. You probably have patients and patient groups whom you find easier to work with, and patients and patient groups who may cause you greater discomfort and anxiety. You probably have cases and illnesses that make you nervous or uncertain.

Ignoring your own feelings and thinking that you must mask them in order to be all things to all people hurts your relationship with patients. In the course of training for medical school, doctors-to-be are often placed in the position of having to suspend their own needs and feelings in order to meet a career goal. Day-to-day patient care requires a certain amount of sublimation of feelings in order to remain objective and decisive. When this sublimation of feelings generalizes to a broad range of patient problems, you risk a breakdown in patient relationships.

If you can accept your feelings and learn to understand them, you can adopt coping strategies that will enable you to function more successfully and comfortably.

Medicine is full of experiences that tug at your feelings. More often than you would like, you are faced with patient hours when the burdens of practice, or perhaps other personal stresses, are subtly with you. Confronted by the patient's needs, personality, and problems, you have the makings of a complicated and often unmapped constellation of feelings.

One of the authors leads a conference for residents and medical students that helps physicians identify their feelings before determining appropriate responses to patients. Year after year, beginning residents have difficulty in this conference for one of two reasons. There are those who are so defensive about their own feelings that they minimize the importance of a conference to talk about feelings at all. These are the technocrats who pride themselves on not letting feelings "interfere" with evaluation and treatment. The other group of residents who misunderstand the early directions to focus on their own feelings by shifting to what the *patient* must be feeling. They are quick to race on to figure out what their patient intervention should be before cataloguing what might be going on with themselves.

As the weeks go by, it is gratifying to see how this all changes as they become more at ease in starting with their own feelings and defenses before analyzing what might be going on inside their patients' minds. What was first frightening becomes fun. What was extra work becomes a way of speeding up their getting to know their patients. What follows are interventions that are more responsive to their patients' needs.

One case presented at one such conference centered on difficulties a male resident was having with a woman slightly older than he. The initial clue to difficulties in their relationship came from his admission that he was avoiding seeing this patient on rounds. He had already decided that he would not follow this patient's case in the outpatient clinic.

Although initial discussion failed to surface immediate reasons for avoiding this patient, a more detailed discussion of his visits with her illuminated the problem. This woman suffered from poorly controlled diabetes. One reason she cited for not feeling well was that she received little help from her husband. She talked of the long hours he worked and his unpredictable schedules as one reason why she could not regulate her food intake. She hardly disguised her anger at her husband.

As the physician presented this case, he became uncomfortable but came to see that the patient's complaints paralleled his own struggle to balance the demands of residency with his home life. Once he gained perspective on the interaction of his problems with this woman, he was able to redefine a more positive approach to working with her.

Besides having your own personal issues triggered by a patient's concern, there are also inherently sticky subjects. Take sexuality, for example.

If you want to engage in open, helpful discussions of sexuality with patients, you must first examine your own attitudes about sexual matters. Until you have, it can be very difficult to talk objectively and openly about such matters with your patients in a nonjudgmental way.

The same can be said for the patient who mentions suicide. As one medical student put it, "If I ask about it, what do I do if the patient answers affirmatively?" Coming to know what you have a tendency to avoid is the first step toward further analysis of your resistances to such discussion. Physicians most able to help patients are generally those who have taken the time to get to know this part of themselves.

Yet another area that can trigger physician discomfort involves how to tell patients when you are limited in what you can do for them. When not handled properly, patients often mistake your avoidance as rejection. On the other hand, an open admission on your part, such as, "This is as far as I can go with your care, but I will help you access the services of someone better equipped in this area, and I will stay in touch with you," can encourage your patient.

Drs. Richard Gotlin and Howard Zucker, from the Departments of Medicine and Psychiatry at Mount Sinai School of Medicine in New York, describe in "Physicians' Reactions to Patients" (*New England Journal of Medicine*, 308,

(18), 1983, pp. 1060–1061), common physician responses to common situations and patient types. They also show coping strategies for physicians who experience these negative emotional responses (see Tables 22-2 and 22–3).

Denying feelings on the part of either patients or physicians will create misunderstandings and frustration and can erode the patient–physician relationship. Although difficult, it is important to realize the impact of feelings on relationships and make them work for you.

Ask yourself:

- Do I think it's important to help patients share their feelings?
- Am I sensitive to what being a patient means to most people?
- Do I want to understand patients' personal views on why they are sick and how they should be treated?
- Do I use direct questions and other techniques to help patients open up?
- Am I able to listen nondefensively to these feelings?
- Am I able to respond with empathy when patients are sharing feelings?
- Can I read people's feelings by listening to the tone of voice a patient uses or choice of words?
- Do I think it's important for me to understand my feelings about patients and diseases in order to remain objective?
- Can I can tell when I am losing my objectivity?
- Do I know how to use various coping strategies in order for me to become more objective?

The result? Closer, more trusting partnerships and patient satisfaction.

Table 22–2. Frequent Physician Responses to Commonly Encountered Situations and Patient Types.

Situation	Physician's Emotional Response	Physician's Behavioral Response
Terminal illness/chronic incurable disease	Sympathetic identification, feelings of inadequacy, impotence, lowered self-esteem, frustration	Denial, reluctance to discuss illness with patient, avoidance of patient and family
Patient in emotional crisis; physician lacks time or skill	Feelings of helpessness, loss of control, inadequacy	Failure to obtain consultation or refer patient
Institutionally determined termination of relationship (rotation or completion of residency)	Guilt, sadness	Procrastination or failure to inform patient

Patient Type	Physicians' Emotional Response	Physicians' Behavioral Response
Organic brain syndrome/dementis; language/cultural differences; inability to understand explanations of disease or treatment	Impatience, frustration	Hostility, rejection, abruptness, avoidance, minimizing seriousness of symptoms
Hostile patient/borderline personality	Taking patient hostility personally; hatred; feeling authority threatened	Reciprocal hostility, rejection (power struggle, derision, forced discharge)
Overly dependent patient	Initial gratification, followed by resentment, anger, impatience, guilt	Hostility, abrupt distancing, coldness

Table 22–2. *(cont.)*

Patient Type	Physicians' Emotional Response	Physicians' Behavioral Response
Hypochondriacal patient	Impatience, frustration, anger	Rejection (derision, avoidance, prescription given out of exasperation)
Antisocial/self-destructive patient	Disapproval, anger	Punitive hostility, rejection (neglect or overtreatment)
Noncompliant patient	Sense of loss of control, threatened authority; frustration; anger	Hostility, rejection, denial (power struggle, loss of interest)

Source: New England Journal of Medicine, May 5, 1983.

Table 22-3. Strategies for Physicians To Cope with Negative Emotional Responses.

Physician's Emotional or Behavioral Reaction	Coping Statements
Avoidance	Analyze why: attempt to understand and master feelings that lead to avoidance; stay with the patient; discuss with colleagues.
Identification with patient	Recognize: avoid tendency to deny seriousness of disease or to give way to despair; stay with the patient.
Hostility/rejection	Acknowledge and analyze: don't attempt to like the unlikable patient; use behavorial approaches; if situation is intolerable, transfer patient to another physician.
Feelings of impotence, inadequacy (e.g., in caring for dying patient)	Discover areas in which help and comfort can be rendered physical and emotional; be realistic about limitations of medicine; give the patient time to go through the stages of bereavement.
Frustration, confusion, uncertainty about dealing with the patient; coping strategies not effective	Request psychiatric consultation/referral.
Anxiety, guilt, and frustration about meeting patient's recognized emotional needs	Allocate time realistically according to need; request consultation/referral.

23

How To Handle Sticky Situations

No matter how polished your basic skills are, some situations with patients require finesse and sensitivity that tax even the most skilled physician. This chapter addresses three of the many sticky situations that inevitably arise in most people's practices:

- Sticky situation #1: People resisting responsible behavior and responsible self-care.
- Sticky situation #2: Dealing with mistakes and disappointments.
- Sticky situation #3: Delivering bad news.

STICKY SITUATION #1: WHEN PATIENTS RESIST RESPONSIBLE BEHAVIOR AND RESPONSIBLE SELF-CARE

Responsible self-care inevitably involves attention to diet, smoking, substance abuse, sexual practices and other behavior related to lifestyle. The responsible physician feels compelled to raise issues that the patient may not want to hear. The result: annoyance, resistance, or even just plain tense moments of truth.

The challenge to the physician is to help patients see ways they can better take care of themselves. This involves trust from the beginning and physician skill in drawing on all he or she knows about the patient in a nonjudgmental, concerned manner. The physician needs to express information in an honest and straightforward fashion and work with the patient to negotiate workable, achievable action plans.

Triggering responsible choices without suggesting blame or guilt

When lifestyle choices interfere with a patient's health, some physicians become blaming or guilt-inducing. In fact, it's hard not to. Physicians can't help but have feelings about patients and their roles in creating health problems for themselves. But the fact is, the physician who is blaming or guilt-inducing tends to work against desired outcomes. These physicians' feelings, if not understood and controlled, can negatively affect your ability to guide patients to care for themselves in a responsible, systematic fashion.

Consider Mrs. Brill, a 66-year old woman with chronic arthritis, who presented to her physician with complaints of progressively increasing knee pain. Her exam confirmed a deteriorating joint that was becoming progressively less tolerant of stress. This was not the first time that Mrs. Brill had come to see her doctor with this complaint.

On prior visits, her physician had advised her to eliminate activities that required walking and a great deal of standing. The physician's advice went unheeded. Mrs. Brill continued to work as a sales clerk to supplement her husband's retirement income. For recreation, she cooked and entertained her children and grandchildren. To her physician, it appeared that Mrs. Brill resisted medical advice. To the patient, the advice given seemed unrealistic and impossible to heed.

What needed to occur in Mrs. Brill's case was first an exchange of feelings and a discussion of choices acceptable to both the patient and the physician. Only after a progressive discussion between the two of them about levels of stress and strain on her knee and how the patient could bring about some relief in the course of her preferred activities was the patient able to take her doctor's advice. The prospect of giving up activities closely associated with her sense of identity in response to someone else's direction created a situation in which she was unlikely to comply. Once her physician realized that she needed to feel that she had options and choices, they were able to move toward a more realistic compromise between activity and rest.

The doctor needed to present his recommendations in the following manner: "The arthritis will continue to be a source of some damage to that knee. Let's look at how you might relieve some of the stress that is adding to that damage.

What are the opportunities in the course of your day to provide a few more moments of relief to that joint?"

Many doctors have complained that patients expect miracles. They want modern science and technology to magically make them well without effort or involvement on their part. This avoidance of responsibility can certainly frustrate physicians, especially since doctors face so many effects of patients' neglect and abuse of their own bodies. At the same time, doctors need to help patients get well as a result of the patient's own efforts. This takes a sense of responsibility and commitment on the part of the patient, and this is not easy.

To increase the probability that patients will act in their own best interests, consider the seven pointers outlined below.

1. *Don't dwell in the past.* When a connection between a patient's behavior and an illness is clear, help the patient understand the connection. Focus on what the patient can now do rather than on past behavior.

2. *Don't preach or moralize.* When you do, you usually make the patient defensive and tense. Avoid *shoulds* and condescending tones. Present the health issues as facts.

3. *Do stress the positive.* Help the patient see the positive benefits of the recommended behavior change or therapy.

4. *Do encourage; don't threaten.* In some cases, the flat-out "You're killing yourself" will work—with some patients. Many times, scare tactics have reverse effects. You need to know the patient and consciously consider whether scare tactics are likely to help or hinder.

5. *Explore the patient's feelings.* If you believe it's best to use a strong, harsh approach, allow the patient room to react. Invite patients to express their feelings. Then, empathize while standing firm on your bottom-line message. Example: "I realize you're skeptical about ever stopping smoking after so many efforts, but the fact is, it's your only hope if you want to extend your life."

6. *Discuss options.* Some patients resist your advice because they have alternative courses of action in their minds. Try to find out what the patient sees as an alternative. Consider it seriously. See whether a compromise course might work better than your recommendations unheeded.

7. *Identify support systems.* Let the patient know of any support groups and services that might help.

To help patients face difficult changes, it may be helpful to include another family member, especially if these changes will affect other people. It is not a good idea, however, to use the family member as an ally, with the patient as the "enemy." Example: "You've got to get your wife to stop smoking" or "You must get your husband to lose weight." This approach removes responsibility from the patient and places it on the family member, where it really doesn't belong.

Patients do need to become responsible for their own treatment. As difficult as it may be, the doctor can never make a patient well without his or her commitment and cooperation.

STICKY SITUATION #2: DEALING WITH MISTAKES AND DISAPPOINTMENTS

In any practice, no matter how stupendous, mistakes and other annoyances are inevitable. Occasional long waits and delays, failure to notice patient needs, insensitivity to patient feelings, office staff inappropriateness, and blatant medical mistakes are a fact of life. Medicine is not an exact science, and even the best physicians can misjudge, misread, misdiagnosed and mislead. Yet, there is a tremendous amount of pressure inside and outside the medical community to "be perfect."

Clearly, the doctor and staff want to work toward eliminating problems and mistakes. In achieving close and successful doctor-patient relationships, how these mistakes are handled becomes pivotal.

Telling a patient about our mistakes can be a very delicate area of information exchange. Doctor and patient alike often become fixed on the notion that physicians are omniscient and can do no harm. Being able to tell a patient, "This is not the result that we had hoped for and I will share in the responsibility for finding a better way to handle this problem," can be a very hard thing to do if you are wedded to the notion that you are not allowed to make any errors in your work.

So, given the delicacy of the situation and your concerns about the scrutinizing patient, what can you do?

Don't offer excuses

A resident is scheduled to clean an infected surgical wound. The doctor was to see that the patient, who was extremely sensitive to pain, had been given pain medication prior to the cleaning. The resident never ordered the medication and, when it came time to clean the wound, made a decision to subject the patient to pain rather than delay the cleaning. While the resident had reasons for this decision, the patient only knew one thing for sure—the procedure was awful. The patient made a point of telling everyone about the doctor's negligence and lack of concern. The resident visited the patient the next day and tried to make her understand that the wound needed cleaning and that had to be the priority. His excuses fell on deaf ears. Later, the resident returned to talk with the patient, but this time sat on the bed and apologized for being insensitive. The doctor displayed a great deal of empathy and agreed that the patient was right, the medicine should have been ordered and the decision to proceed without pain medicine was not a wise one. The patient was appeased.

Be direct

Another doctor tells of having given an incorrect prescription to a patient which resulted in complications. The doctor discovered the mistake, immediately called the patient, admitted the mistake, and corrected the problem. The patient's feelings because of the doctor's directness: "My doctor is only human."

Allow patients to share their feelings

The patient with the infected wound needed an opportunity to vent her frustrations and let off steam before she could accept the doctor's apology. This is an essential step and one often neglected when handling problems or mistakes. Many physicians tend to want to move quickly toward finding solutions and often frustrate the patient's need to share their feelings. The skill needed is active listening (refer to Communication section) and becomes even more critical when a patient is extremely hostile or angry.

The hostility curve

Usually a hostile, angry reaction follows a certain pattern, if it is dealt with skillfully by another person. We can call this pattern the "Hostility Curve." Figure 23–1 shows what it looks like.

- Most people are reasonable a good deal of the time. They function at a *rational level*. At this level, you can talk with them about things reasonably.
- When a pileup of aggravations or one incident provokes a person, he or she will *take-off*, blowing off a lot of steam, possibly becoming abusive to you or whoever is around, and in general expressing a lot of hostility. It may seem to go on quite a while. Once the person leaves the rational level, there is no use trying to get the person to be "reasonable." But this take-off can't last forever. The hostile person just runs out of steam and begins to *slow down* if not provoked by anyone further.

As you see from the figure, when you argue or try to reason with someone (point 4) at the slow-down point, you only produce another take-off, and this can go on and on. You've seen it happen in huge blow-ups, where one person keeps setting off the other, when you hear voices get louder and louder and louder.

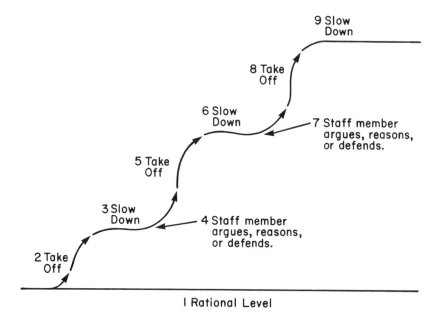

Figure 23–1. The Hostility Curve.

We talked about what not to do; now let's look at what we can do to bring the hostile situation under control.

At this point, the physician who has been listening to this hostile take-off can say something. What you say makes a big difference. If you say something *supportive*, like "I know this has been a very upsetting experience for you," you can be very helpful to that person.

In addition, you must be supportive in your nonverbal behavior. Being supportive does not necessarily mean agreeing, but it does mean letting the other person know that you understand his or her feelings.

- If you do say something supportive, you will usually see the hostile person *cool off*. He or she comes back down to a rational level.

- Once the person has returned to the rational level, you can begin to *problem-solve* with him or her about what caused the anger. People are in a mood to problem-solve when they are rational, not when they are up at the top of the hostility curve.

In addition, here are some *do's* and *don't's* for further background.

Do

Understand that the patient's hostility is directed at the situation, not at you as a person.

Recognize the patient's anger, let him or her know you understand it.

Listen carefully to what the patient says, waiting until the anger is out before responding.

Keep an open mind about who is wrong, what should be done, until you have a chance to investigate the problem.

Help patients save face when they realize they have behaved poorly.

If possible, gently steer the patient to a private area where there will be less outside involvement.

Have both of you sit down. If you need support, lean forward on something (armrest, table).

Keep your tone of voice calm and your pitch low.

Keep to yourself your own judgments about what "should" and "should not" make people angry.

When a patient's anger begins to slow down, support him or her.

Don't

Take hostility personally.

Deny the patient's anger, or tell him or her to "calm down." Refuse to listen to the anger or the reasons for it.

Defend yourself or the angry person until he or she has calmed down and you have investigated the problem.

Embarrass patients by pointing out the foolishness of their behavior.

Have one of you standing and one sitting.

Get caught up in the hysteria by raising your voice to match the hostile person's.

Jump to conclusions about what "should" and "should not" make people angry.

When a patient's anger begins to slow down, take advantage of it by arguing and reasoning.

The threat of malpractice and the dramatic increase in such occurrences certainly makes dealing with mistakes more difficult. Doctors are afraid to admit to even minor problems for fear that it will have major consequences. Most literature on malpractice in medicine, however, emphasizes that problem encounters are more likely to translate into a malpractice suit when *concealed* rather than whey they are openly addressed between patient and physician.

What can help?

Developing a true partnership in the initial stages of your relationship will help. This includes:

- Getting to know your patient's likes and dislikes
- Understanding your patient's feelings
- Being open to alternatives, feedback, and suggestions
- Presenting yourself as human and capable of making mistakes.

STICKY SITUATION #3: DELIVERING BAD NEWS

Nowhere is the doctor's ability to communicate more challenged than in instances when you must deliver bad news. You need to draw on your ability to empathize, clarify, outline, and encourage, and empathize again. Such interactions truly reflect the "art" of medicine. You need to be extremely sensitive to your patient's needs and feelings and, at the same time, be aware of your own behavior and feelings.

The physicians we interviewed shared interesting observations and opinions not only on ways to deliver bad news, but also on how important it is to think through and crystallize in advance a process that works for the doctor and the patient—a process that will ease what is inevitably a difficult and painful event.

The doctors we consulted have given the bad news delivery process considerable thought. Many remembered positive role models whose style helped shape their own responses. Some stated that they have developed greater ease in this area through time and experience. All agreed. In spite of the difficulty and pain involved, many personal rewards stem from helping patients face and cope with emotionally challenging times.

The patients we consulted confirmed the importance of their physicians in coping with bad news. "I couldn't believe how sensitive my doctor was"; "I don't know what I would have done"; "I saw a side of my physician that I never knew existed."

What do patients need?

When we asked our doctors to describe their techniques, we were impressed by the variety of not only styles and behaviors but also philosophies. Yet, at the heart, regardless of style and philosophy, these physicians characterized three basic patient needs that they feel physicians should address when communicating bad news:

1. *Patients need information.* Patients' need for information becomes stronger when they are faced with having severe or terminal illnesses. They feel a powerful need to understand the whys, hows, and whats of their diseases, if not immediately, then eventually.

2. *Patients need control.* The more severe the illness, the more vulnerable and powerless the patient tends to feel. To counter these feelings, patients need to "do something," become involved and regain whatever sense of control is possible.

3. *Patients need comfort, understanding, and support.* Seriously ill patients feel alone and frightened. They need to know that they have support and understanding—that someone has their best interests at heart.

With these three basic needs in mind, we will discuss approaches to sharing bad news, and the pros and cons of each approach.

Preparing a patient

Elizabeth Smith comes in for a check-up. She has been feeling ill and complains of enduring lumps in her neck and groin. During the exam, you notice that her glands are indeed quite swollen, and you suggest a series of blood tests. You suspect cancer, although there are also other possibilities. How much information should you share at this point?

Opinions vary. Some physicians feel that you should tell patients why you are ordering tests. What do you think? Which of the following is most appropriate?

- "Your glands are swollen. This could suggest a simple virus, mononucleosis, or cancer."
- "I won't know anything until we run some tests."
- "These tests will check for _____, _____, and _____."

Some doctors feel that information at this point, especially if cancer is an option, imposes unnecessary stress on patients. They prefer to say, "Your glands are swollen, I'd like to order some tests. This could be nothing, but I'd like to be sure." Others say it all because they want the patient to be aware of the possibilities and not shocked if the results are life-threatening.

Questions to consider are:

1. If the patient does have a serious illness, do you need to begin to prepare the patient early on for it?

2. Should you worry the patient if it might turn out to be a minor problem?

3. How much information about alternative eventualities do you think the patient deserves?

What does the patient think?

Since there can be no hard-and-fast rules to answer these questions, since patients vary and so do physicians, many doctors suggest consulting the patient for cues. For instance, if you ask the patient, "What do you suspect?" you'll often find that the patient already has a theory about what's wrong with him or her. Some people hold back on full information because they're afraid they'll alarm the patient unnecessarily before they have all the facts. But patients have made appointments with you, in most cases, because they already suspect a problem. By finding out what they already think, you can use that information to guide your interaction. "Mrs. Jones, you say you are worried about this lump, especially because your mother had breast cancer. I can't tell you that it's not serious until we do further tests. But I can tell you that there certainly are other possible explanations, including a virus, mononucleosis, and other much less serious possibilities."

Don't leave people wondering

Patients report that the worst part is not knowing *why* they are having tests. What is the doctor looking for? If patients are left wondering, they don't feel good about the interaction with their physician if the doctor has been vague in order to protect the patient. Whatever the outcome, trust between patient and physician is threatened because the physician, from the point of view of the patient, has been tight-lipped and withholding.

Although a great deal depends on your understanding of the patient's needs, a key for preparing patients seems to be this: if you are going to give *any* information, make certain that the patient is clear about what you have said, not left wondering and confused.

Where and how to deliver bad news

Opinions differ here also. Many doctors said they don't like to have patients receive bad news when they are alone, thinking that patients need and deserve the support of people close to them. One doctor reported calling patients at home to give test results, knowing that the patient would be in a supportive environment. This way the doctor could "arrange" for the next meeting very soon which could focus on "what we can do." One solution in your initial interview with a patient—before there is bad news to share—may be to ask the patient how he or she would like to receive bad news if there ever is any. The patient can tell you whether he or she would like to be at home, or in the office, alone or with a support person. Although asking this when the patient is healthy might feel awkward, if the need ever arises to act on the information, you could save patients a great deal of discomfort. Imagine a family doctor saying to a patient, "I hope you keep your health for decades, and I'll certainly do all I can to help. But, I want to ask you this—if the need for me to convey disturbing news to you ever arises, can you tell me your feelings about that and how and when you wish I would do this?"

A very important aspect of sharing bad news with patients involves letting your patients know that you understand their pain and that you are there for them. Your tone of voice, body language, closeness, and touch all need to convey warmth and sensitivity. One patient describes that when her doctor told her she had cancer, he launched immediately into actions to be taken: for instance, "And we'll start with this treatment and this drug, etc." This doctor intended to instill hope by letting the patient know that she could fight the disease. At that moment, however, she said that she needed a hug, a shoulder, and empathy. She wasn't quite ready for tests and she didn't perceive her doctor as sensitive to her needs.

Sharing supports

Of course, often patients' needs for support will go beyond what you can deliver. At this point, you need to be familiar with outside resources, including places or people the patient can turn for more emotional help. We are not in any way suggesting that doctors become the "announcers of news" and turn the job of listening and caring to others, but rather to become familiar with alternatives and options, and to know how and when to use them. Support groups available for patients with cancer, multiple sclerosis, and other debilitating illnesses can do wonders for people when they feel alone with their problem.

Helping patients gain control

Letting patients know what can be done for them medically is certainly a critical part of conveying bad news. If the patient consents, many doctors include other family members when sharing substantive information. When there are options and treatments to consider, your patient alone may be too anxious or upset to comprehend information or weigh the options clearly.

Physicians must maintain a delicate balance between:

1. Presenting options so that patients can understand them.

2. Helping patients make choices without over-directing them.

3. Inviting the patient to include supportive loved ones if they choose to.

4. Monitoring patients' emotional state.

Conveying hope

The physicians we interviewed also stressed the importance of conveying hope and encouragement to patents. They recommend presenting news with a "Here's what we *can* do for you" spirit, even if it's "Here's how we can ease your pain and discomfort." News should never come across as, "We're done. There's nothing left that we can do." It should never be said in a way that makes the patent feel abandoned. This may again be delicate since doctors need to be realistic and help patients accept their illness.

WHAT IS SUCCESS?

In the areas discussed, we stress the need to weigh the options and strike a balance between:

- Too much vs. too little information
- Too much vs. too little encouragement
- Too much vs. too little hand-holding

The key seems to be learning as much as possible about your individual patient and having many options for dealing with patients you deem appropriate. If you only have one way, then you can't adapt to different patients' needs or styles. You need to assess and plan for each situation. A repertoire of alternatives and flexibility enables you to succeed with a greater number of patients.

Whether it is a poor prognosis or the need to talk about difficult treatments, these encounters can shift from being highly aversive and avoided to opportunities to deepen your relationship with your patients. You can make a powerful difference to people. It is these moments that can be meaningful moments in the practice of medicine. In an age when so much change seems to be occurring in practice, this is one enduring part of medicine that makes it different from so many other careers. What is of such great help to patients becomes a moment of meaning for the physician.

STICKY SITUATIONS ABOUND

The three kinds of situations we've mentioned merely scratch the surface of the whole host of unpredictable, uncomfortable and sometimes frightening situations you have to handle routinely. But there are options for handling these and other situations with tact and honesty. The point we want to emphasize is, if you focus on the results you want to achieve with your patients, directness, a non-judgmental attitude, and respect for the patient's right to know seem to be the winning behaviors for patient satisfaction.

V
Innovations in Practice Enhancement

As the medical marketplace becomes more competitive and physicians engage in strategic efforts to heighten patient satisfaction, exciting, often bold, practice enhancement strategies are emerging.

This part is designed to describe a handful of such strategies. Not meant to be in any way exhaustive of the array of exciting experiments happening nationwide, they provide instead a glimpse at the *lengths* and *depths* some physicians are choosing to pursue in order to achieve excellence in their practices and not only satisfy but impress their patients.

Specifically, you'll find described here:

• How to address patients' emotional concerns with the role of the clinical specialist

• How to educate patients for responsibility

• How to fine-tune physician behavior via patient satisfaction surveys and physician development

• How to improve the physician's relationship with the patient via video feedback

As you read, you might think that these innovations are not practical for your practice. That might be so. Our point in presenting these innovations is to make examples of deliberate practice enhancement experiments, experiments that were born of visionary physicians, that consume energy, commitment, and often money; and, despite the commitment they require, are considered powerfully successful and worth perpetuating in the everyday life of a busy practice.

24

Educating Patients for Responsibility

As many consumers become involved in self-care, they want to know more about their own bodies, illnesses, and lifestyle options in order to optimize their own health. More people want to make informed decisions about their own wellness and illness. Information affords today's healthcare consumers a greater sense of control over their own bodies and health options.

But many consumers feel that, in order to learn what they want and deserve to know, they have to subscribe to magazines, go to alternative healthcare providers, or watch television and read the bestselling treatises on everything the medical profession isn't telling them. Unfortunately, many consumers don't even expect their own physicians to educate them thoroughly and open-mindedly about their conditions and options.

The physicians who do take people's needs seriously for education and information stand out in the eyes of the consumer.

But not only that. The physicians who have devoted energy to building substantive patient education into their practices see benefits in increased patient satisfaction, enhanced compliance and more responsible patient decision-making.

ENTER DR. CHERNER

Dr. Rachmel Cherner, M.D., specialist in endocrinology and metabolic diseases, practices in Jenkintown, Pennsylvania. Dr. Cherner has developed what we believe is the "Rolls Royce" model for educating his patients. He graduated from Jefferson Medical College in 1955. He completed his residency at Jefferson Medical College of Thomas Jefferson University Hospital and was NIH (National Institutes of Health) trained in endocrinology and metabolic diseases. He began private practice in 1961, after leaving the United States Air Force. He is currently a Diplomat of the Board of Internal Medicine and Associate Clinical Professor of Medicine at Jefferson Medical College.

Dr. Cherner's interest in patient education originally stemmed from his need to help his diabetic patients take greater personal responsibility for their care. Many of his patients needed to make changes in their daily routines and habits in order to be and stay healthy. While most of these patients did not suffer from life-threatening illnesses, their diseases needed to be managed carefully by the doctor in partnership with the patient.

Dr. Cherner found that the better educated and informed patients were, the easier time they had making the necessary life-shifts and adjustments and adhering to prescribed treatment plans. Thus, he personally began to investigate a series of programs and practices designed to educate his patients about their health problems and possibilities.

At this point, Dr. Cherner's patient education strategy is uniquely comprehensive and effective. It entails seven approaches:

- A complete history, physical examination, and orientation
- Selected books in the waiting area
- Information about their doctor
- Patient handbooks
- Audiovisual resources
- Consultations with specialists
- Monthly support groups

This chapter describes these seven approaches applied to educating patients for responsibility.

APPROACH #1: A COMPLETE HISTORY, PHYSICAL, AND PATIENT ORIENTATION

Although Dr. Cherner is an endocrinologist concerned mainly with the glands and hormones of the endocrine system, his initial approach to his patients resembles that of an old-fashioned general internist. He feels that since he cannot separate the organ or gland from the rest of the body, a complete medical history and physical is essential, so he insists that his staff schedule each new patient for a full hour for the initial visit. He limits the number of new patients seen each week and, when possible, schedules their appointments at the end of his office hours. Dr. Cherner has been known to devote a great deal more time to patients who have had particularly bad experiences with their illness, and who consequently need not only thorough information but also substantial understanding. Dr Cherner's agenda during this initial visit is to:

- Develop a complete medical history with the patient, including educational, social, and emotional attitudes.
- Examine the patient thoroughly.
- Discover what the patient understands about his or her condition and what if anything has already been done medically.
- Give the patient an overview of his or her condition and treatment that's as complete as possible.
- Invite patients to ask questions.

Since, for many patients, this in-depth experience with a physician is new and unexpected, Dr. Cherner's office staff prepares patients for their visits by saying:

> Dr. Cherner feels it's important to have a complete history and physical during your initial visit, and we are setting aside one hour for this appointment. In addition to the examination, you will have an opportunity to spend time with the doctor in his office talking and discussing any questions you might have. We just want you to know what to expect.

A large part of this hour is spent getting to know one another. Dr. Cherner feels that this is the time to let the patient know about his practice, his views on medicine, how he can be used as a resource, his office systems, hours, appointments, and more. Because many of his patients will need to see him regularly, he takes time to set clear ground rules up front.

Because endocrine diseases are generally life-long, it is critically important, he believes, that his patients develop a longitudinal view of their illness. They need to understand the duration and type of therapy the doctor is recommending. They need to become clear about causes of the illness, medications, possible side effects, treatment options, and what they can do to help themselves. This means that the doctor has to supply the patient, over time, with a great deal of information in an easily digestible form. Dr. Cherner lays the groundwork in this initial visit.

APPROACH #2: BOOKS IN THE WAITING ROOM

Dr. Cherner's waiting room is truly a user-friendly medical library for the lay audience. He has carefully selected and sometimes written articles, and makes them available in large loose-leaf binders for his patients to read while they are waiting. These binders contain short, easy-to-read articles on various diseases, diets, medications, and the like.

The following is the opening page of the first volume entitled "A Talk With Your Doctor." It illustrates what Dr. Cherner is trying to achieve.

To All My Patients:

Most of my patients who are old friends are aware of various reading materials that I have scattered about the waiting room. I have attempted to supply the more unusual magazines which I hope you will enjoy. In addition, I have supplied a copy of the *Good Housekeeping Magazine Health Book*, which contains a veritable treasure of medical information. You may be interested in reading my section on endocrinology which was written about two years ago.

What you may not realize is that our office does have additional library facilities. You may notice tucked under the table in the waiting room a large volume with considerable reading material as well as amusing cartoons. I hope in this office not only to educate but also to entertain my patients.

Available for review is an additional volume that I hope will be as entertaining, which mainly presents information on food and nutrition in general. If you ask my staff for access to this book, I am sure that they will comply. Other more specific information is available upon request.

Nonetheless, I have always felt that it might be worthwhile to supply a sort of monthly newspaper, informing you as to the activities in the office such as publications, papers delivered to medical or lay audiences, and supplementary material from magazines, and newspapers which are topical.

So with this thought in mind, I am about to launch an experiment, and would appreciate your suggestions and responses.

Sincerely,

Rachmel Cherner, M.D., F.A.C.P.

Included also in the volume are two short articles that help explain the role/-function of an endocrinologist and an internist (see Figures 24–1 and 24–2).

Included also are short articles, some of which are publications by Dr. Cherner, which help to explain the background of various diseases affecting his patients. Another volume deals strictly with diet and nutrition, and another deals more specifically with drugs and medications—new innovations and break-throughs in the field.

On the use of cartoons

Dr. Cherner includes cartoons from newspapers and magazines in all of his volumes for several reasons.

He feels strongly that humor and levity can counter the seriousness and depression that so often accompany being sick. Since the diseases he treats can, for the most part, be controlled, he wants his patients to know that what they are going through is not the end of the world. Also, many of the cartoons present important points in an entertaining, nonthreatening way (see Figure 24–3).

The volume then presents articles by Dr. Cherner, such as "Diabetic patients: Check *all* the drugs they take" *(Consultant: Journal of Medical Consultation)* which, although written for medical professionals, affords the lay-person clear, plainly stated information about drug interactions and effects on diabetic patients. The following is an excerpt.

> Diabetic patients tend to require many more drugs than other patients, and when you add to those such over-the-counter medications as analgesics and the willingness of some patients to adopt exotic and highly-touted fad diets, you have the groundwork for confusion.
>
> It is essential to take a complete drug history as part of your initial workup and your continuing care of diabetic patients. Particular attention must be paid to the possibility of drug interactions, sensitivity to drugs, and drug-related side-effects. This article updates these important subjects and pinpoints the drugs most likely to enhance hypoglycemia, to antagonize the action of hypoglycemic agents, or to cause an untoward interaction with the sulfonylurea compounds (Box). . . .

What is an endocrinologist?

Endocrinology is the branch of medicine concerned with the glandular internal regulatory system including the pituitary, thyroid, parathyroid, adrenals, ovaries and testes, and the insulin-producing cells of the pancreas. Endocrinology is a subspecialty of internal medicine as are, for example, cardiology and gastroenterology, which deal with the heart and digestive system respectively. An endocrinologist is a specialist who is first broadly trained in internal medicine and subsequently in the diagnosis and treatment of disorders of the endocrine glands. Frequently, an endocrinologist is consulted in cases of severe diabetes or goiter requiring medical treatment and in other situations where a hormonal disorder is suspected or where specialized medical care is needed.

Is an endocrinologist only concerned with hormones?

Metabolic disorders and certain disturbances of body chemistry, as well as some inherited disorders, are also treated by an endocrinologist.

Who needs an endocrinologist?

Not everyone who suffers from diabetes or other endocrine diseases needs an endocrinologist. Many patients can be treated effectively by general practitioners and specialists in internal medicine. A disorder of the sexual glands may be handled by gynecologists or urologists, and sometimes thyroid conditions are treated with surgery. An endocrinologist's skills are most necessary in those cases requiring special knowledge in diagnosis and medical treatment.

Does an endocrinologist perform surgery?

No, an endocrinologist does not perform surgery unless he or she happens to be a gynecological endocrinologist. An endocrinologist's work is limited to diagnosis and medical treatment. However, this type of physician frequently works with surgeons in preoperative evaluation and in postoperative hormonal treatment.

The following are typical questions asked by patients of endocrinologists. The answers given here are meant to be of a general nature only since no medical case is exactly the same as the next.

Will I still need my family doctor?

Yes, you will. Suppose you have a problem that requires continuing treatment by an endocrinologist; your family doctor will still advise and/or treat you when other non-related problems occur and will continue your treatment if and when your problem does not require the attention of your endocrinologist. Your family doctor and endocrinologist often consult each other about your problems and care.

I have been sent by my personal physician for consultation. What happens next?

Following consultation you will go back to your referring doctor for follow-up unless your case requires the continued attention of an endocrinologist. Then, by mutual consent, the latter will administer and supervise treatment until his or her services are no longer necessary.

What about my care when my endocrinologist is away for a weekend or a medical meeting?

In most cases your personal physician will be informed of your condition and be able to manage it while your endocrinologist is away. However, if the endocrinologist has been treating you exclusively, you should contact the office directly for instructions and referral to another physician.

Will my insurance cover the services of an endocrinologist?

Insurance coverage is varied, and each case is handled individually. The medical assistant or office nurse in the endocrinologist's office will be glad to discuss this with you.

What about fees and billing?

Fees will vary with the individual case, but generally reflect the specialized ability and time devoted to each problem. Endocrinologists are glad to discuss the matter of fees with their patients. Physicians usually send out a monthly itemized statement to their patients. Your statement will show any amounts paid by your insurance plan.

What about telephone calls?

Many telephone calls can be avoided by having a member of the family come in with the patient when the physician is ready for a conference to give an opinion and recommendation. Subsequent calls can often be handled by the endocrinologist's medical assistant who either will be able to answer questions directly or relay the physician's answer to the caller.

Can an endocrinologist give me a physical checkup?

Yes. As a broadly trained internist, comprehensive diagnostic work is part of an endocrinologist's everyday practice. Some of them prefer to see patients only after referral by another physician, whereas others may do regular checkups of their own. During the course of an examination, if a condition is found that does not fall within his or her specialty, the endocrinologist may arrange for the services of another physician. Generally, blood counts, urinalyses and X-ray tests will be conducted on most patients undergoing a complete examination in an endocrinologist's office.

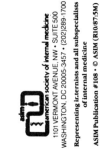

american society of internal medicine
1101 VERMONT AVENUE, NW • SUITE 500
WASHINGTON, DC 20005-3457 • (202)289-1700

Representing internists and all subspecialists of internal medicine

ASIM Publication #108 • © ASIM (R10/87/5M)

Figure 24–1. Your internist is an endocrinologist.

Your doctor is an internist. . . . a physician who specializes in adult medical care and the non-surgical treatment of internal organs and functions of the body; a medical detective and diagnostician; a personal physician, health counselor, educator and consultant. Internists are the major providers of continuing, comprehensive health care to adults and adolescents in the United States.

The internist's training and background

The specialty of internal medicine begins with attaining the degree of Doctor of Medicine (MD), followed by a hospital internship and residency program of several years' duration, working closely with experienced teaching internists.

At this point in his or her career, the internist-in-training may take other special work to gain more expert knowledge in such areas of practice as cardiology, gastroenterology, allergy, and chest diseases.

After formal training come rigorous examinations that qualify him or her as a specialist in internal medicine (and, sometimes, as a subspecialist in a particular type of diagnosis and treatment). He or she is then ready to practice.

Your internist keeps up with modern developments in research and treatment by constant study of medical journals and books, taking postgraduate courses, and attending medical meetings. Continuing education becomes a way of life.

What your doctor does as an internist

An internist, in the role of diagnostician, compiles a comprehensive "case file" on each patient—detailing the present symptoms and a history of physical and emotional difficulties.

The mark of an internist is thoroughness—and the compilation and study of the medical history is done meticulously, taking as much time as the internist deems necessary.

As an historian often predicts crises through knowledge of the past, so an internist diagnoses illness from a patient's medical history and symptoms.

The internist has been described as a "medical detective"—known for physical examination of the entire body, searching for clues to a correct and complete diagnosis. Like today's "scientific" detective, the internist uses the most highly developed scientific tools when they are needed to help the patient—laboratory tests, electrocardiograms, metabolism tests, fluoroscopy, X-ray examinations, CT scans, and radioactive isotopes are among the everyday tools available for use.

Through analysis and interpretation of a patient's medical history, physical condition, and the results of modern scientific tests, the internist is trained to reach a diagnostic conclusion by considering even seemingly unrelated clues.

This knowledge is then applied in a very human way—talking with the patient and weighing first impressions with what is found later. The internist also functions as the patient's health manager, guiding him or her through the course of treatment as well as counseling the patient on appropriate lifestyle and behavior modifications.

Internists and their patients

The practice of internal medicine, of course, varies with the individual interests, training and experience of each internist—and of the community he or she serves.

As a personal physician

Internists establish caring and continuing relationships with their patients, helping them manage their own health to prevent disease, which is why internists are often chosen as personal physicians. The patient may go to see the internist for periodic physical examinations and may call upon him or her during an illness or medical emergency. Often functioning as an interpreter or guide to the patient's condition, the internist may refer the patient for appropriate testing and/or for consultation from a subspecialist in internal medicine or from a physician in another medical specialty.

As a consultant

The internist's special knowledge and background as a diagnostician is most often sought by doctor associates. In this role, he or she provides an opinion, the report of the examination, a diagnosis, and recommendations for treatment to the physician who requested the opinion or referred the patient. As a consultant, the internist will not personally undertake treatment unless the referring physician asks him or her to do so.

If a patient goes directly to an internist whose practice is largely in a consulting capacity, the internist usually advises the patient on the selection of a personal physician.

Nearly all internists are consultants, but most of them are also personal physicians or are associated with other internists who serve their patients as personal physicians.

As a subspecialist

Internists in this category, whose practices are restricted to consultation, devote their special knowledge and skills primarily to helping patients whose problems center on one organ or system of the body, such as the heart, blood vessels, kidneys or lungs. Such subspecialization is a natural and necessary result of the rapid advancement in medical science, diagnosis and treatment that has marked the specialty of internal medicine in the past few decades.

The internist within the medical profession

The internist is often called the "teacher of doctors" in light of the responsibility to train interns and residents in the hospital. Many physicians who teach full time in medical schools received their training as internists.

Figure 24-2. Your doctor is an internist.

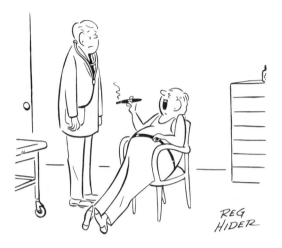

"I know exactly what you're going to say."

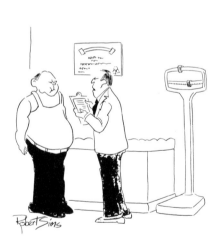

"And for exercise, I want you to talk a long walk every day—while everybody else is eating dinner."

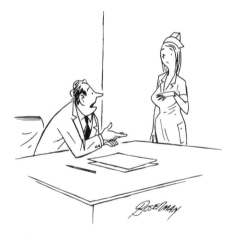

"What they want is for me to make them feel good enough to go back to doing the things that make them feel bad."

Figure 24–3. Selections from Dr. Cherner's collection of cartoons.

APPROACH #3: EDUCATING PATIENTS ABOUT THE PHYSICIAN

Dr. Cherner feels that, in addition to educating his patients about their illness, he has a great deal to gain from educating his patients about himself and his practice. He believes that a positive doctor-patient relationship is built on mutual trust and respect, and he wants to give his patients an opportunity to get to know him professionally.

Aside from inviting patient questions face-to-face, Dr. Cherner writes and distributes medical articles for his patients and also writes and makes available an update on his professional and personal activities.

Authorship

Many of the articles in his "Talks with the Doctor" volumes are written by him, thus affording him a great deal of credibility in the eyes of his patients. Patients are comforted knowing that he is published in his field. And many patients take what he says to them more seriously because he has stated the same message in his written works.

Updates on his activities

Annually, in his "Talk with the Doctor" volume, Dr. Cherner includes a letter to his patients letting them know his recent professional activities and accomplishments during that year. He describes his community involvement, his recent writings, his speeches and presentations, and his professional development. He believes that patients appreciate getting to know their physicians professionally, especially if their physicians are active, always learning, and respected professionals.

The following is an example of Dr. Cherner's annual update.

1986 Activities

As most of you are aware, Dr. Cherner's medical activities do not cease in the evening when office hours are technically over. He remains "on call" for emergency calls, comsultations with his colleagues, plus many other associated medical duties. He has also retained his affiliation with Thomas Jefferson University Hospital and continues to participate, on request, in various teaching and academic activities. He retains his academic title as Associate Clinical Professor of Medicine in the division of Endocrinology, Department of Medicine.

Dr. Cherner was honored to be the keynote speaker at his reunion, Class of 1955, held at Thomas Jefferson University on June 5, 1985. Dr. Cherner reviewed the history of many of Jefferson Medical Colege's best teachers, and was subsequently honored at a dinner held at Carpenters' Hall, downtown Philadelphia in the Independence National Park. His speech was published in the Jefferson Medical College alumni bulletin, summer edition.

Dr. Cherner has also continued as an adjunct participating physician and consultant at Albert Einstein Medical Center, Northern Division. He also continues as an active endocrine consultant at Parkview Hospital Division of the Metropolitan Hospital Center. It goes without saying that Dr. Cherner continues to be active as Attending Endocrinologist at the Rolling Hill Hospital right here in Elkins Park.

His complete review of hyperthyroidism was published in the January 30, 1985, issue of *Consultant Magazine.* An additional article was published in *Consultant Magazine* on March 30, 1985, entitled "Diabetes—When Compliance Is Appalling." An additional brief consultation article on Diabetes and Vitiligo was also published in a later issue.

Dr. Chener attended the sixty-sixth annual session of the American College of Physicians, held in Washington, D.C., from March 28–31, 1985, and intends to attend the next annual session of the American College of Physicians to be held in San Francisco in early April.

Dr. Cherner has also continued as a literature "referee" and as a book reviewer for the *Annals of Internal Medicine,* the prime publication of the American College of Physicians. He also continues to function on the Board of Consultants of *Consultant Magazine,* with particular interest as a consultant in endocrinology and metabolic diseases.

Dr. Cherner has also been honored by being asked to speak at medical conferences both at Rolling Hill Hospital medical staff meetings, as well as to consult to the Temple University Family Medicine Residency Group.

In a more personal vein, Dr. Cherner was honored in publication of a fine article with photographs in the *Times Chronicle Newspaper* group in Montgomery County. More recently he was honored by publication of an extensive article in the "Town and Country Section" of the Sunday *Philadelphia Inquirer* on January 13, 1986.

Most excitingly, Dr. Cherner and office staff have decided to initiate a new endeavor, to commence in this office on or about the first of February, 1986. He is proud to announce the formation of the Pavilion Diabetes Treatment Center, providing diabetic education, therapy, diet review, and diabetic rehabilitation services.

More information will be available concerning the operation of this unit in personal mailings to my patients.

I am sure that you remain interested in my activities in terms of guaranteeing that you are receiving the most excellent medical care. I hope you are reassured also by my desire to contribute my interest to the community at large.

Sincerely,

Rachmel Cherner, M.D., F.A.C.P.
Endocrinology and Diabetes Mellitus

APPROACH #4: PATIENT HANDBOOKS

The most complete source of patient information and education comes from the personal 100-page handbook Dr. Cherner and his staff have developed for patients with diabetes. This handbook, like the "Talk with the Doctor" series, contains many articles that address the background of the disease, information on diet, therapies, and the like. The table of contents illustrates the scope.

Diabetes Handbook Contents

1. What Is Diabetes Mellitus?
2. Juvenile Diabetes Type I
3. Maturity Onset Diabetes Type II
4. Long-Term Effects of Diabetes
5. Dietary Considerations in Diabetes
6. Exercise
7. General Health Care
8. Instructions for Urine Testing and Home Glucose Monitoring
9. Oral Antidiabetic Agents
10. Insulin Administration
11. Sick Days
12. Postscript—The Future

(Reprinted with permission of Rachmel Cherner, M.D.)

And the postscript from this manual highlights Dr. Cherner's underlying personal philosophy and intent.

Postscript: The Future

You have now reached the end of this volume. The journey has been arduous and long. There has been a mountain of necessary facts to learn. You may want to reread sections, or indeed read this book again—cover-to-cover. I hope that it has been valuable. Please keep it for further reference as a courtesy gift from Pavilion Diabetes Treatment Center.

The future looks very bright. An effective insulin pump is just around the corner. It may end the drudgery of insulin "needles." It may afford closer control of hyperglycemia, and prevent diabetic complications.

Remarkable advances in the immunology of diabetes may lead to a vaccine which can prevent juvenile diabetes.

Future genetic research may prevent the development of diabetes in our progeny.

The future looks bright, yet—we must be content with our current knowledge of diabetic control. Normalization of blood glucose, prudent low fat diet, and good body hygiene are still good bets in preventing diabetic complications.

We at Pavilion Diabetes Treatment Center wish you the best. We have tried to show you the right path. It is now up to you to put this information to good use for *your health.*

> *Good luck and good health is our wish!*

Pavilion Diabetes Treatment Center (Reprinted with permission of Dr. Rachmel Cherner, Pavilion Diabetes Treatment Center)

APPROACH #5: AUDIO VISUAL RESOURCES

For patients requesting even more information or information in another medium, Dr. Cherner offers a series of short, easy-to-understand tapes that patients can view in his office. These tapes help patients who have difficulty with written material and support his verbal explanations about diet and nutrition with additional facts in a more entertaining format. Often, Dr. Cherner requests that a patient view certain tapes and then meets with him/her to discuss the information gleaned. That way he can check for understanding and agreement.

Guide to use of educational aids

Dr. Cherner asserts that written and audiovisual material in patient education should be used to support and supplement understanding, but should not be the main source or method of communicating with patients. Written materials that can be taken home are helpful as supplementary material because:

1. Since people tend to forget what they hear, especially when they're nervous, if they have information in writing, they are less likely to call and ask you to repeat your instructions or explanations.

2. They can share the information with family members, achieving the involvement and support of people close to them.

3. Patients may need an initial overview but, generally speaking, most cannot absorb large quantities of information at one sitting. Written support material gives the patient an opportunity to learn, review, and absorb bit by bit at his or her own pace.

APPROACH #6: CONSULTATIONS WITH SPECIALISTS

Many of Dr. Cherner's patients benefit from the support system he provides. He connects his patients to a variety of specialists who provide additional information, support, and consultation. Nutritionists, physical therapists, and nurse specialists are among the resource people he uses on a regular basis. While Dr. Cherner goes to great lengths to provide his patients with rich information, he feels no need to be their *only* information source. When he makes referrals, he believes it builds patient confidence.

APPROACH #7: MONTHLY SUPPORT GROUPS

Dr. Cherner delivers monthly lectures on diabetes at his local hospital. These forums are open to the public, and he encourages his own patients to attend. These monthly lectures address a variety of topics. He also makes available at no cost support materials for those patients who choose not to attend.

More is better

Dr. Cherner has many reasons for dedicating time, energy, and money to this elaborate array of educational opportunities for his patients. He believes:

1. The more educated the patient, the greater the likelihood of successful therapy.
2. The more educated the patient, the less anxiety and stress around the disease.
3. The more educated the family, the more support the patient receives.

And, says Dr. Cherner, he himself benefits, not just the patients. Payoffs for the physician include:

- A more educated patient is more cooperative.

- Patients are grateful for information.
- A more involved patient is less likely to search for another physician.
- Teaching is the best way to build a strong, trusting relationship.
- Grateful, informed, patients *do* spread the good word.
- He feels self-respect and job satisfaction, since he knows he has done all he can for his patients.

IN SUMMARY

Dr. Cherner is a patient education enthusiast and has translated his enthusiasm into a strategic patient education strategy. He is gratified by the results and from the positive feedback from patients and peers. The word is out about this specialist, and patients and referring physicians are grateful for his attention to bridging the information gap.

25

Addressing Your Patients' Emotional Concerns: The Role of the Clinical Specialist

Leila Grant is terrified of anesthesia. The last time Leila was hospitalized, her mother died. Listening and sensitive questioning can help Mrs. Grant become aware of the link between her past experience and her own fears about anesthesia. Once she is listened to and more aware, she is likely to become a little less frightened.

Mr. Levine is a powerhouse in the board room, but in the hospital he's timid and intimidated. He doesn't ask questions. He hopes his wife will think and ask questions for him. A sensitive person attuned to family dynamics can help the physician see this dynamic and involve Mrs. Levine centrally in the communication process.

Mark Haskins has a fused hip and is hospitalized for hip replacement. He has mixed feelings about gaining newfound mobility after surgery. It turns out that Mr. Haskins had endured tuberculosis as a child. He had been advised during his recuperation, "Lie still and don't move." He didn't listen and he did move. From his point of view as a child, this caused his father to become ill and die. Mr.

Haskins had absorbed the message "Don't move." Now, in the face of vastly improved mobility, he is afraid to move. Sensitive listening and questioning reveals the source of his mixed feelings and helps Mr. Haskins address them, so he can help, not impede, his own rehabilitation.

Martha Sherman panics when the nurse raises the bars on her bed. The nurse's explanation that the bars keep the patient safe seem to do nothing to ease Martha Sherman's panic. For good reason, the nurse insists on keeping the bars raised and leaves the room. If someone could take the time to listen and understand, it would become apparent that the bars remind the patient of early trauma in a concentration camp. By bringing this connection to consciousness, by recognizing and talking about the source of her anxiety, Martha Sherman can more readily see the raised bars as security, not as a threat.

In each of these situations (provided by Alice Eiseman of Longwood Orthopedics, Chestnut Hill, Massachusetts), if someone is available to build rapport, listen, and understand, he or she can help the patient and the patient's family prepare for, accept, and assist in their medical treatment and its aftermath. Situations like these are more the norm than the exception. Clearly, they affect the patient's attitude toward healthcare and hospitalization, the experiences surrounding them, and the compliance and recovery process that follows.

But how many doctors singlehandedly have the time to deal with this level of concern? And how many doctors have the skill?

ADDRESSING THE NEEDS OF THE WHOLE PERSON

Emotional concerns can impede the patient's endurance and recovery, as well as interfere with compliance. Not only is it therapeutic to elicit and address the patient's emotional needs and concerns, but it also makes the doctor's job easier.

This point is obviously not new, nor are special people and services available to address it. In many practices, existing physicians and nurses have successfully been able to devote time and attention to addressing patients' emotional concerns. Other practices have expanded their basic staff to include "traditional" professionals (nurses and physicians) who translate into reality the practice's commitment to a comprehensive humanistic approach. In many situations, nurses are the ideal candidates to help with this practical integration of medical treatment with the psychosocial issues stirred by a health encounter.

One such example is the in-vitro fertilization service at the Albert Einstein Medical Center in Philadelphia. The nurse specialist assigned exclusively to this program is the go-between with couples not only for evaluation and treatment issues but also for psychological, financial, and social issues. She has the time and the training to be keenly sensitive to the myriad concerns that infertility triggers. A psychiatrist (one of this book's authors, in fact) is involved as well, first by screening candidates, then by helping them to articulate their questions and concerns. Both the nurse specialist and the psychiatrist then make recommendations to the other staff who interact with the patients.

Increasingly, many specialty practices like renal dialysis, breast cancer, oncology, infertility, in vitro fertilization, and transplant have augmented their staff so that their people can devote substantial attention to supporting the patient in the emotional domain. They find that the more complex the problems related to the patient's condition, the more important it is to have ample resources devoted to it. Core staff attuned to emotional concerns and dynamics start up dialysis treatment, train couples to give Pergonal injections for infertility, and prepare patients for chemotherapy.

Other practices have dedicated entire positions to addressing patients' emotional concerns and providing support throughout every aspect of treatment or care—sometimes in the form of nurse specialists, social workers, rehabilitation psychologists, and psychologists or psychiatrists whom they've integrated into their healthcare team and made available full time to work with patients and their families around special emotional needs, the personal and interpersonal issues triggered by their condition, and their interactions with the healthcare provider. Hopefully, all practices have established referral links, so that they can and do easily refer patients to psychiatrists or other appropriate professionals for certain complex problems.

The concept of dedicating substantial human resources to serve this function—whether full time or part time, whether integrated into core staff or on an adjunct basis—is just beginning to blossom.

TWO SCHOOLS OF THOUGHT

The need to devote attention to the patient and family's emotional concerns and needs is hardly debatable. But what is debatable is whether a practice should have special people whose job it is to address the nonmedical aspects of illness and treatment. There are, in fact, at least two schools of thought. Some people say that a medical practice should *not* hire a special person to cater to the patient's emotional needs, because the physician and other existing staff should be doing it. If they aren't, they should be trained and their capacities expanded, so that they can deal with the whole person.

Others consider that view an idealistic view that would be nice in the best of all possible worlds. But these pragmatists acknowledge that dealing with the whole person as fully as some specialty practices need to is just not feasible for many practicing physicians.

These people believe that systematic, timely attention to patient and family concerns by the physician and existing staff just does not easily fit within many physicians' practices, that it's just not practical. Unavoidable time pressures, increasingly demanding patients and families, shorter hospital stays due to insurance DRG's (diagnosis-related groups), and the nursing shortage frustrate many physicians who feel pressed to become optimally efficient in their interactions with patients. Many feel the time pinch in attending to the patients' medical needs, let alone their emotional needs.

The question is: How can the physician, trained to be expert in a clinical specialty, devote quality attention to the emotional needs and concerns that inevitably arise for patients experiencing health trauma and hospitalization?

Some practices need to devote a position to it.

THE ROLE OF THE CLINICAL SPECIALIST: A ROLE BORN OF EXPERIENCE

To show the power and potential of such a role and how it was defined and became successfully integrated into a medical practice, consider the case of Alice Eiseman.

Alice Eiseman had multiple orthopedic hospitalizations. She knew firsthand about the emotional issues that arise for patients. And she knew firsthand how an orthopedic practice could increase patient satisfaction by increased attention and resources devoted to the patient's emotional needs and concerns.

Alice Eiseman had worked as a child-life therapist whose job it was to provide emotional support to children and their families. She had for years explored creative ways to make hospitalization less traumatic for people, first with children, and later, with indigent adults at the Lemuel Shattuck Hospital in Boston.

To strengthen her background and credentials for pursuing her mission, Ms. Eiseman completed a master's program in Counseling and Consulting Psychology at the Harvard Graduate School of Education. She also devoted substantial time and energy to programs at the Harvard Medical School because she wanted to learn about the educational process of physicians, its strains and challenges. In short, Alice Eiseman wanted to understand both sides of the patient-physician interaction and to be able to empathize with the expectations and issues important to each.

As a result of her repeated experiences as a patient and as a colleague among medical students, Ms. Eiseman concluded that some physicians could greatly enhance their patients' satisfaction, their effectiveness, and their practices' success by teaming up with a psychologically trained clinical specialist. Given the time demands on the physician, most physicians, she felt, could not take the time it might require to identify and address the full gamut of their patients' emotional concerns and needs that impinge on their medical treatment.

In 1983, Ms. Eiseman approached Benjamin Bierbaum who had performed her own hip surgery. She approached Dr. Bierbaum because of her unequivocal respect for his competence and his drive to provide superior medical care and service to his patients. She proposed to develop the position of clinical specialist as an enhancement to his practice.

Case in point: Benjamin Bierbaum, M.D.

Benjamin Bierbaum, M.D., has practiced as an orthopedic surgeon for 20 years. In practice with four other physicians of Longwood Orthopedic Associates, Inc. in Chestnut Hill, Massachusetts, Dr. Bierbaum specializes in reconstructive joint surgery. He is also chairperson of the Department of Orthopedic Surgery at New England Baptist Hospital in Boston, and Clinical Professor of Orthopedic Surgery at Tufts University Medical School. Approximately 70 percent of his work relates to surgery of the hip. Dr. Bierbaum performs approximately 250 operations per year. In addition, he travels extensively, typically twice each month to lecture and provide postgraduate education.

Pressed for time because of his many responsibilities, and dedicated to top-notch patient care, Dr. Bierbaum, in 1983, added a "clinical specialist" to his practice—a clinical specialist who would help him to identify and cater as expertly to the emotional needs and concerns of patients and families, as he caters to his patients' surgical needs. Dr. Bierbaum recognized that patient and family concerns were extensive, especially in his practice that focused largely on out-of-state patients.

What exactly is a clinical specialist?

> *The Clinical Specialist:* a key member of the medical practice team; an adjunct person who listens patiently to the patient and family, figures out what their emotional concerns and needs are, and takes steps to focus their attention, the physician's attention and the hospital's attention on meeting these needs.

The job description

- Meets all new patients with the surgeon, so that patients see the clinical specialist immediately as an extension of the surgeon.
- Stays with the patient after the surgeon leaves the room to make sure all the patient's questions have been answered.

- Takes time to listen; challenges the patient's irrational assumptions; helps overcome or control fear and take action to aid in the patient's own recovery.

- Helps the patient build a solid relationship with the physician so that the patient feels safe and has a positive experience.

- Sees every patient the day before surgery, either at the office or in the hospital.

- Finds out who the patient wants the doctor to contact after surgery.

- Helps the patient face surgery with confidence and strength and consider the strengths (the patient has) that will help endurance and rehabilitation.

- Helps the patient articulate questions and encourages the patient to ask appropriate questions.

- Explains terms and demystifies medical treatments.

- Helps prepare the patient for surgery, provides information, makes sure records are intact, creates checklist for physician alerting him or her to special needs.

- Follows patient after discharge and during follow-up visits, thus providing continuity and familiarity.

- Helps family members express and cope with their own anxiety, so that they can support the patient.

- Helps provide for the patient some privacy or distance in the face of hovering family members, so that the patient can rest and/or cope with emotions—and helps the family understand the importance of this distance.

In short, patients and family members see the clinical specialist—in this case, Alice—as an empowered representative of the physician who extends the physician's ability to provide the care and caring they need. According to Dr. Bierbaum, "She does behind-the-scenes work that makes her indispensable and enables me to do what I do best."

HOW YOUR PRACTICE CAN BENEFIT

According to Dr. Benjamin Bierbaum, his practice and his patients are enhanced by the clinical specialist role.

- The more you educate patients about their own problem and needs, the more you strengthen the relationship between the patient and the physician. And this is certainly important in today's legal environment. Most malpractice suits arise from poor communication, from a feeling patients have of not being tended to by their physician.

- Even though there's no reimbursement for the clinical specialist role and I pay Alice's salary, there's no question about the fact that my practice benefits from her presence.

- Some patients are reluctant to bring up issues: they don't want to bother me, or embarrass me or embarrass themselves. As a hip patient and with a degree in counseling, Alice is better able to gain their confidence, and I can be more effective as a result.

- Now that the nursing shortage is acute, everyone in the hospital has to limit their time with the patient. Alice compensates.

- She helps them become educated, aware of what they feel, and more accepting of what they need to do.

- I practice in a teaching hospital. Fellows and agency nurses rotate through. These changing faces can upset patients and families. Alice provides stability by seeing patients in the office early on, in the hospital, and in the office afterward.

- The most exciting part of this... If you can provide emotional support for patients and their families, everybody feels better for it.

KEY FACTORS IN CAPITALIZING ON THE CLINICAL SPECIALIST ROLE

To make the role of the clinical specialist work, you need to consider three success factors: the physician, the person in the clinical specialist role, and the link with the hospital.

The physician

When asked what kind of physicians can make the role of clinical specialist a far-reaching practice enhancement, both Alice Eiseman and Benjamin Bierbaum cite the same key factors. Physicians must:

- Have a special interest in patients as people and recognize the power of their emotions in the healing process.
- Admit that they can become more efficient without sacrificing quality by extending their staff.
- Empower the clinical specialist to act on the physician's behalf.
- Build a trusting partnership with the clinical specialist.
- Value substantial, enduring involvement with the patient.

The clinical specialist: The person

Who's qualified for the role? According to Ben Bierbaum, you have to look for someone who can work with your type of practice and your type of patients. And these characteristics are important:

- Medical background, familiarity with medical terminology; ability to communicate clearly in plain talk
- Good with people, sensitive, calming, caring
- Understanding of psychological and emotional concerns
- The analytical skills to know what's appropriate for the clinical specialist to address instead of the doctor.
- Respect for and comfort with the physician's competence and style.

Benjamin Bierbaum adds, "What matters most is the person's understanding of what you're trying to accomplish, more than their training background. Find a psychologically skilled person, a sociologist, social worker, or psychologist with some medical background who can learn specifics related to your particular practice."

The link with the hospital

The third key party is the hospital. The physician and clinical specialist need to work out a relationship with the hospital that facilitates actions by the clinical specialist on behalf of the physician.

To help the patient, the family, the physician and hospital staff, the clinical specialist inevitably needs to work closely with hospital staff.

> Ann Williams is 67 years old. She's hospitalized for hip surgery. Her husband is ill. The hospital staff recommends discharge to a rehab hospital. Ann Williams is distraught because she wants to hurry home to her sick husband. Given the circumstances, it seems advisable to opt for physical therapy in the home instead of in-patient rehab. The clinical specialist, who has time to talk at length with the patient, offers staff another perspective on Mrs. Williams, a perspective that results in their making a different recommendation.
>
> While Laura Smythe is hospitalized for joint replacement, she becomes concerned that she has breast cancer. She asks for the appropriate tests but is told that these can wait until her next internist visit. She is upset. The clinical specialist has the time to talk with her at length, and after discussing her findings with the doctor, the doctor sees the value of having the test done immediately.

Jim Bentz is foggy about his physical therapy instructions. The clinical specialist, who had the time to get to know the patient, alerts the therapist to the fact that the patient didn't understand the printed instructions and was too embarrassed to ask because of a reading problem. As a result, the therapist visits the patient to explain and demonstrate what the patient needs to do.

Mr. Slater is not ready to leave when visiting hours are over. He is fearful about leaving his wife whom he has never seen sick before. The hospital is strict about visiting hours, but after speaking with the clinical specialist, they help Mr. Slater to feel comfortable leaving his wife.

The clinical specialist can take the time to provide in-depth patient education. As a result, the patient can better relate to the staff. At the same time, he or she helps staff understand the idiosyncratic behaviors and needs of the patient, so they'll be more attuned to the patient's needs—more quickly.

Since the relationship between hospital staff and the clinical specialist is new and can be delicate, the clinical specialist needs to be a skilled and sensitive person. He or she must respect the hospital staff and their time constraints, offering her extra set of eyes and ears to help everyone provide the quality of care and caring they all want to provide. Also, he or she needs to secure credibility within the hospital structure, perhaps through a position like "clinical assistant" that makes her supportive role legitimate in the eyes of the staff. The clinical specialist, after all, needs access to patient charts and a wide variety of hospital personnel.

A SATISFYING JOB

Here's what Alice Eiseman says about her role:

> I love this job. It's fascinating to see many patients go through essentially the same experience, each uniquely. They go through the same hospital routines, the same tests, the same rehab process, but all experience this in their own way. I am there to recognize each individual's needs and to make the experience easier for patients. I devote all of my time to this, whereas a physician cannot. I help the patient and I enable the physician to do what he does best.

Benjamin Bierbaum is sold on the value of the clinical specialist role for practice enhancement. You can benefit in similar ways. Find a person, whether full or part time, to augment your staff and focus exclusively on providing and helping you provide to patients and their families dedicated attention to their emotional needs and concerns. The result: improved clinical outcomes and heightened patient satisfaction.

26

Strategies to Strengthen Physician Effectiveness at Kaiser Permanente

Many people wonder why some physicians don't behave better toward patients. The fact is that medical schools and most residency programs emphasize clinical knowledge and skills and give short shrift at best to the nonclinical aspects of the doctor-patient relationship. Then, once physicians are in practice, their top-dog status, reticent, nonassertive patients, and the absence of accountability in the practice environment tend to mitigate against receiving frank, specific, constructive feedback about their behavior and its effects on patients. The result: limited opportunities for growth and improvement in the behaviors that constitute "the art of medicine."

PATIENT SATISFACTION PROJECT AT KAISER PERMANENTE MEDICAL CENTER

The Northern California Kaiser Permanente Patient Satisfaction/Art of Medicine Project began in 1985, when the Assistant Physician-in-Chief of Kaiser, San Rafael, surgeon Paul F. Alpert, M.D., became concerned about shaping the nonclinical behavior of his physicians to produce maximum patient satisfaction.

Noting that, "while many of our physicians were clearly excellent in the art of medicine, others were significantly less excellent" (Alpert and Alpert, 1987, 1988), his goal was to raise them all to maximum levels. He began by consulting with his clinical psychologist wife, Geraldine Alpert, Ph.D., a member of the Psychiatry Department of Kaiser, South San Francisco, and a psychotherapist whose daily work requires expertise in designing strategies for behavior change.

Initially, they attempted to delineate the behaviors critical to the art of medicine, and with this in mind, reviewed the relevant literature (DiMatteo, 1979, 1980; Korsch et al., 1968; Ben-Sira, 1976, 1980). The components consistently considered important seemed to include: demonstrating a feeling of caring and concern for the patient; acting interested and seeming involved; being pleasant and socially appropriate; listening attentively; and offering an appropriate level of both social and medical feedback. As they studied their list, they were impressed that "these were all behaviors that already existed within the behavioral repertoires of our physicians." They had watched all of their colleagues (including those who seemed to have the least satisfied patients) display these characteristics at cocktail parties, community gatherings, and a variety of settings in which these behaviors were appropriate and socially mandated. "It, therefore, appeared that the difference between excellence and nonexcellence in the art of medicine was not a lack of appropriate social skill, but failure to appreciate the importance of using these skills in the medical setting. We concluded from this that the task was to raise . . . physicians' level of consciousness to a point where they were aware of the importance of these behaviors and would routinely use them with their patients." They hypothesized that this goal could be accomplished with two essential ingredients: *motivation* on the part of the physician to change and feedback about the requisite behaviors.

The program the Alperts designed to accomplish their goals included five key components:

1. Measurement of physician behavior: creation of a patient satisfaction questionnaire.

2. Designing a method of data collection that would provide adequate numbers of responses for all physicians.

3. Motivation component: sensitizing physicians to the importance of their art of medicine behavior in satisfying patients. This component involves information giving and motivation building.

4. The feedback component: providing feedback to the physicians about the quality of their behavior as perceived by their patients.

5. Announced vs. unannounced tests: Demonstrating to physicians that the requisite behaviors are ones that they already have in their repertoire and over which they have voluntary control.

Measurement of physician behavior: The Patient Satisfaction Questionnaire

Based on the components of patient satisfaction emphasized in the literature, the Alperts created eleven 9-point scales designed to measure the relevant behavior. Of these eleven items, nine emphasized nonmedical aspects of the patient—physician interaction and two queried the patient's perception of the physician's technical skills. The reason for including the two items concerned with perceived skill was to see whether patients differentiated between bedside manner and skill. These eleven items were incorporated into a 19-item questionnaire. The first five items requested demographic data. The last three items sought information on the respondent's attitude toward physicians in general, toward answering the questionnaire, and any additional comments the respondents wished to provide. Only items 6 through 16 were counted toward the physician's scores (see Figure 26–1).

A brief three-item questionnaire was also developed by selecting three items from the original questionnaire which were most highly correlated with the total score (see Figure 26–2).

The correlation between the original questionnaire and the abbreviated version was .88.

The data collection method

At the point of designing the original 19-item questionnaire, the Alperts also grappled with the problem of how expeditiously to obtain a high enough response rate at each data collection to be able to give meaningful data to every doctor on each occasion. With the usual return rate from Kaiser mail surveys running between 20 percent and 30 percent, the time and expense anticipated to get meaningful data for every doctor was enormous. Also, these low return rates always raise questions concerning the portion of the population that is responding and create questions about the meaningfulness of the responses. The Alperts guessed that the primary problem accounting for the low return rates was that surveys arriving with the usual computer generated address label and metered postage qualify as junk mail for most individuals and, therefore, are tossed without being opened. To counteract this problem, they came up with the unique strategy of asking each patient to self-address an envelope at the time of checking in for the day's appointment. Within a week, the questionnaire then arrived in an envelope with a real stamp and hand-addressed in the patient's own writ-

PATIENT CARE QUESTIONNAIRE

KAISER PERMANENTE MEDICAL CENTER • SAN RAFAEL

1. Name of doctor you saw today:_____

        Department:_____

2. Number of previous visits to this doctor:

        ___None   ___1-2   ___3-5   ___6 or more

3. Number of years as a Heath Plan member:

        ___less than 1 year   ___1-3 years   ___4-9 years   ___10 or more

4. Year of Birth _____   ___Male   ___Female

5. How serious do you feel the condition is for which you made this appointment?

        ___Not very serious   ___Moderately serious   ___Extremely serious

---

For the following questions, please circle the number on the scale which best describes how you feel about the doctor you saw today.

---

6. How easy was it to talk to your doctor?

1	2	3	4	5	6	7	8	9

extremely difficult   extremely easy

7. How well do you feel your doctor listened to you?

1	2	3	4	5	6	7	8	9

extremely poorly   extremely well

8. How much did your doctor seem to care about you and your problem?

1	2	3	4	5	6	7	8	9

didn't care at all   cared a great deal

9. To what degree was your doctor's manner of conveying information reassuring and positive (considering the nature of the illness)?

1	2	3	4	5	6	7	8	9

needlessly worrying   appropriately reassuring

(OVER PLEASE)

Figure 26–1. Patient Care Questionnaire.

10. To what degree did your doctor treat you with tact and respect?

1	2	3	4	5	6	7	8	9

extremely low degree — extremely high degree

11. How thorough did you feel your doctor was in evaluating your condition?

1	2	3	4	5	6	7	8	9

not at all thorough — extremely thorough

12. How satisfied are you with the information you received from your doctor about your problem and its treatment?

1	2	3	4	5	6	7	8	9

completey dissatisfied — completely satisfied

13. How would you rate your doctor in terms of training, skill and experience to deal with your medical problem?

1	2	3	4	5	6	7	8	9

very poor — excellent

14. How much confidence do you have in your doctor?

1	2	3	4	5	6	7	8	9

no confidence — total confidence

15. To what extent do you feel the treatment you received was equal to the care your doctor would want for a member of his/her own family?

1	2	3	4	5	6	7	8	9

not at all — entirely

16. Overall, how do you feel about the appointment with your doctor?

1	2	3	4	5	6	7	8	9

very dissatisfied — very satisfied

17. How do you feel in general about the medical profession?

1	2	3	4	5	6	7	8	9

extremely negative — extremely positive

18. How do you feel about being asked to complete this questionnaire?

1	2	3	4	5	6	7	8	9

annoyed — pleased

19. If you have any additional comments, please use the space below.

_____

_____

_____

The doctors of Kaiser San Rafael are seeking feedback on the personal care we are providing our patients. We would appreciate your help. For the following questions, please circle the number on the scale which best describes how you feel about the doctor you saw today. Put the completed card in one of the collection boxes near the elevators and exits. Thank You.

Name of doctor you saw today: _____ **Department:** _____

1. How well do you feel your doctor listened to you?

2. How much did your doctor seem to care about you and your problem?

3. To what degree was your doctor's manner of conveying information reassuring and positive (considering the nature of the illness)?

4. If you have additional comments, please use reverse side.

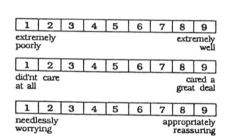

Figure 26–2. The three-item questionnaire.

ing. With this method, the return rate jumped to 60 percent, a staggering improvement at no appreciable cost.

Motivation Component. This component was designed to sensitize physicians to the importance of the art of medicine behavior in satisfying patients.

A series of Grand Rounds presentations was given by Dr. Paul Alpert "to sensitize the physicians to the importance of the nonmedical aspects of the doctor–patient relationship on ultimate patient satisfaction." The material presented included a review of the research on patient satisfaction and a discussion of behaviors that either enhanced or decreased satisfaction. Also important in the Grand Rounds presentation was a reiteration of the already agreed upon facility goal to work toward increased patient satisfaction.

Feedback Component. The fourth step of the project was to design a feedback package that was to be given to each physician after the baseline testing and after each subsequent data collection. The goal of the feedback package was to provide the physician with as much information as possible about how he or she personally was being rated and also about how he or she stacked up in comparison to other doctors in the department and in the facility as a whole. Each doctor was given a packet that contained copies of all of the patients' questionnaires (including the patient comments which were offered by over 67 percent of the patients). In addition, doctors were given their own raw scores, the mean score for their department and graphed distribution of mean scores for the members of their department; they were also provided with the facility mean score and a similar graphed distribution for the facility.

Samples of the data displays are shown in Figures 26–3, 26–4, and 26–5.

With the exception of the physician's own scores, all data were given anonymously. No one other than the investigators had access to individual physician data. Along with the data, at various points in the project, the doctors were given explanatory letters describing changes that were occurring, the implications of these changes, and the need for more response from those physicians showing inadequate improvement. The letters also underlined for those who were not keeping up that they were not doing so while others were.

Announced Vs. Unannounced Tests. These tests demonstrated to physicians that the requisite behaviors are ones that they already have in their repertoire and over which they have voluntary control.

In an attempt to demonstrate vividly to their doctors that "physicians already have within their repertoire the skills needed to be experts in the art of medicine," the final phase of the program was introduced. This phase involved comparing patient satisfaction scores for the physicians obtained on days when physicians knew the testing was being done to scores received on days when testing

	Mean Score	Sample Size
NAME _____		
Collection #6	8.9	6
Cumulative Score (Collections #1–6)	8.4	33
DEPARTMENT _____		
Collection #6	8.1	26
FACILITY — Collection #6	8.0	1,467

Figure 26–3. Art of Medicine/Patient Satisfaction Project: Summary scores. Reprinted with permission of Kaiser Permanente Medical Center.

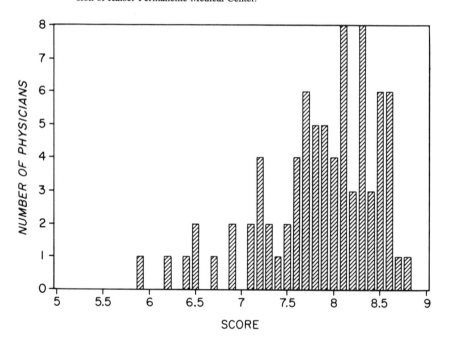

Figure 26–4. Distribution of physician mean scores, October 1985.

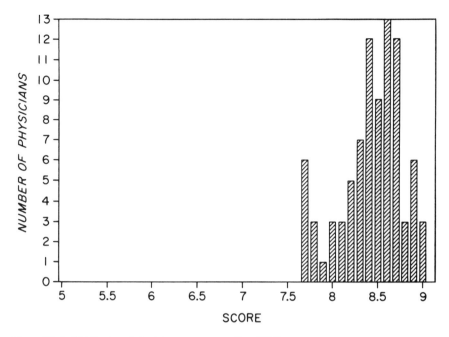

Figure 26–5. Distribution of physician mean scores, June 1987.

was done without the physicians' knowledge. Blind testing was done with the long questionnaire using the mail-in procedure already described. The procedure for the announced testing utilized the abbreviated three-item questionnaire, which each patient received on checking in (and which served as a reminder to the physician, as it was often in the patient's hand when greeting the doctor). The doctors were told in advance that patients would be receiving questionnaires on the announced days and that they were being asked to complete them before leaving the facility.

Results

According to the Doctors Alpert (personal communication, August 19, 1987), after repeated assessment and feedback to physicians:

- The facility's patient satisfaction mean increased significantly.
- The lowest score in the facility rose from 5.4 to 7.4.
- Of the 21 physicians who were the lowest scorers initially, all moved well into the satisfactory range.
- The number of patients who gave their physicians low scores decreased by 55 percent.

- During a period of 12 months in which no testing or feedback occurred, the facility mean dropped somewhat, but not to the original baseline levels. Most important, the doctors who were originally the lowest scorers were the ones who best maintained their levels of improvement.

- Most impressive of all, and clear confirmation of the Alperts' thesis that "these behaviors already exist within our physicians' repertoire" is the remarkable increase in scores when physicians know they are being evaluated. On the 9-point scale, the facility score moved from a mean of 8.0 when the physicians did not know they were being evaluated to a high of 8.4 when they did know they were being evaluated. Considering that a score of 9 is perfect, the move from 8.0 to 8.4 is enormous. Ninety percent of the physicians showed improvement just knowing that they were being evaluated, and the 10 percent who didn't were already very high scorers.

Contagious effects

As the Alperts refined these techniques and began to share their preliminary findings with their colleagues at other Kaiser facilities, offspring projects were instituted at every Kaiser facility in the Northern California region. Most used either the Alperts' Patient Satisfaction Questionnaire or some variant of it to measure physician behavior and, as in their project, also used feedback as the primary change agent.

KAISER—SANTA CLARA TRIES A DIFFERENT APPROACH

Another Northern California Kaiser facility, in Santa Clara, chose a significantly different approach. In March 1987, Assistant Physician-in-Chief Robert Pearl, M.D., and Organizational Development Specialist Joyce Reynolds, Ph.D., decided to institute Satisfaction Survey Cards focused on physician behavior and to provide training in the art of medicine to physicians to help them examine and expand their behavioral repertoires. The Santa Clara facility focused on physician effectiveness in acute appointments, because patients in these appointments are likely to have only one or a very small number of appointments annually, and the impressions made during those appointments color their perceptions of the overall medical plan. Such patients constitute approximately half of the Santa Clara facility's appointments.

The Santa Clara facility instituted the survey card shown in Figure 26–6 to solicit patient feedback about physician behavior.

After receiving feedback, a few low-scoring physicians and several others whose scores were lower than desired expressed interest in patient interaction skills training to help them raise their scores. So, Drs. Pearl and Reynolds developed a pilot program to raise physician awareness and build their skills in

Patient Care Survey

Kaiser Permanente Medical Center—Santa Clara

What is the name and department of the physician you saw today?

1. Name: ———————————— 2. Department: ————————————

3. Is he or she your regular personal physician?   □ YES[1]   □ NO[2]   □ NOT SURE[3]

4. What is the main reason for your visit today? (Please check one.)

    □ 1. Urgent Care/Same Day

    □ 2. Return Visit/Continuing Care

    □ 3. Routine Exam (physical, check-up, pap & pelvic, first prenatal, etc.)

    □ 4. Consultation

    □ 5. Other: ————————————————————————

5. Is this your first appointment at this facility?   □ YES[1]   □ NQ[2]

• PLEASE COMPLETE OTHER SIDE •

How would you evaluate the physician that you saw today? (Please circle one.)

	A=Great	B=Good	C=Fair	D=Poor
6. Showed concern for your needs:	A	B	C	D
7. Answered all your questions	A	B	C	D
8. Gave you clear information and explanations:	A	B	C	D
9. Spent enough time with you:	A	B	C	D
10. Was knowledgeable and competent:	A	B	C	D
11. Your overall impression:	A	B	C	D

12. Would you want to see this physician again?

    □ YES[1]   □ NO[2]   □ NOT SURE[3]

13. Comments or suggestions about your physician based on above questions.

————————————————————————————————

————————————————————————————————

————————————————————————————————

**As you leave, please return this survey card in the sealed envelope
to the receptionist or nurse who gave it to you. Thank you.**

DL 6/88

Figure 26–6. Patient Care Survey.

behaviors key to patient satisfaction. Low, medium, and high scorers participated, since it was felt that people could pool their knowledge and learn from one another. Participating physicians were from primary care as well as surgical departments, and met monthly on their lunch hours for six consecutive months (from December 1987 to March 1988).

The training program was built on these underlying assumptions:

1. The right diagnosis is necessary and not sufficient for patient satisfaction. Patients assume we will deliver high quality care and judge us on the quality of our relations with them.

2. There exists a variety of behaviors and techniques which can lead to a positive patient-physician interaction. We need to increase our repertoire of communication skills if we want to improve. Patients want a compassionate, caring individual who will be their ally and will serve as their resource for them.

3. Time spent on communication and relationship building is an investment more than an expenditure.

4. In order to increase our relations with our patients, we must develop a better understanding of the key phases of physician-patient interaction, and change our behaviors to better conform to our members' expectations. These behaviors have to be practiced until they become part of our daily routine.

5. Underlying all else, there must be a genuine and personal interest in our members and maximizing what we can do to decrease their discomfort.

6. Physicians all too frequently focus on the occasional difficult patient, rather than attempting to increase the satisfaction of the typical member. (Reprinted with permission, Kaiser Permanente Medical Center, Santa Clara, California.)

Interaction skill training

The educational program for physicians focused on the doctor–patient interaction, problem patients and difficult medical situations. The sessions were based on five key phases in the physician–patient interaction, including:

- Meeting and greeting the patient
- Establishing rapport and listening to the patient's chief complaint
- Conducting the physical examination
- Communicating the diagnosis and treatment
- Committing to being the patient's ally and advocate for follow-up.

Related to each phase in the physician–patient interaction, the seminar helped physicians expand their individual repertoire of skills by brainstorming ideas and options and then practicing them. The following worksheet (see Figure 26–7) demonstrates one example of an exercise used to focus physicians on specific behavior improvement experiments. Physicians selected three to five new behaviors from their brainstormed lists to try as homework during the intervening month and then report later about the impact they perceived on their patients.

After four sessions, the instructors scheduled practice sessions with trios of physicians. In these practice sessions, participants alternately played the roles of physician, patient, and observer. Finally, in the last session, the instructors and physicians made and reviewed videotapes in which the physicians could observe their own behavior and their effectiveness in applying the skills developed within the training program. Follow-up to the program will involve addressing systems issues within each specialty that physicians became aware of as impediments to physician effectiveness and patient satisfaction.

UNREALISTIC? NOT REALLY!

You can institute a system to provide physicians in your practice with feedback about their behavior and its effects on patients.

- Develop your own survey and give it to your patients with a self-addressed return envelope. Peruse the returns and learn from them.
- Take initiative to strengthen your own behavior toward patients so that you achieve optimal patient satisfaction. If you're in a small or large practice, you might:
- Attend a one- or two-day training program on patient relations skills. These are often available at hospitals or through commercial training companies.
- Do you have a co-worker who is present when you're interacting with patients (e.g., a nurse)? Have the guts to invite this person to give you feedback on your behavior and suggest ways you might show greater attention, responsiveness, and empathy in your interactions with patients.
  If you're in a larger practice, you have two additional alternatives:
- Initiate a mutually instructive support/co-training arena in which you and your physician colleagues help each other examine patient relationship objectives and problems, and swap and practice behavioral alternatives that might increase patient satisfaction.
- Hire a training professional or consultant expert in patient–physician relationships to provide training for the physicians in your practice. A periodic "briefing" on physician effectiveness in their relationships with patients or a skillbuilding refresher provides a professional shot-in-the-arm.

Name _____

Dept. _____

PHASE & Intended Outcome	3–5 EXAMPLES OF BEHAVIORS AND TECHNIQUES THAT YOU WILL TRY IN THE FUTURE.
I. *MEET & GREET THE PA-TIENT* so that the patient knows who you are and that you know who they are.	
II. *ESTABLISH RAPPORT & LISTEN TO PATIENT'S CHIEF COMPLAINT* so that the patient experiences you as interested in him/her as an individual.	
III. *CONDUCT PHYSICAL EX-AMINATION* so that patient has confidence in your clinical ability.	
IV. *COMMUNICATE THE DIAG-NOSIS & TREATMENT* so that the patient experiences your concern and fully understands the condition, follow-up steps, & responsibility.	
V. *COMMIT TO BE THE PA-TIENT'S ALLY & ADVOCATE FOR FOLLOW-UP* so that the patient trusts you will be there for him/her whenever needed.	

GENERAL BEHAVIORS & TECHNIQUES THAT WORK FOR ALL PHASES:

Figure 26–7. Physician–Patient Interaction Worksheet.

IN SHORT

For Kaiser Permanente in Northern California, Drs. Alpert, Alpert, Pearl and Reynolds developed and established innovative approaches to strengthening physician behavior toward patients. In one case they invited feedback from patients on the relationship and communication skills of their physicians. In a second case, they invited feedback, then engaged physicians in learning opportunities to improve. Their approaches are, unfortunately, rare. Admittedly, the thought of hearing patient feedback might be unnerving, but the alternative—no feedback—can mean blind spots that, if confronted, do strengthen patient satisfaction.

No doubt, following the lead of the Kaiser Permanente innovators, the enlightened, marketing-oriented physicians will increasingly take the courageous steps necessary to check out patient perceptions of their behavior and do all they can to improve it.

NOTE: The San Rafael, South San Francisco and Santa Clara facilities are three of the medical centers in Kaiser Permanente of Northern California, an HMO with more than 2 million members.

REFERENCES

Alpert, Geraldine, and Alpert, Paul, All information on the Kaiser San Rafael Patient Satisfaction Project, including direct quotes, is from personal communications in 1987, and unpublished manuscripts, 1985–1988.

Ben-Sira, Z. "The function of the professional's affective behavior in client satisfaction: A revised approach to social interaction theory." *J. Health and Social Behavior*, 1976, *17*, 3–11.

Ben-Sira, Z. "Affective and instrumental component in the physician-patient relationship: An additional dimension of interaction theory." *J. Health and Social Behavior*, 1980, *21*, 170–180.

DiMatteo, M.R. "A social-psychological analysis of physician-patient rapport: Toward a science of the art of medicine." *J. Social Issues*, 1979, *35*, 1233.

DiMatteo, M.R. "The significance of patients' perceptions of physician conduct: A study of patient satisfaction in a family practice center." *J. Community Health*, 1980, *1*, 18–22.

Korsch, B.M., Gozzi, E.K., and Francis, V. "Gaps in doctor–patient communication." *Pediatrics*, 1968, *42*, 855–871.

Pearl, Robert, and Reynolds, Joyce, "Physician–patient interaction skill training program." Kaiser Permanente Medical Center; Santa Clara, California, 1988.

27

Fine-Tuning the Physician–Patient Relationship through Video Feedback

Most people acknowledge the importance of physician behavior in establishing a satisfying doctor–patient relationship, but some physicians claim that physicians with excellent skills are born, not made. Some, in fact, assert that, as much as they would like to strengthen their interpersonal skills with patients, they wonder if change is really possible for them.

When we asked this question to physicians with mixed years of experience, most said that warm, compassionate relating to patients is something that some people are just naturally good at. However, all agreed that physicians who are not "naturals" can learn key behaviors and build a repertoire of effective patient communication and relationship skills, if they are committed to and motivated to do so, and if they work at it. The physicians we interviewed certainly acknowledged the importance of personality and natural style, but they pointed also to physician peers who had dramatically improved their behavior with patients when they realized that their practice's success was impeded by inferior or mediocre relationship skills.

HOW DOES THE MOTIVATED PHYSICIAN CHANGE?

When we asked how motivated physicians can make these behavioral and perhaps even attitudinal changes, the answers boiled down to two key strategies: feedback and options.

First of all, physicians need to know what they already do behaviorally and its effects on or consequences for patient satisfaction. This calls for feedback. The patient surveys discussed in Chapter 26 are one way to solicit and receive feedback. But, a more powerful tool is specific behavioral feedback—the kind made possible by direct observation. When you or people with an understanding of your objectives watch your behavior, they can help you see what you already do and its effects. And, they can expand your behavioral repertoire, so you can have choices and alternatives when you're interacting with patients. The combination of feedback and options constitutes an unbeatable and powerful personal change strategy for the physician motivated to change.

The Cadillac feedback model

How can feedback and options be orchestrated, in an effort to produce desired changes in your behavior? The Cadillac model, from our point of view, is that used in many family practice, pediatric, and psychiatric residency programs. After describing it, we will suggest ways the crux of this model can be built, not only into residency programs but also into ongoing medical practices in a cost-effective way.

The description that follows is based on a visit to the Tatem-Brown Family Practice Center located in Voorhees, New Jersey, where Robert DiTomasso, Ph.D. (Associate Director for Behavioral Medicine), and Charles "Dick" Almond, M.D. (Associate Director in charge of Curriculum), gave us the grand tour of their impressive facility and sophisticated behavioral feedback system. Part of the West Jersey Health System, the Tatem-Brown Center is a combination of a Southern New Jersey physician group practice and a family practice residency program affiliated with the University of Pennsylvania. The physician staff of the center includes five family physicians and 18 family practice residents.

Video feedback system

The Tatem-Brown Center has an extensive video feedback capability which they use daily as part of their Behavioral Medicine Program under the direction of Robert DiTomasso, Ph.D. Five exam rooms and one minor surgery room have video cameras that can film patient–physician interactions. In a viewing room, the six monitors are available for the faculty preceptor interested in viewing what's happening at the time it's happening or reviewing tapes hours or days later. Nurses explain the taping process to patients before they enter the exam room. Emphasizing that the focus is on the physician's behavior, the nurse secures informed consent from the patient beforehand, using the form excerpted below:

Videotaping/Observation Consent Form (Revised 6/16/88)

As a family medicine center and medical education site, affiliated with the University of Pennsylvania School of Medicine, we are devoted to providing both excellence in medical care and educating physicians in the specialty of family practice. A major goal of our program is to evaluate the physician-patient encounter with actual patients like yourself and to provide our physicians with feedback. Our focus in observing is upon the physician. In order to accomplish this goal, we are requesting your permission to allow us to observe and/or videotape your interaction with your physician. The observation and/or videotape will be used solely for the purposes of professional education and research.

These are some points which you should understand in granting your permission:

1. Our goals in observing and reviewing the encounter with your physician involve *educational* and *professional* purposes only.

2. We have the utmost respect for your rights to *privacy* and *confidentiality* about matters you may choose to discuss with your physician. Therefore, we *guarantee* that only qualified professionals on the staff of the center will observe your interaction. We are strongly bound by a code of professional ethics to protect your confidentiality by not revealing any personal information that you may disclose to your doctor (unless you were a danger to yourself and others).

3. We respect your right to participate in this project. If you decide to participate and then at the conclusion of the encounter decide that no one should see the tape we will erase it immediately. Finally, you may choose at any point during the course of the encounter to decline your participation.

Thank you.
Mary A. Willard, M.D.
Robert A. DiTomasso, Ph.D.
Charles R. Almond, M.D.
David K. Dovnarsky, M.D.
Gloria S. Durelli, M.D.

I have carefully read the above information.

I understand the goals and purposes for observation and videotaping as well as the terms of my participation.

I give my permission for my tapes to be used for training purposes.

Date	Patient Signature	Nurse Signature
_____	_____	_____

(Reprinted with Permission. Tatem-Brown Family Practice Center.)

To protect patient privacy, the cameras are turned off during any physical exams, and the patient can ask to have the tape turned off at any other time as well. Drs. DiTomasso and Almond report that patients very quickly forget that the tape is on.

At least weekly, each physician's interactions with patients are observed and reviewed. Two senior faculty each day are committed to video-precepting. Residents look at their own tapes, discuss them with peer feedback or review them with a faculty member. While the taping system is used for teaching on a wide range of clinical issues, its main purpose is to provide the kind of ongoing feedback and coaching needed to help the physician excel at the physician-patient relationship. While ethical issues, medical-legal issues, practice management issues related to time and efficiency, and patient care issues are all explored, the emphasis is on what might be the most elusive aspects of patient care—physician *behavior*. The taping starts as soon as the doctor enters the room. The observer can see graphically how physicians build rapport, what their questioning techniques are, what their sensitivity is to the patient's verbal and nonverbal cues, how well they show empathy and understanding, how they show respect for the patient (and family), how well they elicit the person's agenda, and more. The form that follows is used initially to help faculty and residents become astute observers. The form shows the kinds of behaviors that the Tatem-Brown physicians have found to be not only important to the patient, but also subject to change when feedback and coaching are provided to shape behavior.

As Drs. DiTomasso and Almond told us of the learning that takes place from this process, they gave many examples of language skills. Dr. Almond talked, for instance, about the importance of ongoing patter and chatter which tends to ease patients' anxieties and also gives them the perception that the doctor is really engaging with them. Also, through observations and feedback, physicians can develop a vast repertoire of words to use upon entering a room, starting conversation with the patient, filling time gaps, and ending the appointment.

Let's see. Now, I'm going to take a look at your ears . . . Now, I'd like you to schedule an appointment for six weeks from now. But you know if you have any concerns between now and then, I want

Interview Process Behavior Checklist

Instructions: Place a check mark in the appropriate box to the left
of each item. Provide comments and suggestions as
appropriate.

Resident: _____

Date: _____

Reviewer: _____

Tape Ft.: _____

Interview Behaviors

YES	NO		Comments	Suggestions
☐	☐	Maintained appropriate eye contact with patient		
☐	☐	Facial expressions reflected mood of patient		
☐	☐	Displayed appropriate head movements		
☐	☐	Displayed a relaxed body position		
☐	☐	Body posture is appropriate (e.g. leaned forward but not imposing		
☐	☐	Faced patient fully		
☐	☐	Used intermittent one-word vocalizations ("mm-hmm") or verbalizations		
☐	☐	Spoke clearly and audibly		
☐	☐	Spoke at a moderate pace		
☐	☐	Pursued important topics (themes) introduced by patient or at least acknowledged them as worth pursuing		

Figure 27–1. Tatem-Brown Observation Form.

☐ ☐	Helped patient to remain at ease by reassuring attitude		
☐ ☐	Asked single questions		
☐ ☐	Used open ended questions (probes) to elicit information		
☐ ☐	Used logical sequence (flow) in questioning		
☐ ☐	Used jargon-free, non-technical language		
☐ ☐	Checked to determine if patient understood what was explained		
☐ ☐	Listened carefully to what patient said rather than jumping to conclusions		
☐ ☐	Elicited relevant psycho-social data (family, social sexual, education, work)		
☐ ☐	Accurately reflected (paraphrased) the patient's verbalizations (cognitive content)		
☐ ☐	Accurately reflected (mirrored) the patient's feelings		
☐ ☐	Accurately summarized (two or more feelings) what patient was feeling		
☐ ☐	Accurately summarized (two or more patient verbaliza-tions) what patient said (cognitive content)		
☐ ☐	Used clarifying questions (Do you mean...?, "Are you saying...?)		

		Provided support and reassurance		
❏	☐	Appropriately confronted patient with discrepancies in behaviors (verbal, non-verbal, and feeling)		
❏	☐	Suggested appropriate alternatives to patient		
❏	☐	Recognized and responded to nonverbal cues of patient		
❏	☐	Resisted distractions		
❏	☐	Provided positive feedback (reinforcement) for specific and appropriate behavior on part of patient		
❏	☐	Used self-disclosure (sharing) appropriately		
❏	☐	Used transitional statements when changing topics		

Instructions: Please check to determine if resident appropriately addressed the issues listed below.

		Medical Patient Care Issues		
❏	☐	Resident Learning Objectives		
❏	☐	Patient Education Issues		
❏	☐	Psychosocial Issues		

you to feel free to call me anytime. If I'm not here or not available, I'll call you as soon as I can. And, if Frank or June has any questions, please tell them to call me, too. You and your family shouldn't hesitate to call if you have any questions or concerns.

Dr. Almond points out that some people have a hard time making small talk, but that you can certainly learn to get much better at it, when you hear the language of others who are good at it and have the chance to see the positive effects on the patient. That's what the video feedback system provides.

The taping makes feedback and coaching possible immediately after the patient–physician interaction, but before the patient leaves, so gaps in information or understanding can even be remedied on the spot. During the visit, we saw a demonstration that worked like this:

- We watched on a TV monitor as the physician entered the exam room, greeted the patient and conducted the initial diagnostic interview. After the physician talked with the patient about the problem as diagnosed, the physician asked the patient to wait a few minutes while the physician stepped out (to prepare a prescription, check the chart more thoroughly, etc.).

- The physician stepped into the video room and talked with Drs. DiTomasso and Almond, who replayed a bit of the video and offered immediate feedback on what they observed during the initial interaction with the patient. They described what they had seen, and they offered suggestions about how to make the interaction better. In this case, they suggested additional open-ended questions that would help the patient reveal barriers to compliance. They pointed out medical jargon and plain-English alternatives. They pointed out opportunities to reflect back the feeling coming from the patient to check its accuracy. They pointed out nonverbal gestures that would place the physician's focus more on the patient, less on her mother. And they suggested two or three specific ways the physician could strengthen the interaction right away upon reentering the exam room to complete the patient's visit.

- Later, the physician and preceptors, and sometimes the entire group of physicians, watched the tape together and discussed in even greater detail what the physician did (or didn't do), its apparent consequences for the patient, and behavioral options for the future that would lead to greater effectiveness. The rules for giving feedback in this hot-seat situation are that the giver must be constructive and behavioral. Anyone can stop the tape at any time to reexamine a key part, describe behavior, and suggest alternatives.

The philosophy expressed repeatedly is that by seeing interactions with all kinds of patients (e.g., hostile, angry, depressed, and withdrawn), the physician develops a vast repertoire of ways to behave to maximize his or her effectiveness with the patients, *and* to tailor his or her behavior to different kinds of patients.

BACK TO REALITY

Impressed by the obvious power of the system at Tatem-Brown, we pushed ourselves to confront the questions we anticipate from pragmatic skeptics.

Q: Can you really change doctors' behavior? Aren't patient interaction styles a matter of personality?

A: Personality is, of course, powerful. but, we have absolute evidence of the ability of behavioral feedback to make physicians much more effective, much more sensitive to behavioral and feeling cues, and much more versatile in the use of appropriate behavior suited to the patient's needs. The results are dramatic, but it takes ongoing feedback and coaching and motivation, not a one-shot training experience.

Q: Can you really teach empathy? Lack of empathy is at the heart of patient dissatisfaction with their doctors.

A: You certainly can, to a degree. But the learner has to have a stake in learning to be more empathetic. If the motivation is there, a person can learn to behave much more empathetically.

Q: The priority on coaching and feedback is understandable within a residency program. But how about in an ongoing medical practice where experienced physicians deliver care, and where time is of the essence? This kind of system would be completely unrealistic except in a teaching setting.

A: This elaborate video system—perhaps so. But, there is no question that this kind of system presses for a standard of care that is really excellent. Perhaps, to a practicing physician or group practice, the question is whether they are open enough to help each other excel— whether they place such a priority on the quality of the relationship that they're willing to make the time and energy available for some kind of modified system. You know, even a $60 tape recorder in an exam room can provide the material for excellent feedback and improvement. It's just that most doctors wouldn't go to the trouble, or perhaps be open to making conscious improvements.

Q: I am who I am. The way I practice medicine is fine.

A: You may be right that the way you practice medicine is fine. Certainly, if you feel no impetus to examine your behavior, this is irrelevant to you. If, however, you have the slightest doubt about your style, you can use periodic behavioral feedback to reassure yourself—

or pinpoint needs for behavioral fine-tuning.

APPLIED TO REALITY

Not many physicians would need or want the Cadillac video model just described, although large, forward-thinking group practices shouldn't rule it out. It would support consistent standards of behavioral excellence among all of your physicians and would sustain your practice's competitive advantage.

But there are alternatives to this Cadillac model that are more affordable and less elaborate.

Starting with the simplest, try taping physician–patient interactions with a $50 tape recorder. Listen to the tape and let others listen to it and make suggestions. Or develop a buddy system in which one physician observes another and afterward makes behavioral suggestions. Or videotape role-play situations in which staff play patients of various kinds with various interaction styles, providing the physician with feedback and a chance to fine-tune his or her behavior in a replay situation.

The point is that feedback is a powerful, constructive shaper of behavior. And video feedback is not only the most graphic feedback available; it also allows you to play and replay the interaction so you can identify nuances and alternatives. If you're committed to fine-tuning your relationships with patients in clinical interactions, you too can set up systems to ensure that your people give you the benefit of seeing your behavior as others see it and becoming more effective with your patients as a result of that experience.

28

Innovation: The Philosophy of Quality Not Quantity

In an age of increasing attention to patient satisfaction, more physicians are looking and listening hard to their patients to identify their desires and preferences as to how healthcare providers can, in the face of treatment alternatives, provide what the patient wants. When physicians really listen, some are finding that what patients really want might fly in the face of state-of-the-art medical technique.

We talked with Dr. Charles H. Ewing, Medical Director at Rydal Park Complete Care Facility in Rydal, Pennsylvania, about this controversial issue.

We consulted Dr. Ewing because many of his patients and physician colleagues recommended him to us as a person who had really thought through this issue and had developed, as a result, a philosophy grounded in his patients' preference for quality over quantity of life.

At the core of Dr. Ewing's philosophy is the belief that doctoring with older people is fundamentally different from doctoring with younger people.

HOW WILL I DIE?

Generally, according to Dr. Ewing, older patients are preoccupied with how they are going to die, not *whether* they are going to die. Most are aware that they are nearing the end of their life and are not frightened by that. They have seen friends and acquaintances die or become disabled, the latter being worse, as they fear being severely impaired, damaged, and dependent. They are afraid of pain and suffering. As they grow less able, most become resigned and ready to die. According to Dr. Ewing, most have come to terms with this and can look back on a relatively happy, productive existence. Of course, if they can, this makes it easier for the patient and the physician. Very few ask their physicians to make them well or make them live longer. Instead, they want their physicians to help them make the inevitable easier and less painful. They are truly concerned with comfort and the quality of their lives.

Dr. Ewing believes that the doctor's role becomes one of providing comfort and solace, not only medical expertise. The doctor has to weigh the medical options at all times, trying to create a balance between too much and too little. The doctor must avoid tough treatment modalities and surgical procedures that will upset the patient, preferring preventive programs geared to prevent disabling and unpleasant side effects. This means a shift in emphasis from extending life at any cost to maintaining quality of one's experience and optimal comfort.

For a 55-year-old patient with angina, you would consider angioplasty or bypass surgery. An 89-year-old patient with angina and severe cardiac disease probably merits a different approach. Is the likelihood that the patient may die in peace worth the risk of what the patient dreads most—a disabling stroke?

CREATING THE BALANCE

Says Dr. Ewing, since each case is unique, you need to take your cue from the patient. How strong is the patient physically and emotionally? Can the patient accept treatment and therapy? Some patients have an incredible will to survive and want and deserve all that science and technology can provide. For others, the more aggressive choices are medically and ethically wrong.

So, Dr. Ewing believes that the doctor is always juggling options—which diseases to attack (since in most cases many are occurring simultaneously) and how to treat them. The key, he says, is to consult your most important diagnostic resource—the patient.

BUILDING TRUST

In order to use this important resource, Dr. Ewing says you must first establish a trusting relationship with the patient, letting the patient know that you understand their fears and concerns and that you will do everything humanly possible to address them. This is the pivotal issue at the crux of all else. Dr. Ewing believes that the most important way the doctor can communicate this is through listening—listening to the patient's

1. Fears about being sick
2. Fears about being disabled
3. Descriptions of their symptoms
4. Understanding of why they are sick.

How do patients know you are listening? By letting the patients talk and not interrupting, and by being open to their ideas.

Contact

Building trust with the sick elderly also includes lots of eye contact, head-nodding, smiling, and touching. This contact is far more important with older patients than others. Elderly people need to know that their *friend* (you, the doctor) has their best interests at heart, that you care about them as a person and will make decisions based on this caring and understanding.

Honesty

Another key ingredient involves being straight with older patients. Again, their fear is not of death—they know they have illnesses, that they are sick—they want to know what it means and what can be done not to make them well but comfortable. If you are vague, thinking that you are thereby protecting the patient, this may actually erode trust and create a barrier to communication and cooperation.

> *Example:* A patient has undergone surgery for colon cancer and the surgeons were not able to remove all of the tumor. The patient needs to understand that one day the tumor will reappear and take his life. The doctor's role, then, is to comfort and assure the patient that everything will be done to make the patient comfortable. The overarching message: "I will always be here for you—until the end."

No false promises

Of course, you must mean it! Elderly patients really need to know that you are not going to abandon them even if you're busy.

Giving choices

Often doctors do not include the elderly in their care assuming, incorrectly, that the patients don't want choices, or aren't competent enough to make them.

Dr. Ewing believes that patients need to and can be meaningfully involved in decisions about their health and illnesses. The challenge for the doctor is to be clear and present the options in ways that patients can understand, remembering that they are primarily concerned with immediate outcomes that do not jeopardize their chances for a peaceful, dignified death.

A patient considering a pacemaker needs to be helped to think through two options and their consequences for his style of life and mode of dying. The pacemaker may prolong his life, but leave him open to other problems and uncertainties. Without a pacemaker, his heart, which is quite weak now, may simply stop one day, providing him with the peaceful, easy death the patient has often hoped for.

Dr. Ewing claims that a major key to his success with his patients stems from his comfort in dealing with death. He knows that his patients are going to die and, while he wants them all to have as healthy a life as possible, he is not preoccupied with extending their lives. He feels that many doctors believe that their role is to do everything medically possible to keep their patients alive, whereas Dr. Ewing believes that he must do everything medically possible to make his patients comfortable. Unlike many physicians who feel helpless if they cannot "cure the disease" and, in fact, distance themselves from patients, Dr. Ewing feels close to his patients and connected to them in the dying process. He describes one woman who was being treated around the time of our interview. The patient was nearing death. Her heart was very weak. Surgery as a viable alternative for this 95-year-old woman was ruled out. Instead, she was being treated with medication. Dr. Ewing had been completely honest with the patient. When she asked, "How long?" he responded, "I honestly don't know. I've done everything I can do. I can continue to monitor the medications which have some effect, but this may only be for a few days or weeks. I can't see much longer than that." He added, "You mean a great deal to me. I've grown very fond of you. You really are one of my favorite patients, and when I lose you, I know that I'm going to lose a friend." And Dr. Ewing means it.

Epilogue

In this book, we've presented options for rethinking the way you manage your practice and the services, ambience, and amenities you afford your patients. We want to close with the following bottom-line points:

1. Patient satisfaction is a result of intelligent effort. If you want to heighten satisfaction among your patients and attract more patients, you can do so by taking strategic action.

2. Start anywhere. We tried to present a comprehensive approach to practice enhancement with enough options to enable you to find options consistent with your practice philosophy. As a result of exposure to these options, you might be thinking (in fact, we hope you're thinking), "So many possibilities and so little time."

To that, we say, start anywhere. Albert Einstein said, "God is in the details." Every enhancement you make triggers an incremental improvement in patient satisfaction; and with enough small, incremental changes, you begin to see breakthroughs in patient appreciation and recognition of your patient focus.

3. Beware of stagnation and complacency. Some physicians think their practices are A-OK and they stop paying attention to the fine points in catering to patients. But inattention is dangerous. In fact, some physicians say that inattention means inevitable complacency and even stagnation as you bask in the glory of a successful practice without enough attention to the ways you can make it better and stronger.

4. There are no recipes that work for everyone. You might have thought that some of the options we described are too elaborate, expensive, or ambitious for the kind of practice you have. Perhaps so. Certainly, since practices differ in size, volume, growth goals, patient population, resources, and specialty, you need to pick and choose enhancements appropriate to the kind of practice you have. And only you are the expert on that. There are no recipes that work for everyone.

5. A practice that's user-friendly for patients relieves your management burdens in the long run. Many physicians find management burdensome—management of staff and management of the myriad operational details involved in running a medical practice. The fact is, if you set up sensible, easy-to-use systems and staff management practices in the first place or fix once and for all the inadequate ones you've been tolerating, you can trim the energy and frustration you devote to practice management. It takes more time to fix problems once they've occurred than to set up systems, procedures, and staff expectations that make things work right in the first place. And, when you make things right and reduce people's complaints and frustrations, you liberate your own energies for practicing medicine.

It's up to you. You have options and the power to make conscious choices among an array of alternatives. Who wins?—your patients, your staff, your practice's success, and you. Because when you have a patient-oriented practice in which you, your staff, your office systems, and procedures all cater to the patient, you have an atmosphere in which you can practice medicine and provide the quality of care and caring that you know patients expect and deserve.

Index